305
Current Topics in Microbiology and Immunology

Editors

R.W. Compans, Atlanta/Georgia
M.D. Cooper, Birmingham/Alabama
T. Honjo, Kyoto · H. Koprowski, Philadelphia/Pennsylvania
F. Melchers, Basel · M.B.A. Oldstone, La Jolla/California
S. Olsnes, Oslo · M. Potter, Bethesda/Maryland
P.K. Vogt, La Jolla/California · H. Wagner, Munich

A. Radbruch and P. E. Lipsky (Eds.)

Current Concepts in Autoimmunity and Chronic Inflammation

With 29 Figures and 18 Tables

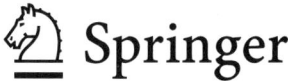

Andreas Radbruch, Ph.D.
Deutsches Rheumaforschungszentrum Berlin (DRFZ)
Schumannstr. 21/22
10117 Berlin
Germany
e-mail: radbruch@drfz.de

Peter E. Lipsky, MD
National Institute of Arthritis and Musculoskeletal and Skin Diseases
9000 Rockville Pike
Bethesda, MD 20892-1560
USA
e-mail: lipskyp@mail.nih.gov

Cover figures by Katrin Moser (chapter Manz et al., this volume):
BrdU (green) labeled long-lived and BrdU-negative short-lived plasma cells (blue) in the spleen of NZB/W mice. B cells are shown in red.

Library of Congress Catalog Number 72-152360

ISSN 0070-217X
ISBN-10 3-540-29713-8 Springer Berlin Heidelberg New York
ISBN-13 978-3-540-29713-0 Springer Berlin Heidelberg New York

This work is subject to copyright. All rights reserved, whether the whole or part of the material is concerned, specifically the rights of translation, reprinting, reuse of illustrations, recitation, broadcasting, reproduction on microfilm or in any other way, and storage in data banks. Duplication of this publication or parts thereof is permitted only under the provisions of the German Copyright Law of September, 9, 1965, in its current version, and permission for use must always be obtained from Springer-Verlag. Violations are liable for prosecution under the German Copyright Law.

Springer is a part of Springer Science+Business Media
springeronline.com
© Springer-Verlag Berlin Heidelberg 2006
Printed in Germany

The use of general descriptive names, registered names, trademarks, etc. in this publication does not imply, even in the absence of a specific statement, that such names are exempt from the relevant protective laws and regulations and therefore free for general use.
Product liability: The publisher cannot guarantee the accuracy of any information about dosage and application contained in this book. In every individual case the user must check such information by consulting the relevant literature.

Editor: Simon Rallison, Heidelberg
Desk editor: Anne Clauss, Heidelberg
Production editor: Nadja Kroke, Leipzig
Cover design: design & production GmbH, Heidelberg
Typesetting: LE-TEX Jelonek, Schmidt & Vöckler GbR, Leipzig
Printed on acid-free paper   SPIN 11560074   27/3150/YL – 5 4 3 2 1 0

Preface

The immune system has been known to be capable of distinguishing self from non-self since the pioneering work of Paul Erhlich more than a century ago. Originally described in experiments studying blood transfusion compatibility, the principle of "horror autotoxicus" is still valid, although today the phenomenon is usually described in terms of tolerance or ignorance. A great deal has been learned about the various processes preventing self-reactivity normally. These include processes that operate during immune cell ontogeny and subsequently on reactivity of mature lymphocytes in the periphery. They encompass mechanisms that are intrinsic to potentially reactive lymphocytes and can result in central or peripheral deletion or the alteration of functional potential. In addition, there are influences that are extrinsic to potentially auto-reactive lymphocytes, including the function of regulatory cells, differentiation state of antigen-presenting cells, availability of self-antigen, the cytokine and chemokine milieu, as well as the trafficking patterns involved in generating productive immune interactions. It is clear that the immune system devotes a considerable effort to the avoidance of the development of potentially pathogenic self-reactivity.

Despite this, the development of self-reactivity is relatively common. Although the development of autoimmune disease is less frequent, autoimmune diseases, such as rheumatoid arthritis, multiple sclerosis, systemic lupus erythematosus, psoriasis, thyroiditis, and myasthenia gravis, are all too common, and can cause considerable morbidity and even mortality. That the breakdown of self/non-self discrimination can result in autoimmunity and in some circumstances autoimmune disease has been known for more that 50years. In most circumstances, however, the precise mechanism underlying the development of autoimmune disease is unknown. Although many elegant animal models of autoimmune disease have been developed, some of which result from a single genetic defect, in most circumstances the relevance of these animal models to human autoimmune disease remains uncertain.

There has been great progress in the last few years in the development of more precise knowledge of the control of the function of the immune system. Awareness of the complex interactions of the innate and the adaptive immune system, the role of apoptosis in regulating the evolution of immune reactivity, as well as the role of various regulatory cells in shaping and limiting immune reactivity has permitted the development of a better understanding of immune system biology. New insights have not only come from traditional immunologic studies, but also from genetic analyses of both immune responsiveness and autoimmune disease. In addition, new insights have emerged from studies of the control of cell signaling, biochemical analysis of the regulation of cellular differentiation, as well as the detailed analysis of the biology and biochemistry of the plethora of effector molecules involved in regulating the expression of immune reactivity.

The wealth of new insights has prompted a re-assessment of the mechanisms controlling self/non-self discrimination and the specific abnormalities that result in a breakdown of this fundamental and essential protective property of animals. The goal of this volume is to utilize the wealth of new information to re-assess self/non-self discrimination with the expectation that viewing this old challenge with more modern eyes may generate novel insights. It is anticipated that new hypotheses may emerge about the control of autoimmunity, and that novel potential targets may be recognized as potential points of intervention to treat or even prevent autoimmune disease.

December 2005 *Peter E. Lipsky and Andreas Radbruch*

List of Contents

B Cell Tolerance—How to Make It and How to Break It 1
    F. Melchers and A. R. Rolink

Breaking Ignorance: The Case of the Brain 25
    H. Wekerle

Naturally Arising Foxp3-Expressing $CD25^+CD4^+$ Regulatory T Cells
in Self-Tolerance and Autoimmune Disease 51
    S. Sakaguchi, R. Setoguchi, H. Yagi, and T. Nomura

Sex Hormones and SLE: Influencing the Fate of Autoreactive B Cells 67
    J. F. G. Cohen-Solal, V. Jeganathan, C. M. Grimaldi, E. Peeva, and
    B. Diamond

Innate (Over)immunity and Adaptive Autoimmune Disease 89
    M. Recher and K. S. Lang

Can Unresolved Infection Precipitate Autoimmune Disease? 105
    D. J. B. Marks, N. A. Mitchison, A. W. Segal, and J. Sieper

The Systemic Autoinflammatory Diseases:
Inborn Errors of the Innate Immune System 127
    S. Brydges and D. L. Kastner

Inefficient Clearance of Dying Cells and Autoreactivity 161
    U. S. Gaipl, A. Sheriff, S. Franz, L. E. Munoz, R. E. Voll, J. R. Kalden, and
    M. Herrmann

The Importance of T Cell Interactions with Macrophages
in Rheumatoid Cytokine Production 177
    F. M. Brennan, A. D. Foey, and M. Feldmann

T Cell Activation as Starter and Motor of Rheumatic Inflammation 195
    A. Skapenko, P. E. Lipsky, and H. Schulze-Koops

Signalling Pathways in B Cells: Implications for Autoimmunity 213
  T. Dörner and P. E. Lipsky

Immunological Memory Stabilizing Autoreactivity 241
  R. A. Manz, K. Moser, G.-R. Burmester, A. Radbruch, and F. Hiepe

Genetics of Autoimmune Diseases: A Multistep Process 259
  M. Johannesson, M. Hultqvist, and R. Holmdahl

Subject Index 277

List of Contributors

(Addresses stated at the beginning of respective chapters)

Brennan, F. M.   177
Brydges, S.   127
Burmester, G.-R.   241

Cohen-Solal, J. F. G.   67

Dörner, T.   213
Diamond, B.   67

Feldmann, M.   177
Foey, A. D.   177
Franz, S.   161

Gaipl, U. S.   161
Grimaldi, C. M.   67

Herrmann, M.   161
Hiepe, F.   241
Holmdahl, R.   259
Hultqvist, M.   259

Jeganathan, V.   67
Johannesson, M.   259

Kalden, J. R.   161
Kastner, D. L.   127

Lang, K. S.   89
Lipsky, P. E.   195, 213

Manz, R. A.   241
Marks, D. J. B.   105
Melchers, F.   1
Mitchison, N. A.   105
Moser, K.   241
Munoz, L. E.   161

Nomura, T.   51

Peeva, E.   67

Radbruch, A.   241
Recher, M.   89
Rolink, A. R.   1

Sakaguchi, S.   51
Schulze-Koops, H.   195
Segal, A. W.   105
Setoguchi, R.   51
Sheriff, A.   161
Sieper, J.   105
Skapenko, A.   195

Voll, R. E.   161

Wekerle, H.   25

Yagi, H.   51

B Cell Tolerance—How to Make It and How to Break It

F. Melchers[1,2] (✉) · A. R. Rolink[3]

[1]Department of Cell Biology, Biozentrum, University of Basel,
Klingelbergstrasse 50–70, 4056, Basel, Switzerland
fritz.melchers@unibas.ch; melchers@mpiib-berlin.mpg.de
[2]Campus Charite, Max Planck Institute for Infection Biology,
Schumannstrasse 21–22, 10117 Berlin, Germany
[3]Center for Biomedicine, University of Basel, DKBW,
Developmental and Molecular Immunology,
Mattenstrasse 28, 4058 Basel, Switzerland

1	Introduction	2
2	Repertoire Selections by the pre-B Cell Receptor	6
3	Generation of Immature, sIgM$^+$ B Cells	7
4	Negative and Positive Selection, and Ignorance of the Developing Immature B Cell Repertoires	9
5	Negative Selection and Editing	10
6	Ignorance	12
7	Positive Selection	13
8	Peripheral B Cells Without sIg Expression	14
9	Rescue of Autoreactive B Cells by T Cell-Independent Antigens of Type I, TLR–Ligand–Antigen-Complexes	15
10	Autoreaction Rescued by Ignorance	16
11	Breaking the Tolerance of Mature, Peripheral B Cell Repertoires	17
12	Consequences of Breaking B Cell Tolerance—Autoimmune Diseases	19
References		20

Abstract A series of checkpoints for antigen receptor fitness and specificity during B cell development ensures the elimination or anergy of primary, high-avidity – autoantigen-reactive B cells. Defects in genes encoding molecules with which this purging of the original B cell repertoires is achieved may break this B cell tolerance, allowing the development of B cell- and autoantibody-mediated immune diseases. Furthermore, whenever tolerance of helper T cells to a part of an autoantigen is broken, a T cell-dependent germinal center-type response of the remaining low – or no – autoreactive B cells is activated. It induces longevity of these B cells, and expression of AiD, which effects Ig class switching and IgV-region hypermutation. The development of V-region-mutant B cells and the selections of high-avidity – autoantigen-reactive antibodies producing B cells by autoantigens from them, again, can lead to the development and propagation of autoimmune diseases such as lupus erythematosus or chronic inflammatory rheumatoid arthritis by the autoantibody BcR-expressing B cells and their secreted autoantibodies.

1
Introduction

It has long been clear that tolerance, unresponsiveness to autoantigens, exists in the mature B cell compartments. Major mechanisms to achieve such unresponsiveness include clonal deletion by apoptosis of autoreactive B cells, either generated de novo from pluripotent hematopoietic stem cells and early lymphoid progenitorsm modulated by receptor editing to rescue cells from death, anergy through receptor downregulation, followed by apoptosis often induced by T cells, and suppressive regulation, acting via regulatory T cells indirectly, or by cytokines directly, to eliminate or silence autoreactive B cells (Chiller et al. 1970; Nossal and Pike 1980; Nossal 1992; Goodnow et al. 1988; Nemazee and Bürki 1989a, b; Klinman 1996).

The repertoires of immunoglobulin (Ig) -, antigen-specific receptor (B cell receptor, BcR) -expressing B lymphocytes are generated by stepwise rearrangements of the IgH (first D_H to J_H, then V_H to $D_H J_H$ segments), followed by the IgL (V_L to J_L segments on κL and λL chain loci) chain gene rearrangements. If the IgH chain and L-chain gene rearrangements are in-frame, i.e., capable of generating IgH and L chains by translation of the transcribed rearranged genes, and if the IgH and L chains are capable of pairing, i.e., of forming IgH/L-chain tetramers, the BcRs are expressed at the surface of first an immature B cell, then virgin mature B cell and, finally, after a response to antigen, of a memory B cell population (for reviews see Melchers and Rolink 1998; Rajewsky 1996; Schlissel 2003).

At least two major subcompartments of mature, BcR-expressing B lymphocytes are generated (Fig. 1). Approximately half of them are found in the follicular regions of spleen and lymph nodes and in the recirculating blood and lymph. They are often called conventional, or B2-type B cells. The other half is mainly found in the gut-associated lymphoid tissues, e.g., in Peyer's patches, in follicular structures near the M cell regions of the gut epithelia, and often as single intraepithelial lymphocytes in the lamina propria of the gut. At least a majority of these B cells appear to belong to these so-called BI subpopulations. (Craig and Cebra 1971). In addition, B cells in the spleen are found in the marginal zone (MZ) surrounding the T cell-rich periarteriolar regions (PALS) and the B cell-rich follicular regions. They appear to be mainly of the B2-type conventional B cells.

While conventional, B2-type B cells appear truly resting, i.e., in the Go phase of the cell cycle, ignorant of autoantigens in their environment, BI cells appear slightly activated, "tickled," by autoantigens as well as by antigens present in the gut. These antigens can access the lymphoid follicles in the epithelia lining the gut by penetration through flat epithelial M cells, so that food antigens as well as antigens of the indigenous bacterial flora of the gut might be recognized (Backhead et al. 2005; Fagarason and Honjo 2003; Hooper and Gordon 2001).

Conventional, B2-type B cells are most often triggered into responses by helper T cell-dependent antigens, i.e., by foreign antigens that also stimulate helper T cells to cooperate with the follicular B cells in a response, which takes place mainly in germinal centers. This induces B cells in a CD40 (B)–CD40 ligand (T) cell, cytokine (e.g., IL4- or TGF-α-) -dependent fashion to switch to IgG, IgE, and IgA, and to hypermutate preferentially the V regions of the rearranged IgH- and L-chain genes, leading to affinity maturation of B cells. These switched, hypermutated BcR-expressing B cells have the choice to mature to Ig-secreting plasma cells or to BcR-expressing memory cells, both of them having gained longevity with half lives changed from a few days to weeks and months of survival in the immune system. The memory B cells and the long-lived plasma cells appear to leave the germinal centers to lodge in special niches in the bone marrow until recall by a secondary challenge of the same antigen.

In contrast, gut-associated, maybe B1-type B cells can respond to antigen even in the absence of helper T cells, with Ig class switching mainly to IgA production. Hence, IgA-secreting plasma cells are abundant in the lamina propria. The IgA can transmigrate into the lumen of the gut and may bind to food-derived and to indigenous bacterial antigens. As much as one-third of the IgA levels found in the serum may be derived from T cell-independent stimulation of such gut-associated B cells.

In mice and humans, the generation of B cell repertoires is continuous throughout life, fed from the pools of pluripotent hematopoietic progenitor cells, lymphoid and B-lineage-committed progenitors and precursors, and—perhaps especially strongly in the BI compartment—from BcR-expressing, i.e., fully Ig gene-rearranged B cells. During embryonic development, B cell

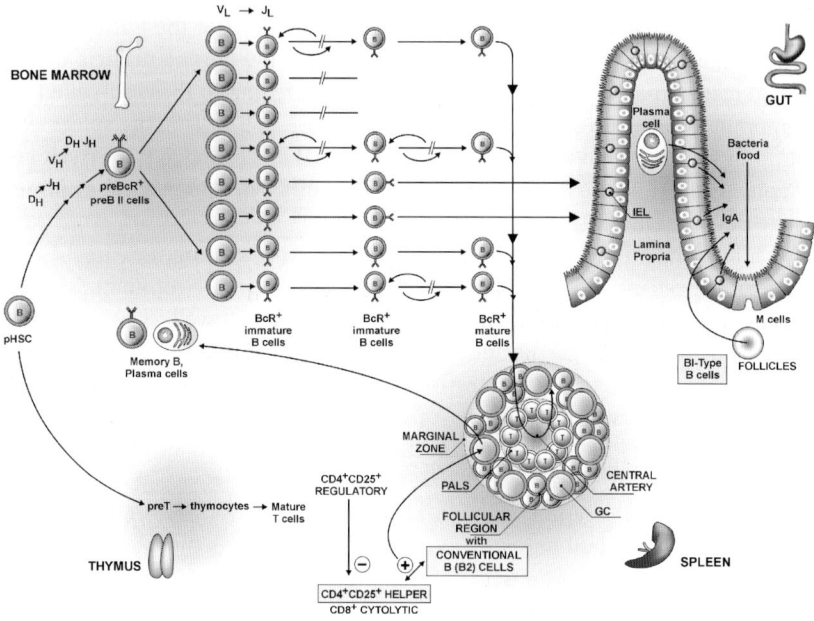

generation occurs in waves at different sites. The first progenitors originate from the aorta-gonad mesonephros area of the embryo, seeding the omentum and the fetal liver, before bone marrow takes over as a continuous site of B cell generation throughout adult life. During life, the B-lineage-committed progenitor and precursor compartments appear to decrease by at least 100-fold, but never cease completely to generate B cells. Therefore, the establishment of an unresponsive state to autoantigens should be achieved by mechanisms that remain operative throughout life.

V(D)J rearrangements of the IgH- and L-chain loci generate a diversity of antigen-binding BcRs, during embryonic development in omentum and fetal liver without, and in adult bone marrow, with N-region diversity introduced by the enzyme terminal-deoxynucleotidyl-transferase (TdT) at the V_H to D_H-, D_H to J_H and V_L to J_L joints. The generated repertoire of IgH/IgL-chain combinations, i.e., of BcRs, is limited by the number of cells generated per day, approximately 5% of the total B cell pool in a young adult, possibly decreasing with increasing age as the frequencies of IL-7/sromal cell-clonable precursors have been seen to decrease 20- to 100-fold within a few months in mice and from birth to 10 years of age in humans (Ghia et al. 1998, 2000).

This means that in adult mice, with 5×10^8 B cells, 2×10^7 B cells may be generated per day. Humans, showing striking similarities in the generation

Fig. 1 Development of B lymphocytes in bone marrow and their partners, T lymphocytes in the thymus. Pluripotent hematopoietic stem cells are the origins of B and T lymphocytes. In the B lineage, precursor B cells rearrange D to J, and then V to DJ segments on the H chain loci and then express pre-B cell receptors (preBcR) as H chain surrogate L (SL) chain heterodimeric receptors. Immature B cells develop thereafter from V to J rearrangements. They express a wide variety of antigen-binding V-region combinations, which include specificities to foreign and autoantigens. If the avidity to autoantigens present in the bone marrow is high, they may be arrested and die by apoptosis, unless they can edit their H and/or L chains by secondary replacements or rearrangements, respectively, and might thereby be allowed to proceed to the mature pools. Low avidity interactions with autoantigens mildly activate and positively select cells as B1 types into the gut-associated lymphoid tissues where they can either lodge as isolated single intraepithelial lymphocytes (IEL), or where they can form follicles underneath the flat epithelial M cells. Stimulated B cells, perhaps under the influence of bacterial and food antigens traversing the M cells to reach the follicles, may give rise to IgM- and IgA-secreting plasma cells, which are found in the lamina propria. IgA is transported through the epithelium to reach the luminal side of the gut to interact with the indigenous bacteria, food, and other antigens. Immature B cells with no avidity to autoantigens are allowed to enter the spleen through the central artery, traverse the T cell-rich periarteriolar sheet (PALS) and aggregate in the follicular regions as B2-type conventional B cells. B cells are also found in the marginal zone surrounding the follicular region. T cells are generated in the thymus and mature to $CD4^+$ $CD25^-$ helper, $CD 8^+$ cytolytic and $CD4^+$ $CD25^+$ regulatory T cells. As in B cell development, immature thymocytes with high-avidity autoantigen-specific T cell receptors are negatively selected to die by apoptosis before reaching the mature cell pools. In addition, regulatory T cells negatively control the differentiation of autoantigen-specific mature effector helper and cytolytic T cells. Foreign antigen-reactive helper T cells cooperate with B2-type conventional B cells either in extrafollicular areas or in the follicular regions to form germinal centers, in which AiD is induced, leading to IgH chain gene class switching and V-region hypermutation, as well as to B cell longevity. Helper T cell responses to autoantigens appear to occur outside germinal centers (William et al. 2002). Long-lived memory B cells and plasma cells migrate out of the germinal centers and back into the bone marrow (Kunkel and Butcher 2003; Manz et al. 2005; Hoyer et al. 2005)

of B cells in bone marrow, have approximately 1,000 times more B cells and should, therefore, also generate 1,000 times more B cells with newly formed BcRs.

It has been estimated that a large part—perhaps more than 60%–80%—of the newly generated repertoires of B cells, both of mice and humans, can bind autoantigens (Ait-Azzuzene et al. 2004). In this chapter, we review the influences on this emergence and on the mature B cell repertoires that contribute to the apparent unresponsiveness of the selected, mature, resting B cell repertoires toward immunogenic stimulation by autoantigens, which could lead to pathological B cell responses resulting in autoimmune diseases.

2
Repertoire Selections by the pre-B Cell Receptor

In the developmental pathway of B lymphocytes from pluripotent hematopoietic stem cells, commitment to the lymphoid cell lineages is marked by the expression of the rearrangement machinery, i.e., the *RAG1* and *RAG2* genes, as well as the IL-7 receptor, which controls much of the cytokine responsiveness of early B- as well as T-lineage progenitors and precursors (Melchers and Kincade 2004) (Fig. 1). Surrogate light (SL) chain and pre-Tα chain are expressed in the early lymphoid progenitors, before they express the IgH chain in B lineage and the TcRα chain in α/β TcR-T-lineage cells. The transcription factors E2A, EBF, and Pax5 control the entry of lymphoid-committed cells into the B-lineage pathway, so that a pre-BI cell develops in which both IgH chain alleles are $D_H J_H$-rearranged. V_H to $D_H J_H$ rearrangements are initiated at the transition from pre-BI to large pre-BII cells. Whenever these rearrangements occur in-frame, and whenever the H chains produced from such a productively rearranged IgH chain allele can pair with an SL chain, pre-B cell receptors (preBcR) are deposited at the cell surface. If the rearrangement at the first $D_H J_H$ allele is productive, rearrangement at the second allele is turned off, securing allelic exclusion at the IgH chain locus, so that one B cell produces only one type of H chain. Membrane-bound Ig H chains signal the cell to turn off the rearrangement machinery and make the second, $D_H J_H$-rearranged IgH chain allele inaccessible for further rearrangements (Melchers et al. 2000). However, the classical preBcR with SL chain appears not to be involved in signaling for this allelic exclusion (Shimizu et al. 2002; Melchers 2005).

On the other hand, the preBcR signals proliferation, so that the pre-BII cells are in the cell cycle, i.e., large. At the same time, the preBcR signals the pre-BII cell to turn off SL chain expression, thereby limiting the amount of SL chain available for preBcR formation. Hence, proliferative expansion of large pre-BII cells is limited, as SL chains are diluted out by cell division. An individual V_H domain of an H chain appears to be probed for pairing by the V_{preB} subunit of the SL chain, and this interaction may display different avidities, depending on the structure of the V_H domain, thereby perhaps expanding different individual Ig H chains in large pre-BII cells to different extents, i.e., for different numbers of divisions.

It appears that the non-Ig-portion of the λ5-subunit of SL chain is mandatory for the capacity of preBcRs to stimulate pre-BII cell proliferation (Ohnishi and Melchers 2004). Since this proliferation appears to be cell-autonomous, preBcRs on the surface of pre-BII cells could be either self-crosslinked, or could be crosslinked by a linker molecule, made by the pre-BII cells, inducing cross-linking of preBcRs via the non-Ig-portions of the λ5 subunit of the SL chain. As SL chains become limiting in the proliferative expansion, pre-BII cells exit the cell cycle and fall into a resting state into the small pre-BII cell stage.

In this view of B cell development, the preBcR does not use the complementarity-determining regions (CDRs) of the V_H domain of its H chain to bind ligands that could induce proliferation. Therefore, the newly generated V_H domain repertoire is not screened for antigen, i.e., autoantigen binding, but merely for fitness to pair, eventually with conventional L chains. In this way, unfit H chains that may have other unwanted properties, such as the formation of self-aggregating immune complexes that might bear the danger of glomerulonephritis and vasculitis, are excluded (Melchers 2005).

In conclusion, the IgH chain repertoire emerging from pre-BII cell expansion and entering L-chain gene rearrangements should be fully autoreactive. This conclusion is also warranted by the observation that in vivo or in vitro administrations of either autoantigens or IgH-chain- and SL-chain-specific monoclonal antibodies do not disturb—positively or negatively—the development of pre-B cells to the stage of an immature, $sIgM^+B$ cell (Ceredig et al. 2000).

3
Generation of Immature, sIgM$^+$B Cells

When large pre-BII cells cease to express preBcRs, they begin to re-express the rearrangement machinery, i.e., RAG1 and RAG2. In human but not in mouse development, they also re-express TdT. Hence the emerging L-chain repertoire can be expected to contain N-region sequences, that is, be more diverse than that of mice. The cells open the L-chain gene loci, first detectable by the production of sterile transcripts. However, the $D_H J_H$-rearranged H chain alleles remain inaccessible for the rearrangement machinery, thus securing allelic exclusion of the H chain locus.

When large pre-BII cells finally exit the cell cycle and become small, V_L to J_L rearrangements become detectable (Yamagami et al. 1999). Hence, the small pre-BII compartment contains cells that have rearranged the L-chain gene loci but do not express L chains, hence do not express IgM on their surface. A part of them appear to be nonproductively rearranged, another part were found to express L chains in their cytoplasm, but not (yet) on the surface, some of them because the pre-existing H chain may not have been able to pair with the L chain; and yet another part may already have expressed L chains on their surface but may have been exposed to autoantigens, downregulating the surface expression (see below). In fact, single-cell PcR analyses and analyses of subcellular L-chain expression of this small pre-BII cell compartment indicate that all of these different types of precursor B cells may be present in this compartment.

In the small pre-BII cell compartment, as well as in the immature, sIgM$^+$B cell compartment, the rearrangement machinery remains expressed, i.e., active. In the mouse, nearly 100 functional V segments can rearrange to four J segments by either deletion or inversion of the intervening sequences, and multiple rearrangements on one allele are possible as long as J elements remain unrearranged. In a large proportion of the small pre-BII cells, multiple L-chain gene rearrangements have been, and still are taking place, and more frequently so than in the immature IgM$^+$B cell compartment. Furthermore, productive rearrangements are often seen to be followed by nonproductive rearrangements, suggesting that the L chains produced from the productive rearrangements were either incapable of pairing or led to the expression of sIgM on an immature B cell, with specificity for an autoantigen present in the environment of the primary lymphoid organ. The reactions of the autoreactive sIgM on immature B cells stimulates a sustained expression of the rearrangement machinery and thereby allows editing of the autoreactive IgM by a second L chain, with the possibility of changing its specificity away from autoreactivity (Gay et al. 1993; Rolink et al. 1993; Tiegs et al. 1995; Melamed and Nemazee 1997; Casellas et al. 2001). As a consequence, some small pre-BII cells are not the precursors, but the products of immature sIgM$^+$B cells.

Initially, only one of the two IgL alleles appears to be usable for V_L to J_L rearrangements, reflected in a differential chromatin methylation and acetylation state of the two alleles (Mostoslavsky et al. 2003). For nearly two-thirds of all emerging B cells, this is sufficient to generate a sIgM$^+$B cell for the peripheral, mature pools of cells. Hence, for two-thirds of the developing and mature B cell repertoires, allelic exclusion at the L chain loci is achieved by an apparent positive selection of an H chain–L chain combination that terminates the expression of the rearrangement machinery. These cells in the repertoires have only one V_L to J_L rearrangement, usually to the must proximal J_L segment on one allele, while the second allele remains in germ line configuration. It is not yet clear how sIgM signals the termination of secondary rearrangements in these cells and whether occupancy by antigen is required for it, but it is reasonable to expect that surface deposition of the IgM is an essential part of this signal (Monroe 2004; Dal Porto et al. 2004).

The role of sIgM on immature B cells appears to be quite different, whenever that sIgM$^+$B cell encounters an autoantigen in the primary lymphoid organ. The rearrangement machinery is kept active, and the cell appears to open the second L chain allele for rearrangements. Hence, the single-cell BcR analyses of wild type B-lineage cells with two rearrangement-competent L-chain alleles have shown that only a minority (i.e., approximately 5%) of all pre-BII cells containing secondary rearrangements retain this second allele in germ line configuration (Yamagami et al. 1999). This suggests the possibility, and danger, that a B cell could produce two L chains from two productively rearranged L chain alleles.

4
Negative and Positive Selection, and Ignorance of the Developing Immature B Cell Repertoires

The large numbers of immature sIgM$^+$B cells that develop from H chain-expressing pre-BII cells with autoreactivity for autoantigens are first screened in the primary lymphoid organs, and later at second checkpoints in spleen (where immature B cells are found). The strength of the signal through the BcR, thought to be a consequence of the avidity of the autoantigen toward the corresponding sIgM-expressing B cell, the environment and the form of the antigen, appear to determine the fate of a B cell at these earliest repertoire checkpoints (Casola et al. 2004; Carroll 2004a, b).

Genetic deficiencies in complement components such as C1q, C4, serum amyloid protein, and complement receptor 2 (CR2), as well as secreted natural serum IgM (Boes et al. 1998, 2000; Chan et al. 1999), lead to systemic autoimmune disease (systemic lupus erythematosus, SLE) with a preponderance of autoantibodies against single- and double-stranded DNA and a variety of other nuclear antigens. Such high avidity autoantibodies are not found in normal, nondiseased individuals.

From these observations two models for the selection of the emerging B cell repertoires have been proposed (Carroll 2004a). In one model, the maturing B cells are protected from the stimulatory influence of autoantigens released from apoptosing, blebbing cells in the primary lymphoid organ because macrophages expressing complement receptors (C1qR for C1q, CRI for C4) efficiently take up, and thereby remove, apoptosing cells bound by natural serum IgM and complexed with C1q and C4b. This model does not explain how the developing repertoire of immature B cells is purged of autoreactive cells, and does not take into account that immature B cells are sensitive to being induced to apoptosis rather than to proliferation and to the development of Ig-secreting plasma cells and memory B cells.

5
Negative Selection and Editing

The second model, by contrast, proposes that autoantigens from dying cells are presented to the emerging repertoire of B cells by stromal cells in the primary lymphoid organs. These autoantigen-presenting cells are suggested to express CIq receptor and CRI, to bind CIq or C4, respectively, which, in turn bind to surface IgM occupied by autoantigens on autoreactive B cells. Depending on the strength of the interaction of the BcRs with autoantigens, and possibly also on the nature of the stroma cell (in bone marrow or spleen), this autoantigen-induced signaling can have different outcomes. It can lead to apoptosis of the B cell, if the avidity of autoantigen-BcR binding is high, leading to negative selection of the B cell repertoire. Such negative selection has been documented in a variety of experimental settings. If BcR downregulation and re-expression

Fig. 2 A hypothesis for the modes of selection of the developing B cell repertoires in the primary lymphoid organs for B cell development, e.g., bone marrow. B cells first express BcRs on their surface as immature cells. Autoantigens can bind to those B cells which express BcRs with sufficient avidities as complexes with natural antibody-type serum IgM, possibly produced mainly by B1 cells. The antigen–antibody complexes can bind C1q and C4, activating the classical complement activation pathway. It is proposed that stromal cells in the microenvironment of the primary B cell-generating organ express Fc mu receptors, C1q receptors (*C1qR*) and C4 receptors (*CR1*), which bring the autoantigen-complement IgM-loaded B cells near these stromal cells to establish B cell–stromal cell contacts and expose the B cells to cytokines produced by the stromal cells. The avidity of the BcR–antigen interaction modulates the actions of these contacts and cytokines to be, for high avidity, negative (to apoptosis), and for low avidity, positive (mild activation). Autoantigens with polyclonal B cell activators, e.g., TLR2, TLR4, or TLR9 ligands can replace cytokines and cell contacts and signal B cells. Genetic defects in serum IgM, C1q, C4, C1qR, CR1, and possibly Fc mu R all inactivate this mechanism of repertoire screening and predispose to B cell/autoantibody-mediated autoimmune disease. Those B cells not recognized by autoantigens can be exposed to BAFF via BAFF receptors (*BAFF-R*), produced by cooperating cells such as dendritic cells (DCs), also activatable by TLR ligands. BAFF induces polyclonal, BcR-independent maturation of BcR^+ immature B cells without proliferation to mature, B2-type conventional B cells. BAFF thereby competes for positive B cell repertoire selection. Excessive BAFF production, for example, can rescue autoantigen-reactive B cells from deletion, while deficiencies in BAFF and/or its receptor results in defective development of B2-type conventional, but not of B1 B cells

of a secondary BcR due to editing of a new L chain, thus leading to a new, nonautoreactive BcR, occurs fast enough, this apoptosis may be avoided.

As an extension of this model, one could propose that the stromal cells also express receptors for natural serum IgM (Fc receptors) to include serum IgM in these processes (Fig. 2). In this way, the serum IgM could also bind to autoantigens, and then be able to fix CIq, creating a multiple bridge between the CIqR, CRI, and FcR on stromal cells and the autoreactive BcR on the immature B cell, brought together by CIq, C4, serum IgM, and autoantigens. Approximately 90% of the 2×10^7 sIgM$^+$ immature B cells that are made each day in the bone marrow of a mouse never arrive at the immature sIgM$^+$B cell pool of the spleen, suggesting that most of the negative selection of the B cell repertoires occurs at the transit from bone marrow to spleen (Rolink et al. 1999).

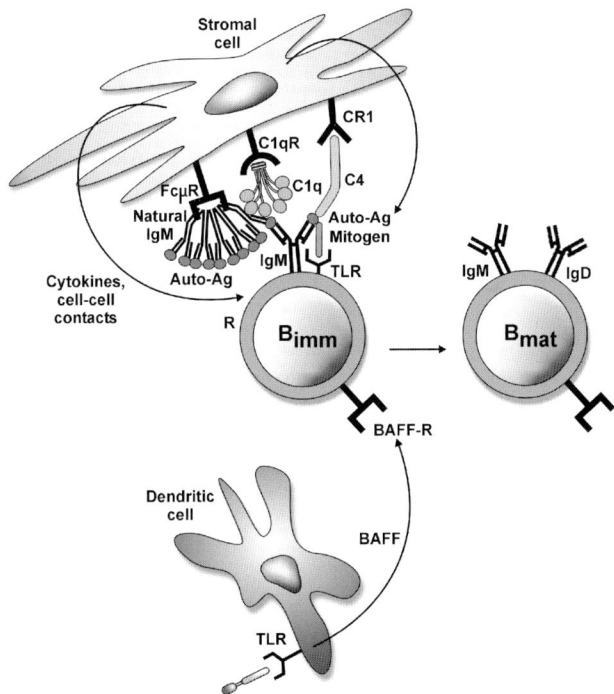

6
Ignorance

Emerging B cells with no apparent autoreactivity pass the two checkpoints in bone marrow and spleen, as long as they express a surface membrane-deposited BcR. A variety of Ig-transgenic mouse models support this view (Fields and Erikson 2004). The ignored B cells enter the spleen via the terminal branches of the central arterioles and populate the follicular regions as conventional, B2-type B cells. Initially they are short-lived, with half-lives of 2–4 days. They then mature to longer-lived B cells, with half-lives longer than 6 weeks. The BcR complex with Ig and Ig is mandatory for transition to the peripheral sIgM$^+$B cell pools; no sIg$^-$ B cells survive normally. The transition from short-lived to long-lived, from AA4.1$^+$ to AA4.1$^-$, CD21$^-$/CD23$^-$ to CD21$^+$/CD23$^+$ cells is controlled by a series of genes, including OBF, bt, and CD40. Thus, bt$^-$/CD40$^-$-, or bt$^-$/OBF$^-$ double-deficient mice have a strong defect at the transition from the immature, transitional T1- and T2-type B cells to mature B cells (Rolink et al. 2001). In addition, crosslinking of surface IgM by anti-IgM-antibodies (possibly a polyclonal example of a crosslinking autoantigen) induces immature B cells of bone marrow as well as spleen (T1 and T2) to apoptosis. This apoptosis can be prevented by the transgenic expression of the anti-apoptotic transgene *bcl-2*, and is circumvented by polyclonal activation with LPS, and with CD40-specific antibodies, or CD40 ligand.

Deficiency in the expression of the TNF family member, BAFF (also called B-lys), or its receptor, BAFF-R blocks the maturation of immature B cells into conventional, B2-type B cells, but not to B1-type B cells (Schneider et al. 1999; Moore et al. 1999; Gross al. 2001; Schiemann et al. 2001; Rolink and Melchers 2002; Ng et al. 2005). In vitro BAFF induces polyclonal maturation of immature B cells from bone marrow and from spleen (T1, T2) without proliferation (Rolink et al. 2002). BAFF has been found in the sera of some lupus erythematosus patients, as well as in the sera of NZBxNZW SLE autoimmune disease-prone mice. In these mice, administration of BAFF-specific antibodies prevents, or at least delays the development of SLE disease. Therefore, excessive production of BAFF, administered at the sites of negative selection of immature B cells, could rescue autoreactive B cells from deletion, leading to autoimmune reactivities in the peripheral mature conventional B cell repertoires (Fig. 2). One major site of BAFF production has been found to be dendritic cells. Hence, in order to interfere with the deletion of autoreactive immature B cells, such dendritic cells would have to be located near the sites of B cell deletion in bone marrow or spleen, and would have to be strongly activated to BAFF production to effect rapid maturation of autoreactive immature B cells before they are subjected to negative selection. Such a scenario still needs to be investigated, and the observed partial rescue of B cell tolerance by T-cell independent antigens may be one experimental way to probe the molecular and cellular requirements for such competition with clonal deletion.

7
Positive Selection

Autoreactive, in fact often polyreactive B cells (Leslie et al. 2001) can be positively selected, and appear to accumulate in the BI compartments of the gut-associated lymphoid tissues, i.e., in the follicles below the M cells of the flat epithelium of the gut (Fig. 1). They are also found as single, intraepithelial cells. B cells within the marginal zone of the spleen also appear to be positively selected. However, it remains to be seen whether this major traffic intersection of newly generated (as well as possibly of recirculating) B cells, in contact with cellular debris of dying blood cells and of killed bacteria about to be removed from the circulation in the spleen, are the sites of positive selection into the BI compartments, which are later predominantly found in the gut.

B cells in the gut-associated lymphoid tissues (GALT), including the lamina propria, produce IgM, and predominantly switch to IgA (Fig. 1). Secreted IgA traverses the epithelia associated with the secretory piece that it acquires during the migration through the epithelial layer. On the luminal side, it binds with low affinity and high crossreactivity to bacteria of the endogenous flora and to food antigens. Hence, the low-avidity positive selection of these (eventually IgA-producing and secreting) BI cells appears to possible be useful for neutralizing interactions of the secreted antibodies with potentially infectious bacteria of the gut flora. At least in parts, this IgA production appears to be quite distinct from the Ig production elicited in a helper T cell-dependent, inflammatory response of B cells in germinal centers of peripheral lymph nodes and the spleen. First, while the follicular B cell response beneath the M cells may be helper T cell-dependent, germinal center-derived, the submucosal, intraepithelial response in the lamina propria can be helper T cell-independent. One-third of the IgA might derive from such T cell-independent B cell responses in these T cell-independent responses. The expression of the Ig class switch-inducing AiD gene could be induced by a CD40 ligand–CD40 interaction, in which the cooperating cell providing the CD40 ligand is not known and must not be a helper T cell. Furthermore, these B cell responses could be co-stimulated by other cell–cell contacts and cytokines, which might not be typical for a T cell-dependent, germinal center response of B cells. Hypermutation of the V regions of the IgM, and later IgA, expressed and secreted by the lamina propria of the intestine BI cells could well occur in the AiD-expressing,

IgA class switching cells, but the lack of the selection of better fitting V-region mutants by bacterial antigens and the lack of germinal center formation, i.e., exclusive B cell proliferation, may decrease the probability to generate and select better-fitting antibacterial antibodies, as much as that should also decrease the probability of generating high-affinity autoreactive antibodies.

8
Peripheral B Cells Without sIg Expression

The Epstein-Barr lines (EBV) encodes latent membrane proteins (LMP), of which LMP 2A, a multispanning transmembrane protein, expressed in B lymphocytes, can associate with Igα and Igβ and share with these two anchor proteins an ITAM motif (Gross et al. 2005; Fruehling and Longnecker 1997; Miller et al. 1995; Caldwell et al. 1998). In fact, the phosphorylated form of the ITAM motif of LAMP 2A recruits tyrosine kinases and adaptor proteins that are also used by the BcR complex for signaling. In this way, LMP 2A acts as a BcR analog, supporting the selection into the peripheral mature B cell compartments of B cells lacking BcRs. High-level transgenic expression of LMP 2A selectively recruits cells into the BI compartments, e.g., into the gut and intestine, while low-level expression promotes development of conventional, B2-type and marginal zone B cells (Casola et al. 2004). Neither of these B cell populations can be stimulated by T cell-dependent antigens to develop germinal centers in peripheral lymphoid organs, indicating that BcRs on the surface of B cells are needed for peripheral germinal center responses. By contrast, the low-level, but not the high-level, i.e., the conventional B2, but not the B1 cell-directed LMP 2A expression allows germinal centers to be formed in the gut. Hence, the role of BcRs in germinal center formation in the gut might be replaced by an antigen-unspecific mechanism antigen uptake, which allows processing and presentation by MHC class II molecules to helper T cells. Alternatively, these gut-associated BcR-deficient B cells might be stimulated by bystander helper T cells activated with bacteria of the gut, or by bacteria-derived polyclonal activators, such as LPS, lipoprotein, etc., in the latter case via TLR2, TLR4 and others, or by other T-lineage cells or NK cells not restricted by the recognition of MHC class–peptide complexes. In summary, T cell (or NK cell) -dependent, BcR-independent (perhaps MHC class II-independent) activation of B cells in germinal centers can lead to GC responses, in which the activated B cells (as well as T or NK cells) can be expected to secrete pro-inflammatory cytokines—such as IFN, IL-1, IL-4, IL-5, IL-6, and TNF—which can lead to systemic manifestations of autoimmune-like reactions, in severe cases to bowel disease. It remains to be seen how strong the contributions of the BcR-independent responses of GALT-associated B cells are in BcR-proficient immune systems.

Furthermore it has been observed in pre-BI cell-transplanted RAG-deficient mice, containing only pre-BI cell-derived BI cells, but no T cells, that one-third of the normal levels of IgA can be produced, apparently T cell-independently, mainly by cells in the intestinal lamina propria, without the formation of germinal centers (Rolink et al. 2001). It is likely that these cells are also present in BcR-deficient, high-level LMP 2A-expressing lamina propria BI cells. Obviously, they cannot produce IgA, but they can be expected, again, to respond to bacteria by the secretion of cytokines that might be of the pro- or anti-inflammatory types.

In conclusion, the GALT-associated B cell compartments can develop even when the B cells do not express BcRs (and possibly also not MHC class II), i.e., they can function in cellular responses of proliferation and differentiation to effector functions in an antigen-independent, perhaps bacteria-dependent way, leading to pro-inflammatory (and perhaps also anti-inflammatory) responses that could manifest themselves as quasi-autoimmune.

9
Rescue of Autoreactive B Cells by T Cell-Independent Antigens of Type I, TLR–Ligand–Antigen-Complexes

Immature and mature B cells express Toll-like receptors (TLR) (Akira and Takeda 2004) such as TLR2 (for bacterial lipoprotein), TLR4 (for bacterial LPS), and TLR9 (for bacterial CpG). It has long been known that these bacteria-derived TLR ligands can act as polyclonal activators for both stages of B cell development, inducing the B cells to proliferation and maturation to Ig secreting cells. At limiting, nonpolyclonally activating concentrations of these TLR ligands, hapten-TLR ligand conjugates can induce hapten-specific B cell proliferation and maturation. In this way, conjugates of CpG with double-stranded (ds) DNA, as well as chromatin–IgG complexes, can activate dsDNA-specific IgG or chromatin-specific IgG, respectively, i.e., autoantigen-reactive B cells to autoantibody production. Initially, and perhaps normally, the peripheral B cell repertoires might not contain high-avidity autoantigen-reactive B cells, therefore limiting these TLR-dependent, initially T cell-independent responses to low-affinity autoantibodies. However, high-affinity autoantibodies might develop with these T cell-independent antigens in at least two possible ways. In one, helper T cells or N cells may take over the stimulation of the activated B cells. In the former case, this induces AiD expression, i.e., Ig class switching and hypermutation, as well as longevity of B cells leading to high-affinity autoantibody production. However, tolerance to autoantigens has to be broken in the helper T cell compartment.

In the other way, autoantigen–TLR–ligand complexes might activate immature B cells to proliferation, rather than to apoptosis of the autoantigen-specific B cells, as, for example, LPS has been seen to induce such responses on a polyclonal level with immature B cells. Thereby, autoantigen–TLR–ligand complexes could compete with autoantigen–natural IgM–complement complexes for reactions leading either to survival and proliferation or to apoptosis of the autoantigen-reactive cells. This may well occur during the peak of a bacterial infection and might become chronic if the infection is chronic. A real danger of autoimmune disease (in the case of dsDNA IgG or chromatin to SLE) should only arise if the response of the rescued, matured, activated autoreactive B cells is taken over by a helper T cell-dependent, or otherwise AiD-inducing action of the immune system.

10
Autoreaction Rescued by Ignorance

A mouse strain has been generated by transplantation of a nucleus from a peripheral sIg$^+$B cell into an enucleated embryonic stem (ES) cell, followed by implantation of the nucleus-altered ES cell into a foster mother to develop the new mouse strain (Hochedlinger and Jaenisch 2002). The mouse strain carries one productively $V_H D_H J_H$-rearranged H chain allele and, surprisingly, two productively $V_L J_L$-rearranged L chain alleles. Hence, its B cells express Ig receptors with two different L chains. To study the two IgM receptors independently of each other, two mouse substrains were bred in which only one of the two L chain alleles is carried and expressed, each together with the H chain (Gerdes and Wabl 2004). One L chain allele (cu2) contributes to an IgM on B cells that leads to the rapid and efficient selection of the (monoclonal cu2 L chain/H chain) expressing B cells into the follicular, originally short-lived, conventional, B2-type B cell compartments, which are not impeded by high- or low-affinity reactions with autoantigens. Hence they are ignored during their development, similar to the two-thirds of B cells that a normal mouse generates as cells with one productive $V_L J_L$ rearrangement on the first allele, while retaining the second allele in germ-line configuration.

However, the other L chain allele (b4) of the nuclear transplant mouse makes an autoreactive IgM with the same H chain. It recognizes an unidentified autoantigen on apoptotic cells in the nearby environment of the primary lymphoid organ. Consequently, a large fraction, but not all of the developing B cells at the transition from immature to mature cells from bone marrow to spleen are deleted, i.e., negatively selected. Since the deletion is more extensive when the B cells cannot edit the b4-L chain by secondary V_L to J_L rearrangements, i.e., on a RAG-deficient background, the b4-L chain /H chain-containing IgM induces editing.

This suggests the following scenario for the generation of the original B cell from which the nucleus was isolated and used to generate the mouse strain by nuclear transplantation (Melchers 2004). At the transition from pre-BI to large pre-BII cells, one productive $V_H D_H J_H$ rearrangement led to the formation of a preBcR, which expanded the pre-BII cell population by proliferation. One of the resting small pre-BII cells then rearranged the V(b4) segment to J on the first allele and in-frame. The sIgM on the resulting sIgM$^+$ immature B cell then recognized the autoantigen, and this recognition signaled the cell to open the second allele and rearrange V (cu2) to J. Again, the rearrangement was productive, and the expression of the second IgM and of IgM molecules with mixed L chains allowed the cell to shut down the rearrangement machinery and to enter one of the mature pools of B cells. Ignorance appears to have dominated over self-recognition.

These results raise many questions. How frequently are double producers selected into the BI or the conventional B cell compartments? Do double producers also emerge from V_H to DHJH rearrangements and are they positively selectable by mixtures of ignorant and autoreactive V_H domains? It also remains to be seen whether such double BcR-producers constitute a potential danger for autoimmune reactions and autoimmune diseases.

11
Breaking the Tolerance of Mature, Peripheral B Cell Repertoires

After the selections of the repertoires of BI and of conventional (B2) cells, we expect these repertoires to be essentially devoid, because purged, of high-affinity autoantigen-reactive BcR-expressing B cells, unless such autoantigens did not have a chance to be exposed to the developing B cells in the primary lymphoid organs (i.e., in bone marrow) and in spleen. Hence, all stimulatory actions on these B cells that do not activate AiD should not generate high-affinity, autoantigen-reactive B cells and autoantibody secretion. Such B cell-activating actions include the ways in which T cell-independent antigens are expected to stimulate B cells. Such T cell-independent antigens, e.g., of type 1, are known to use the receptors of polyclonal activators such as TLR4, -2 or -9.

Furthermore, continuous exposure to soluble antigens (hence, also autoantigens) can induce a state of anergy in mature B cells trough continuous downregulation of BcRs from the surface. This induces, or keeps, a short half-life of such B cells. In addition, helper T cells specific for the processed form of the anergizing antigen recognize the peptide–MHC class II complexes and co-stimulate the now Fas-expressing B cells via Fas-ligand expressed on the T cells. Fas-induced apoptosis of the specific B cells is initiated, while all other B cells not recognizing any soluble (auto)antigens are not stimulated and survive.

Most importantly, helper T cell repertoires are purged of autoreactive cells at comparable stages of their development in the thymus, with much the same result of negative selection by high-avidity interactions of autoreactive TcR-expressing T cells by autoantigen-MHC-presenting cells in the thymus. Furthermore, the development and maturation of autoreactive helper T cells is suppressed by autoantigen-specific suppressor T cells, today called $CD4^+$ $CD25^+$ regulatory T cells. It remains to be investigated whether these regulatory T cells also have direct suppressive interactions with mature B cells in autoantigen-specific ways.

However, whenever these B cell repertoires can be initially activated by helper T cells—and viral as well as bacterial infections are suspected of doing that through release of sequestered autoantigen, through molecular mimicry of TcR- and/or BcR-directed epitopes of infection antigens with autoantigens, or through polyclonal activation of T and/or B cells—in CD40 ligand-CD40-dependent ways, or whenever T cell-independently activated B cells can be restimulated with the help of T cells, AiD can be induced. The resulting hypermutation of Ig variable-region genes can then generate high affinity, autoantigen-reactive B cells, and autoantibody secretion. Whenever the autoantigen is present in this—usually germinal center-located, T cell -dependent antigen and autoantigen-dependent response—this should favor the positive selection of such high-affinity autoantibody-producing B cell clones, much in the same way in which a foreign antigen selects high-affinity antibody-producing cells specific for the foreign antigen in a normal immune response. Therefore, breaking of the B cell compartment tolerance is often achieved by breaking this tolerance with a helper T cell capable of recognizing a peptide on self-MHC processed from an autoantigen taken up through a low-avidity autoantigen-specific BcR-expressing B cell. These helper T cells then induce CD40 L- CD40-dependent AiD activation and, hence, V-region hypermutation in the autoantigen-reactive B cells. Thereafter the autoantigen selects hypermutated BcR-expressing B cells with higher avidities toward the autoantigen. This leads to clonal expansions and eventual high-avidity autoantibody secretion of BcR-mutant B cells that have also gained longevity, hence, are long-lived memory B and plasma cells.

As a consequence of such an autoantigen-driven-, high-avidity antibody-selecting response, two major players of autoimmune disease are generated:

1. Autoantibodies with the capacity to form large immune complexes are secreted into the blood stream. Bound to Fc receptors on reticuloendothelial cells in the kidney and the blood vessels and thus activating complement, they destroy the tissues and, hence, induce glomerulonephritis and vasculitis.
2. Expanded numbers of long-lived B cells with high-avidity autoantigen-specific BcRs can cooperate much more efficiently with helper T cells in inflammatory germinal center B cell responses because their high-avidity, autoantigen-specific receptors allow the uptake, processing, and MHC class II presentation of autoantigen peptides at concentrations that might be 10e22–10e33-fold lower than the antigen-presenting capacity of a dendritic or a macrophage cell that can take up such autoantigens only by autoantigen-unspecific endocytosis at much higher concentrations (Lanzavecchia 1987; Coutinho, Gronowicz and Möller 1975).

It remains surprising that autoimmune reactions resulting in chronically altered, deregulated responses are not more frequent, given the many genes that must function in stimulatory and suppressive ways to effect immune protection against the wide world of foreign invaders and to maintain nonresponsiveness and suppression to the equally wide world of autoantigens.

12
Consequences of Breaking B Cell Tolerance—Autoimmune Diseases

In at least two major types of autoimmune diseases, autoantibodies, and B cells producing them, contribute to the pathophysiology of the disease. In both cases, somatically hypermutated autoantibodies have been identified, and some of them have been shown to possibly induce, but certainly propagate factors in the destruction of cells and tissues generating the disease phenotypes. A characteristic spectrum of autoantigens appears to be connected with the induction and/or propagation of these autoimmune diseases. In systemic lupus erythematosus (SLE), nuclear antigens, especially double-stranded DNA, histones, and nucleoprotein complexes such as the ss- and Rho-antigens, are recognized by the somatically mutated autoantibodies. In chronic inflammatory rheumatoid arthritis (RA) posttranslationally modified proteins of cells in the target tissues, e.g., citrullinated proteins of the tissues of the synovialis, characterize some of the autoantigens recognized by the autoantibodies. In SLE viral antigens, for example, those encoded by Epstein-Barr virus and antigens of other infectious agents have been implied in breaking T cell tolerance, thereby setting the stage for B cell activation,

V-region hypermutation, and selection of B cells with hypermutated, nuclear antigen-specific BcRs. In RA, breaking of tolerance may initially involve helper T cell activation by peptides containing posttranslationally modified peptides of autoantigens in MHC class II complexes, followed by activation of B cell-specific for the same, or similarly modified proteins, with the positive selection of hypermutated, high-avidity autoantibody-producing cells. Again, the autoantibodies can form immune complexes and can participate in the destruction of tissue, in this case in the synovialis.

For both diseases, secreted autoantibodies were long suspected to be major disease-propagating factors. However, recent evidence from clinical trials with a B cell-specific monoclonal antibody, i.e., against the B cell-associated surface marker CD20, have shifted the focus of interest to B cells and cells expressing the hypermutated, autoantigen-specific BcRs on their surface as major contributors to the acute disease manifestations. Within 2 weeks, two doses of the CD20-specific mAb nearly abolish major disease manifestations—in a time period in which the autoantibody detectable in the patient's blood stream are hardly reduced. The CD20-specific mAb that induces a strong B cell cytopenia in circulating blood might, therefore, remove the inflammation-inducing cooperators from the autoantigen-peptide-MHCII-specific helper T cells which normally produce inflammatory cytokines such as TNF in the autoimmune response.

Acknowledgements A.R.R. is supported by a grant from the Swiss National Funds No. 3100–066692, F.M. by a grant from the Swiss National Funds No. 3100–066682.

References

Ait-Azzouzene D, Skog P, Retter M, Kouskoff V, Hertz M, Lang J, Kench J,Chumley M, Melamed D, Sudaria J, Gavin A, Martensson A, Verkoczy L, Duong B,Vela J, Nemazee D, Alfonso C (2004) Tolerance-induced receptor selection: scope, sensitivity, locus specificity, and relationship to lymphocyte-positive selection. Immunol Rev 197:219–230

Akira S, Takeda K (2004) Toll-like receptor signalling. Nat Rev Immunol 4:499–511

Backhed F, Ley RE, Sonnenburg JL, Peterson DA, Gordon JI (2005) Host-bacterial mutualism in the human intestine. Science 307:1915–1920

Caldwell RG, Wilson JB, Anderson SJ, Longnecker R (1998) Epstein-Barr virus LMP2A drives B cell development and survival in the absence of normal B cell receptor signals. Immunity 9:405–411

Carroll MC (2004a) A protective role for innate immunity in systemic lupus erythematosus. Nat Rev Immunol 4:825–831

Carroll MC (2004b) The complement system in regulation of adaptive immunity. Nat Immunol 5:981–986

Casellas R, Shih TA, Kleinewietfeld M, Rakonjac J, Nemazee D, Rajewsky K, Nussenzweig MC (2001). Contribution of receptor editing to the antibody repertoire. Science 291:1541–1544

Casola S, Otipoby KL, Alimzhanov M, Humme S, Uyttersprot N, Kutok JL, Carroll MC, Rajewsky K (2004) B cell receptor signal strength determines B cell fate. Nat Immunol 5:317–327

Ceredig R, Rolink AG, Melchers F, Andersson J (2000) The B cell receptor, but not the pre-B cell receptor, mediates arrest of B cell differentiation. Eur J Immunol 30:759–767

Chiller JM, Habicht GS, Weigle WO (1970) Cellular sites of immunologic unresponsiveness. Proc Natl Acad Sci U S A 65:551–556

Coutinho A, Gronowicz E, Moller G (1975) Mechanism of B-cell activation and paralysis by thymus-independent antigens. Additive effects between NNP-LPS and LPS in the specific response to the hapten. Scand J Immunol 4:89–94

Craig SW, Cebra JJ (1971) Peyer's patches: an enriched source of precursors for IgA-producing immunocytes in the rabbit. J Exp Med 134:188–200

Dal Porto JM, Gauld SB, Merrell KT, Mills D, Pugh-Bernard AE, Cambier J (2004) B cell antigen receptor signaling 101. Mol Immunol 41:599–613

Fagarason S, Honjo T (2003) Intestinal IgA synthesis: regulation of front-line body defenses. Nat Rev Immunol 3:63–72

Fields ML, Erikson J (2003) The regulation of lupus-associated autoantibodies: immunoglobulin transgenic models. Curr Opin Immunol 15:709–717

Fields ML, Nish SA, Hondowicz BD, Metzgar MH, Wharton GN, Caton AJ, Erikson J (2005) The influence of effector T cells and Fas ligand on lupus-associated B cells. J Immunol 175:104–111

Fruehling S, Longnecker R (1997) The immunoreceptor tyrosine-based activation motif of Epstein-Barr virus LMP2A is essential for blocking BCR-mediated signal transduction. Virology 235:241–251

Gay D, Saunders D, Camper S, Weigert M (1995) Receptor editing: an approach by autoreactive B cells to escape tolerance. J Exper Med 4:999–1008

Gerdes T, Wabl M (2004) Autoreactivity and allelic inclusion in a B cell nuclear transfer mouse. Nat Immunol 5:1282–1287

Ghia P, ten Boekel E, Rolink AG, Melchers F (1998) B-cell development: a comparison between mouse and man. Immunol Today 19:480–485

Ghia P, Melchers F, Rolink AG (2000) Age-dependent changes in B lymphocyte development in man and mouse. Exp Gerontol 35:159–165

Goodnow CC, Crosbie J, Adelstein S, Lavoie TB, Smith-Gill SJ, Brink RA, Pritchard-Briscoe H, Wotherspoon JS, Loblay RH, Raphael K, Trent RS, Basten A (1988) Altered immunoglobulin expression and functional silencing of self-reactive B lymphocytes in transgenic mice. Nature 334:676–682

Gross JA, Dillon SR, Mudri S, Johnston J, Littau A, Roque R, Rixon M, Schou O, Foley KP, Haugen H, McMillen S, Waggie K, Schreckhise RW, Shoemaker K, Vu T, Moore M, Grossman A, Clegg CH (2001) TACI-Ig neutralizes molecules critical for B cell development and autoimmune disease. Impaired B cell maturation in mice lacking BLyS. Immunity 15:289–302

Gross AJ, Hochberg D, Rand WM, Thorley-Lawson DA (2005) EBV and systemic lupus erythematosus: a new perspective. J Immunol 174:6599–6607

Hochedlinger K, Jaenisch R (2002) Monoclonal mice generated by nuclear transfer from mature B and T donor cells. Nature 415:1035–1038

Hooper LV, Gordon JI (2001) Commensal host-bacterial relationships in the gut. Science 292:1115–1118

Hoyer BF, Manz RA, Radbruch A, Hiepe F (2005) Long-lived plasma cells and their contribution to autoimmunity. Ann N Y Acad Sci 1050:124–133

Klinman NR (1996) The "clonal selection hypothesis" and current concepts of B cell tolerance. Immunity 5:189–195

Kunkel EJ, Butcher EC (2003) Plasma-cell homing. Nat Rev Immunol 3:822–829

Lanzavecchia A (1987) Antigen uptake and accumulation in antigen-specific B cells. Immunol Rev 99:39–51

Leslie D, Lipsky P, Notkins AL (2001) Autoantibodies as predictors of disease. J Clin Invest 108:1417–1422

Manz RA, Hauser AE, Hiepe F, Radbruch A (2005) Maintenance of serum antibody levels. Annu Rev Immunol 223:367–386

Melchers F (2004) The death of a dogma? Nat Immunol 5:1199–1201

Melchers F (2005) The pre-B-cell receptor: selector of fitting immunoglobulin heavy chains for the B-cell repertoire. Nat Rev Immunol 5:578–584

Melchers F, Kincade P (2004) Early B cell development to a mature, antigen-sensitive cell. In: Honjo T, Alt FW (eds) Molecular biology of B cells. Elsevier Science, Amsterdam, pp 101–126

Melchers F, Rolink A (1999) B lymphocyte development and biology. In: Paul WE (ed) Fundamental immunology, 4th edn. Lippincott-Raven, Philadelphia, pp 183–224

Melchers F, ten Boekel E, Seidl T, Kong XC, Yamagami T, Onishi K, Shimizu T, Rolink AG, Andersson J (2000) Repertoire selection by pre-B-cell receptors and B-cell receptors, and genetic control of B-cell development from immature to mature B cells. Immunol Rev 175:33–46

Monroe JG (2004) B-cell positive selection and peripheral homeostasis. Immunol Rev 197:5–9

Moore PA, Belvedere O, Orr A, Pieri K, LaFleur DW, Feng P, Soppet D, Charters M, Gentz R, Parmelee D, Li Y, Galperina O, Giri J, Roschke V, Nardelli B, Carrell J, Sosnovtseva S, Greenfield W, Ruben SM, Olsen HS, Fikes J, Hilbert DM (1999) BLyS: member of the tumor necrosis factor family and B lymphocyte stimulator. Science 285:260–263

Mostoslavsky R, Alt FW, Bassing CH (2003) Chromatin dynamics and locus accessibility in the immune system. Nat Immunol 4:603–606

Nemazee DA, Burki K (1989a) Clonal deletion of autoreactive B lymphocytes in bone marrow chimeras. Proc Natl Acad Sci U S A 86:8039

Nemazee DA, Burki K (1989b) Clonal deletion of B lymphocytes in a transgenic mouse bearing anti-MHC class I antibody genes. Nature 337:562–566

Rolink A, Grawunder U, Haasner D, Strasser A, Melchers F (1993) Immature surface Ig+ B cells can continue to rearrange kappa and lambda L chain gene loci. J Exp Med 178:1263–1270

Rolink AG, Brocker T, Bluethmann H, Kosco-Vilbois MH, Andersson J, Melchers F (1999) Mutations affecting either generation or survival of cells influence the pool size of mature B cells. Immunity 10:619–628

Rolink AG, Schaniel C, Andersson J, Melchers F (2001) Selection events operating at various stages in B cell development. Curr Opin Immunol 13:202–207

Rolink AG, Tschopp J, Schneider P, Melchers F (2002) BAFF is a survival and maturation factor for mouse B cells. Eur J Immunol 32:2004–2010

Tiegs SL, Russell DM, Nemazee D (1993) Receptor editing in self-reactive bone marrow B cells. J Exp Med 177:1009–1020

Schiemann B, Gommerman JL, Vora K, Cachero TG, Shulga-Morskaya S, Dobles M, Frew E, Scott ML (2001) An essential role for BAFF in the normal development of B cells through a BCMA-independent pathway. Science 293:2111–2114

Schlissel MS (2003) Regulating antigen-receptor gene assembly. Nat Rev Immunol 3:890–899

Shimizu T, Mundt C, Licence S, Melchers F, Martensson IL (2002) VpreB1/VpreB2/lambda 5 triple-deficient mice show impaired B cell development but functional allelic exclusion of the IgH locus. J Immunol 168:6286–6293

William J, Euler C, Christensen S, Shlomchik MJ (2002) Evolution of autoantibody responses via somatic hypermutation outside of germinal centers. Science 297:2066–2070

Yamagami T, ten Boekel E, Andersson J, Rolink A, Melchers F (1999) Frequencies of multiple IgL chain gene rearrangements in single normal or kappaL chain-deficient B lineage cells. Immunity 11:317–127

Breaking Ignorance: The Case of the Brain

H. Wekerle (✉)

MPI Neuroimmunology, Martinsried, Germany
hwekerle@neuro.mpg.de

1	Introduction	26
2	Brain Autoantigens in the Immune System	27
3	B Cell Ignorance?	30
4	Activation of Ignorant Autoreactive T Cells—The Transition from Auto*reactive* to Auto*aggressive*	32
4.1	Molecular Mimicry, Duped Ignorance?	32
4.2	Microbial Superantigens	34
4.3	T Cells with Two Antigen Receptors	36
4.4	The Inflammatory Milieu—Link to Innate Immunity	36
5	Regulatory Suppression of Autoimmune T Cells—But How Do Suppressor T Cells Know?	38
5.1	Autoantigen *Retrouvé*: Recognition/Presentation in the Target Organ	39
6	Conclusion	44
	References	45

Abstract Immunological self-tolerance is maintained through diverse mechanisms, including deletion of autoreactive immune cells following confrontation with autoantigen in the thymus or in the periphery and active suppression by regulatory cells. A third way to prevent autoimmunity is by hiding self tissues behind a tissue barrier impermeable for circulating immune cells. The latter mechanism has been held responsible for self-tolerance within the nervous tissue. Indeed, the nervous tissues enjoy a conditionally privileged immune status: they are normally unreachable for self-reactive T and B cells, they lack lymphatic drainage, and they are deficient in local antigen-presenting cells. Yet the immune system is by no means fully ignorant of the nervous structures. An ever-growing number of brain specific autoantigens is expressed within the thymus, which ensures an early confrontation with the unfolding T cell repertoire, and there is evidence that B cells also contact CNS-like structures outside of the brain. Then pathological processes such as neurodegeneration commonly lift the brain's immune privilege, shifting the local milieus from immune-hostile to immune-friendly. Finally, brain-reactive T cells, which abound in the healthy immune repertoire, but remain innocuous throughout life, can be activated and gain access to their target tissues. On their way, they take an ordered migration through peripheral lymphoid tissues and blood circulation, and undergo a profound reprogramming of their gene expression profile, which renders them fit to enter the nervous system and to interact with local cellule elements.

1
Introduction

The brain is generally reputed to be the body's site of intelligence, not of ignorance. An aberrant view has been held by the community of neuroimmunologists. Indeed, from an immunological point of view, the brain has long enjoyed the status of a *terra incognita*. The traditional dogma of neuroimmunology had it that the central nervous system (CNS: brain and spinal cord) is out of reach of the prospecting and protecting mechanisms of immune surveillance. Accordingly, immune cells would ignore the CNS, a state commonly referred to as immune privilege.

The concept of central nervous immune privilege classically rests on several structural peculiarities that set the brain apart from other tissues. These include, first of all, a tight endothelial blood–brain barrier (BBB), which blocks free exchange of cells and macromolecules between blood flow and the CNS parenchyma. Second, the CNS lacks a fully differentiated lymphatic drainage, which would connect the brain with local peripheral immune organs, and, finally, at least under normal conditions, CNS tissues neither express substantial levels of MHC proteins, nor do they harbor specialized antigen-presenting cells (APCs) such as dendritic cells (DCs) (Wekerle et al. 1986; Hickey 2001).

Functionally, immune privilege and ignorance were thought to act on two separate levels. Brain-specific protein structures were supposed to be hidden behind the BBB, without access to immune organs. The immune cell lineages newly arising within thymus and bone marrow would differentiate without any possible contact with CNS components. At least in theory, there could be some positive, but certainly no negative selection (deletion) of CNS-specific T or B cell clones. T and B cell repertoires would be formed without censure by CNS autoantigens. Hence, CNS-specific lymphocytes could be introduced into the repertoires, but they could not reach their target tissues, again due the tight BBB, and the lack of local MHC.

Thus goes theory, but it has not been supported by clinical experience. In fact, immune privilege and ignorance are by no means absolute; there are numerous pathological CNS conditions that involve intracerebral immune reactions. These include responses to microbial infections, neoplasias, and even degenerative disorders are often accompanied by immune cell infiltrations. Most spectacular are, however, the inflammatory processes noted in multiple sclerosis (MS), where immune cells invade the tissue and produce response patterns only seen in established cases of other autoimmune diseases (Lassmann et al. 2001).

How could immune cells gain access to the secluded CNS and respond not only to microbes, or tumors, but perhaps even to autoantigenic components of the tissue? The answer is that separation between CNS and the immune system is not as strict as described until here. In fact, as has been recognized quite recently, there are indeed connections between both organ systems, and, as will be shown, these are numerous and complex. We will see that an ever-increasing number of putative brain autoantigens are produced and also exposed within immune organs (central as well as peripheral), and that particular immune cells are able to gain access to the CNS, where MHC antigens can be induced under certain favorable conditions.

2
Brain Autoantigens in the Immune System

Myelin basic protein (MBP) is the classical brain-specific autoantigen. In many species and strains of animals, immunization against MBP in suitable immune adjuvants almost unfailingly results in the development of experimental autoimmune encephalomyelitis (EAE), a T cell-mediated autoimmune disease targeted exclusively against CNS white matter. The exquisite tissue specificity has been traditionally explained by a correspondingly restricted tissue distribution. Indeed, MBP is produced at the highest level in CNS myelin sheaths, where it is positioned on the inner membrane leaflets, not on the surface (Campagnoni and Macklin 1988).

However, quite unexpectedly, several observations showed that CNS-specific autoantigens were also produced within the immune system, most prominently by thymus cells, mainly stroma, and that these ectopic autoantigens actively influenced the generation of the autoimmune T cell repertoire. At about the same time, two laboratories described a whole family of MBP and MBP-related genes in the immune cells (Pribyl et al. 1993; Grima et al. 1992). Both groups described MBP-like sequences in the thymus as well as in lymph nodes and the spleen. In particular, MBP expression by thymus stroma cells was unexpected. Then Kojima et al. showed directly for the first time the co-existence of CNS autoantigen and specific autoreactive T cells in the same rodent thymus. The autoantigen was the calcium binding protein S-100β, which is expressed in astrocytes, rather than in myelin and myelin-binding oligodendrocytes. S-100β autoreactive T cells transfer inflammation in the CNS, as well as in the eye (Kojima et al. 1994). Besides astrocytes, however, S-100β is lavishly produced by certain thymus stroma cells, located preferentially in the thymic medulla (Kojima et al. 1997).

Would ectopically expressed CNS-specific autoantigen affect the distribution of encephalitogenic T lymphocyte clones within the newly generated immune repertoire? Again, almost simultaneously, two groups independently reported that indeed myelin autoantigens produced in the thymus robustly affect the generation of the myelin-specific, encephalitogenic T cell repertoire. The investigators compared immune reactivity against myelin proteins in normal mice with mutant mice lacking the myelin component in question. They found that myelin protein-deficient mice generally possess many more myelin autoreactive T cells than their wild type counterparts (Anderson et al. 2000; Klein et al. 2000). Complex cell and organ transfer experiments supported the initial suspicion that myelin proteins produced by thymus medullary stroma cells helped remove most of the complementary autoimmune T cells freshly formed in the thymus cortex. Even more, myelin protein portions that may be formed by some strains, but not in others, appeared to reciprocally control the formation of region-specific T cell clones.

Is expression of (myelin-specific) autoantigens in the thymus a singular caprice of nature, is it the exception or the rule? The latter may be the case. A look into another important autoimmune paradigm, type 1, autoimmune diabetes mellitus will make the case. About 10 years ago, a group of diabetologists was interested in producing tumors derived from insulin-producing β cells. To reach this goal, they first linked the gene for the oncogenic T antigen controlled to the pancreas islet-specific insulin promoter, and then inserted this construct into the germ line of transgenic mice. These mice indeed developed, and as expected they showed the transgene in their pancreas islets. It was unexpected, however, that in addition the transgene also showed up in the thymus (Jolicoeur et al. 1994). Subsequent investigations showed that not only insulin promoter-driven transgenes were expressed both in islets and thymus, but that the same was true for insulin itself. An ever-increasing number of autoantigens followed this pattern: they were found not only in the expected specific organ, but in also in the thymus. In the case of CNS autoantigens, the examples include, except myelin components (MBP, PLP, MOG), other proteins such as S100β (Table 1) (Derbinski et al. 2001).

Very recent observations indicate that the *Aire* gene, whose mutated form was discovered in patients with the poly-endocrine autoimmune syndrome APECED, has a role in thymic presentation of some, though not all organ-specific autoantigens. The protein is produced mainly by medullary epithelium, but is also demonstrable in thymic DCs (Zuklys et al. 2000). Its ex-

Table 1 Organ-specific autoantigen expression in the thymus (modified from Kyewski and Derbinski 2004)

Autoantigen	Thymic components				Disease model	Animals
	Macrophage	DC	MTEC	CTEC		
(Golli)MBP	+/−	+/−	+	+/−	EAE	Lewis rat
PLP	+/−	+/−	+	+	EAE	SJL/J mouse
MOG	−	−	+	−	EAE	C57BL mouse
S100β	+	+	+	−	EAE	Lewis rat
AChR	−	−	+	−	EAMG	C57BL mouse
GAD67	−	−	+	−	T1D	NOD mouse
Insulin	−	−	+	−	T1D	NOD mouse
Amylase1	+/−	−	+	+/−	Autoimmune pancreatitis	Lewis rat
A1-crystallin	+/−	+	+	+	EAE	Biozzi mouse
Retinal S antigen	+	−	+	+	EAU	Lewis rat
IRBP	−	−	+	−	EAU	Lewis rat
H/K ATPase-β	−	−	+	+/−	Gastritis	C3H/HeJ mouse
Thyroglobulin	−	−	+	+	EAT	Lewis rat, C3H mouse

EAE, experimental autoimmune encephalomyelitis; *EAMG*, experimental autoimmune myasthenia gravis; *T1D*, Type-1 diabetes mellitus; *EAU*, experimental autoimmune uveitis; *EAT* experimental autoimmune thyroiditis

pression is not autonomous, but regulated by lymphotoxin and its receptor (Boehm et al. 2003; Chin et al. 2003). Much of the Aire protein sits in the nucleus, where it may act on nuclear transcription. Intriguingly, there is recent evidence that, in addition, Aire may act as a ubiquitin ligase, which would involve the protein in processing of intracellular (auto-) antigens and their presentation in the MHC context (Uchida et al. 2004). There are several mechanism(s) by which Aire might control self-tolerance. They may include physical deletion of freshly emerging self-reactive T cell clones, but generation of regulatory T cells is another viable possibility (Mathis and Benoist 2004).

A word of caution seems to be appropriate. Expression of organ-specific autoantigens within the thymic medulla is by no means a guarantee of self-tolerance. This is documented by the existence of the millions of organ-specific autoreactive T cells in the healthy immune repertoire. However, it should be mentioned that thymic autoantigen expression may even have a role in the initiation and maintenance of autoimmune disease. Most prominently, the most common form of human myasthenia gravis goes along with thymic hyperplastic changes, which characteristically include expression of the established target autoantigen, the nicotinic acetylcholine receptor (AChR). AChR-bearing myoid cells, often tightly surrounded by DCs, are typically found in the thymic medulla, which contains substantial numbers of AChR autoreactive CD4 mature T cells (Melms et al. 1988). There is reason to assume that processing and presentation of medullary AChR does not prevent anti-AChR reactions in MG, but rather may be the trigger of the disease (Wekerle and Ketelsen 1977).

3
B Cell Ignorance?

B cell response to antigen differs fundamentally from the T cell counterpart. In contrast to the T cell receptor, the B cell antigen receptor, immunoglobulin, binds to native soluble or membrane proteins and does not need their processing by special APC and embedding on MHC products for successful presentation. Second, while the TCR remains unmodified throughout primary and secondary immune responses, the B cell receptor undergoes drastic changes which form the basis of affinity maturation. During a B cell response, the immunoglobulins are modified by somatic mutations of the antigen binding CDR regions.

This is of importance for understanding B cell autoimmunity. While in the case of T cells, each autoreactive T cell is derived from a progenitor with exactly identical TCR, a high-affinity autoreactive B lymphocyte may have acquired its autoreactivity during a pathological autoimmune response via affinity maturation. Encounter of a developing autoreactive B cell with its autoantigen in the bone marrow (the primary B cell organ) results in the physical elimination of the cell, functional silencing, or, unique to B cells, to the replacement of one autoreactive immunoglobulin chain by another, one with non-self specificity (B cell receptor editing) (Nemazee and Hogquist 2003). Generation of high-affinity autoreactive B cells in the bone marrow therefore is not a prerequisite of a B cell autoimmune response.

There are very few studies investigating the generation of CNS-specific B cell repertoire. One of the few relevant insights comes from the work of Litzenburger and Iglesias (Litzenburger et al. 1998), who produced a knock-in transgenic mouse, whose immunoglobulin (Ig) germline J(H) locus was replaced with the rearranged Ig H chain V gene of a pathogenic MOG-specific mouse MAb (8–18C5) (Linington et al. 1984). As expected, in these single-transgenic mice all B cells expressed the transgenic H chain. It was, however, surprising that about 30% of all recirculating immunoglobulin and about 30% of all B cells specifically bound the autoantigen MOG. These animals never developed spontaneous EAE. However, when sensitized to the encephalitogenic protein PLP, the clinical signs of the resulting EAE were dramatically enhanced. The lesions, which in wild-type mice were almost exclusively inflammatory, showed large confluent foci of demyelination, changes produced by the autoreactive immunoglobulins that attach to the myelin surface and, together with complement and/or phagocytes, cause myelin destruction.

More directly relevant to the repertoire question was a second, double transgenic mouse strain created by the same investigators. This mouse had, in addition to the knocked-in MOG-specific H chain gene, a second transgene encoding the anti-MOG MAb (8–18C5) L chain. These double transgenic mice did not display 100% MOG-binding B cells, as one might have expected, but only approximately 30%, like their single H chain transgenic counterparts (Litzenburger et al. 2000). As it turned out, during development, B cells expressing both transgenic Ig chains were either deleted from the bone marrow or they were forced to replace their transgenic L chain by another, endogenous L chain, a process termed B cell receptor (BCR) editing. BCR cell receptor editing is the well-known result of a confrontation of immature autoreactive B cells with their nominal autoantigen during differentiation in the bone marrow (Nussenzweig 1998).

In analogy to T cell differentiation, the most obvious candidate autoantigen to enforce tolerogenic BCR editing would be classical MOG, expressed on the surface of one of the stroma cells. But this does not seem to be the case. Litzenburger and Iglesias crossed the double transgenic anti-MOG B cell mice on a background lacking MOG autoantigen. Unexpectedly, deprivation of MOG autoantigen in the organism did not affect BCR editing in any demonstrable fashion. So, which self structure, if not MOG, acts as censuring structure in the bone marrow? Is it an antigen, which, from a B cell's point-of view closely resembles MOG but is encoded by a distinct gene?

This raises the question of the origin of the anti-MOG MAb (8–18C5). Obviously, this hybridoma has been created by fusion of a B cell occurring in the spleen of the donor mouse with the neoplastic lymphoma partner cell (Linington et al. 1984). The donor, a BALB/c mouse repeatedly immunized with cerebellar glycoproteins, must have escaped self-tolerance in vivo. How this may have happened is unclear; as one possibility, the B cell may have been a member of the B-1 population, a subset of B cells that preferentially resides in the peritoneal space and produces many of the natural low-affinity polyreactive autoantibodies (Su and Tarakhovsky 2000). Autoreactive antibodies produced by B-1 cells are normally of too low affinity to be pathogenic. Could it be that the anti-MOG MAb is a polyreactive antibody selected for low-affinity binding to an unknown bone marrow structure, and which happens to display heteroclitic high reactivity to the CNS component MOG?

4
Activation of Ignorant Autoreactive T Cells— The Transition from Auto*reactive* to Auto*aggressive*

Now that it is clear that the immune repertoire contains millions of potentially autoreactive T (and B) lymphocyte clones, one may certainly wonder why so few people (and animals) actually develop autoimmune disease. The answer is that auto*reactive* T cells are not automatically pathogenic, i.e., auto*aggressive*. In order to become able to attack their autologous target tissues, an autoreactive T cell must be activated. But activation is not easy to achieve, since there seem to be several tiers of regulatory controls that safeguard the non-pathogenic status of the autoreactive T cells. Breakage of these controls seems to occur only under very special circumstances, as is the case with immunization of animals with autoantigens in complete Freund's adjuvant.

Traditional concepts list four activation mechanisms that may break tissue-specific autoimmunity, most of these related to concurrent microbial immune responses. These are:

1. Molecular mimicry
2. Activation by microbial superantigens
3. Bystander activation in hyperinflammatory microenvironments
4. Utilization of dual T cell receptors, one set specific for microbial antigen, the other one for a true autoantigen.

A fifth mechanism would result from weakened down-regulatory control loops, for example, after loss of suppressor T cells.

4.1
Molecular Mimicry, Duped Ignorance?

Historically, molecular mimicry was the first, and over a long period of time the most attractive concept of organ-specific autoimmune disease. In 1985, Fujinami and Oldstone identified a viral peptide sequence (from the hepatitis B virus polymerase) that shares sequence identity of six contiguous amino acids with the classical encephalitogen, MBP. Immunization of outbred rabbits with the viral decapeptide resulted in histological EAE in some of the animals, going along with MBP-specific T cell proliferation and MBP-binding autoantibodies (Fujinami and Oldstone 1985). This work marked the birth of the mimicry concept of autoimmunity, a concept that engendered a flurry of investigations and published papers.

Subsequent investigations revealed that contiguous sequence identity between microbial and autoantigenic epitopes is not required for cross-activation of autoreactive T cells. With increasing insights into the molecular events of antigen presentation and recognition, it became clear that similarity of amino acid motifs, rather than compete identity is essential in T cell cross-reactivity. This involves motifs required for peptide binding to appropriate MHC class II proteins (anchoring positions), as well as motifs needed for binding the specific T cell receptor surface. It turned out that in some cases only very limited sequence identity of a microbial peptide is sufficient to activate a CNS-specific T cell clone, which implies a large number of bacterial or viral peptide sequences qualifying as potential mimicry partners (Wucherpfennig and Strominger 1995). At the same time, it was recognized that variations of peptide sequences may result in highly variant activation results upon confrontation. While recognition of some of the artificially permutated altered peptide ligands (APL) causes an activation response higher than the one provoked by the original epitope (hyperagonist), others drive the T cell into nonreactivity (antagonists), or divert the cytokine pattern from the original Th1-like to a Th2-like profile (partial antagonists).

Most investigations into mimicry reactions compare mimicking peptides presented by the same MHC protein, but this is a simplification. T cells of a given specificity can be activated by peptides presented in the context of completely different MHC products. A spectacular example was provided by Lang et al. who investigated the peptide reactivity of a human T cell clone specific for the human MBP peptide p85–99 in context of DRB1*1501 (DR15). It was known before that this clone cross-reacted with a related sequence of EBV DNA polymerase p627–641. Studies using monospecific transfected APCs established, however, that, contrary to previous tacit assumption, the mimicking virus peptide was presented by DRB5*0101, a distinct, nonallelic product of the DR2 locus (Lang et al. 2002).

While the mimicry concept, which has mainly been focused on comparing the immunogenicity of synthetic short peptides has led to important therapeutic strategies, its value for understating the pathogenesis of spontaneous autoimmune diseases has remained limited to date. Most mimicry studies ignore that, under in vivo conditions, (auto-)antigenic *proteins* are picked up by antigen-presenting cells and that these proteins are then degraded by intracellular proteases to short peptides, which are fitted into MHC class I or class II proteins before being presented on the cell surface to a specific T cell receptors. Depending on the particular APC, and on the nature of the antigenic protein, individual molecules are cleaved into a limited set of peptides, which may or may not include the cross-reacting epitope sequences identified by screenings of synthetic peptide panels. Thus, future mimicry screenings should go for cross-reacting proteins, rather than for peptides.

Thus it is not surprising that to date there is little cogent evidence that mimicry responses really trigger encephalitogenic responses in real life. While there are numberless studies showing cross-reactivity of myelin-specific T cells with microbial *peptides*, there are extremely few experiments showing such cross-reactivity with microbially infected APC, or APC processing intact microbial protein components.

4.2
Microbial Superantigens

Bacteria and viruses can be spotted by the innate and adaptive immune systems, either via pattern receptors or specific T and B cell receptors. But some of the organisms can fight back. One way is via superantigens, secreted proteins that activate large groups of T cells and thus make them produce pro-inflammatory cytokines in amounts big enough to flood a patient's body and cause severe disease. Toxic shock syndrome was widely publicized some years ago as an example of superantigen-mediated pathogenesis. One version is caused in people by the toxic shock syndrome toxin-1 (TSST-1), a superantigen released from *Staphylococcus aureus* (Llewelyn and Cohen 2003). Apart from producing acute disease, superantigens were credited with shaping the immune repertoire, and, most important in our context, with triggering autoimmune disease.

Like recognition of specific peptide antigen by T cells, superantigens must be presented by APCs in the context of MHC class II proteins. But in contrast to specific antigen presentation, superantigens do not bind into the central peptide groove of MHC proteins, but to the outside. Superantigens do not engage the antigen-recognizing CDR3 regions of the T cell receptor, but bind to variable (V) regions of the TCR β-chain (Marrack and Kappler 1990).

Depending on the number of different Vβ chains targeted, superantigens can activate between 1% and 30% of all accessible T cells. At least in theory, the set of T cell populations selected by a particular superantigen may contain an especially high proportion of autoreactive T cells. Their activation would then kick off autoimmune disease. Such a situation is given in the case of EAE in certain rats and mice. In the Lewis rat and in mice with the MHC H-2u haplotype, autoimmunization with MBP results in an EAE, which is mediated largely by CD4$^+$ T cells utilizing the Vβ8.2 gene for their T cell receptor (TCR) (Heber-Katz and Acha-Orbea 1989).

One could expect that in these animals, superantigens specific for Vβ8.2$^+$ TCRs could well activate MBP-specific, Vβ8.2 utilizing T cells in numbers sufficient to cause EAE. But the experimental results reflected a more complex situation. Superantigen treatment of naïve rodents not only failed to produce EAE, but in most cases even rendered the treated animals resistant against later encephalitogenic treatments (Rott et al. 1992; Gaur et al. 1993). EAE could only be triggered in animals containing an expanded clonal contribution of encephalitogenic T cell clones. This was the case in rodents that had gone through a previous anti-MBP immunization, or in recipients of MBP-specific T cell transfers (Brocke et al. 1993), and superantigens can precipitate EAE relapses in animals that recovered from a previous disease bout (Schiffenbauer et al. 1993). Apparently, in naïve animals, superantigen treatment leads to the depletion of specific TCR carrying clones. Further, there must be a minimal number of autoimmune T cell clones required for triggering of EAE by superantigens, and these T cells should express the memory phenotype.

Do microbial superantigens have a role in human CNS immune disease, especially in MS? Do they have a role starting the disease or can they kick off relapses? Shortly after demonstration of biased Vβ usage in T cells causing EAE in rodents, there were reports that, also in human MS, myelin autoreactive T cells utilized only very few Vβ species. As in other supposed human autoimmune diseases, such as type 1 diabetes and psoriasis, the biased TCR usage by potentially disease-related T cells in MS raised the possibility of microbial superantigens as disease triggers (Brocke et al. 1998). Much of the original enthusiasm has, however, evaporated. First, only in rare cases is there a notable expansion of individual Vβs among MS-related CD4 T cells, and, second, in spite of intensive search, so far no superantigenic microbe has been associated with MS.

There remains, however, a particular class of endogenous superantigens to be considered. Human endogenous retroviruses (HERVs) are integrated in multiple loci of the human genome, where they occupy up to 10% of the entire sequence. According to a recent report, HERV activation can be observed in astrocytes located in MS lesions. These glia cells express a HERV protein, which triggers the release of demyelinating toxic factors (Antony et al. 2004). Alternatively, MS-associated HERVs (Perron et al. 1997) (whose existence does not seem to be globally accepted [Brahic and Bureau 1997]) might activate CNS autoimmune T cells or shape the immune repertoire so as to facilitate anti-CNS autoimmunity, as has been proposed as a general scenario of autoimmunity(Posnett and Yarilina 2001).

4.3
T Cells with Two Antigen Receptors

As a hallmark of the antigen-specific immune response, T cells (and B cells, too) normally express only one particular antigen receptor. This phenomenon, termed allelic exclusion, is noteworthy, as, in principle, receptor genes of both alleles could rearrange T and B cell receptor genes and thus provide one T cell with more than one, perhaps up to four distinct receptor species. During generation of the diversified T cell receptor repertoire in the thymus, recombination of the complete T cell receptor β chain leads to the almost unfailing repression of a second β chain—the other allele is excluded from expression. A similar, though less stringent exclusion is the case with the other T cell receptor chain, the alpha chain (Schlissel 2003).

But even if allelic exclusion is strict, it is not unfailing. As hinted, especially in the case of the TCR alpha chain, rearrangement of one alpha chain may be followed by a rearrangement of a second one, and both chains may make it to the T cell surface (Hinz et al. 2001). Thus in exceptional cases, one T cell may express two distinct sets of T cell receptors, one specific for an autoantigen, the other against a foreign, microbial protein. Theory would predict that in these dual-receptor T cells, recognition of a microbial by one TCR set would co-activate the autoimmune potential represented by the second TCR. This idea has been examined experimentally in EAE, for example by crossing two TCR (one of the receptors specific for CNS autoantigen) transgenic strains of mice. So far, *repression* of autoimmune reactivity by engagement of anti-foreign receptors has been reported, but not *activation* of autoimmune T cells (Dittel et al. 1999).

4.4
The Inflammatory Milieu—Link to Innate Immunity

According to current theory, recognition of antigen by specific T cells may lead to radically different results. Depending on the circumstances of antigen presentation and recognition, the T cell can be either activated, or tolerized, i.e., pushed into a state of non-reactivity. The circumstances involve nature of APCs (including the number and spectrum of co-stimulatory molecules used) and the surrounding microenvironment (cytokines, cell adhesion molecules, etc.) (Walker and Abbas 2002). These rules apply not only to T cells specific for foreign antigens, but also to autoreactive T cells.

Thus, mere presentation of an autoantigen by an APC is not sufficient to trigger a pathogenic autoimmune response; the antigen recognizing T cell must receive an additional stimulus to be fully activated, to start to divide. This second signal comes from the T cell's immediate microenvironment, often from the APC itself, and the second signal is often communicated as a result of an innate immune response. In extreme cases, autoimmune T cells may even be activated in the absence of the specific autoantigen, by especially strong inflammatory stimuli, called bystander activation.

The earliest observations of EAE indicated, by hindsight, a link between CNS autoimmunity and innate immune reactivity. It has been known for decades that EAE can be readily induced by immunizing susceptible animals with autoantigen (MBP, or other CNS proteins) immersed in complete Freund's adjuvant (an oil-in-water emulsion containing strongly pro-inflammatory mycobacterial proteins) (Freund et al. 1953). Adjuvant emulsions without bacterial material, such as *incomplete* Freund's adjuvant, not only failed to produce disease but even conferred protection from induction of autoimmunity.

As has been recognized in the meantime, it is the microbial component that activates APCs close to the immunization site and within the local lymph tissues by binding to toll-like receptors. This response makes the APCs produce a spectrum of pro-inflammatory mediators, which together signal the autoreactive T cell (which may have recognized its autoantigen in proper MHC context on the surface of the APC) to become autoaggressive, to produce disease (Lanzavecchia and Sallusto 2001).

As mentioned, pro-inflammatory signals alone may be sufficient to trigger the autoimmune potential of T cells, even in the absence of concomitant autoantigen presentation. T cells isolated from mice primed with IFA, which by themselves were unable to transfer EAE. They became, however, pathogenic when cultured either with agonist MAbs against CD40 (a strong second signal receptor) or with CpG oligonucleotides, which represent bacterial nucleic acids and activate APCs via the TLR-9 innate immune receptor (Ichikawa et al. 2002). Also, transgenic mice having myelin-specific TCR on all of their CD4 T cells may nevertheless fail to develop spontaneous EAE throughout a long phase of their life. Injection of microbial material (e.g., CpG-containing oligonucleotides, which act via TLR-9) readily precipitate autoantigen-independent T cell activation, and EAE (Waldner et al. 2004).

Thus, a microenvironment which accumulates a sufficient number of autoreactive T cells and at the same time produces a high level of pro-inflammatory mediators, due to innate response to microbes, may activate the autoaggressive potential even in the absence of formal presentation of autoantigens. The pro-inflammatory mediators, which may include IL-23 (or IL-12, as traditionally assumed [Segal and Shevach 1996]) deviate the CD4 T cells from a neutral or Th2-like phenotype to the pathogenic Th1 lineage (Langrish et al. 2005).

5
Regulatory Suppression of Autoimmune T Cells— But How Do Suppressor T Cells Know?

If activation is the prime prerequisite for autoreactive T cells to become autoaggressive, it should be asked why such activation happens that rarely in real life. The answer is that autoimmune T cells are not completely free in their response to activating stimuli, but that they are subject to efficient regulatory mechanisms, often referred to as tolerogenic. Thus effector T cell activation is the result of positive, activating stimuli interacting with counter-regulatory signals. In the presence of intact counter-regulation, this means that the positive activating signal must be much stronger than in an individual with compromised regulation.

In the case of CNS autoimmune T cells, first evidence for counter-regulatory cell loops came from early studies inoculating animals with incomplete Freund's adjuvant, a treatment that protected from autoimmune disease, rather than inducing it. The protective effect could not be transferred to naïve recipients by serum, but by MBP-specific lymphocytes from spleen or other immune tissues (Bernard 1977; Swierkosz and Swanborg 1977). These studies marked the birth of the suppressor cell in EAE, a capricious cell that thereafter submerged for decades until its recent reappearance in a new guise, as Tregs.

Regulatory T cells became visible in transgenic mice that had an MBP-specific T cell receptor in their germline, but lacked recombinase RAG-1, a protein critically required for the generation of endogenous T (and B) cell repertoires. In these mice, without exception, all T cells bear the MBP-specific transgenic T cell receptor on their surface. Most, if not all of the double-transgenic $RAG^{-/-}$, $TCR^{+/+}$ mice develop spontaneous CNS inflammation, most probably as a consequence to the unfettered activation of the autoimmune transgenic T cells. Complex transfer experiments using cells from transgenic mice lacking circumscript immune populations revealed that the salient factor in allowing spontaneous development of EAE was the lack of a regulatory class of CD4 T cells(Olivares-Villagómez et al. 1998; Van de Keere and Tonegawa 1998). Perhaps not too surprisingly, the suppressor cell responsible displayed some key features of $CD4^+CD25^+$ Tregs (Furtado et al. 2002).

What is the target epitope recognized by regulatory T cells? The early experiments isolating regulatory T cells from rodents immunized with MBP in CFA seemed to indicate that the regulatory T cells themselves were specific for the relevant autoantigen. This has not been confirmed by the more recent investigations using TCR transgenic mice. Wild type regulatory T cells of random antigen specificity seem to suppress EAE induction more efficiently than autoreactive T cells (Olivares-Villagómez et al. 1998; Van de Keere and Tonegawa 1998; Hori et al. 2002).

Another type of regulatory T cells were detected soon after the first isolation of MBP specific encephalitogenic T cell lines, when Ben-Nun et al. observed that transfer of the cell not only mediated EAE, but in addition protected animals that had survived disease from renewed attempts to transfer EAE with the same cell line (Ben-Nun et al. 1981). This protection effect was not only seen after transfer of viable T cells, but even after transfer of inactivated T cells. The latter failed to transfer disease, but still procured protection, a phenomenon that laid the basis for T cell vaccination strategies. Later work showed that protection was mediated mainly by CD8 T cells, which recognized clone-specific structures on the surface of the vaccinating CD4 T cells (Lider et al. 1988; Sun et al. 1988).

The importance of CD8 T cells as counter-regulatory cells has been stressed by several groups who depleted CD8 T cell from rodents in vivo, and by such treatment ablated protection against repeated EAE induction (Jiang et al. 1992). Others observed that transgenic mice lacking CD8 T cells develop more severe EAE than their intact counterparts (Koh et al. 1992). It appears now that at least a substantial part of the regulatory CD8 T cells recognize peptide epitopes on the autoimmune T cell receptor, some apparently derived from the β chain's V region. Intriguingly, and against intuition, the receptor-derived peptides are not presented in the context of classical MHC class I molecules, as in the case of most CD8 T cells, but in the context of atypical class Ib, Qa molecules (Jiang et al. 1995). The mechanism of how the regulatory CD8 T cells regulate EAE susceptibility is not clear at all. As mentioned, vaccination with live or attenuated T cell lines induces CD8 T cells, which act by killing their CD4 target cells. Alternatively, CD8 T cells may act on CD4 T cells by diverting them from a pathogenic (Th1) to a nonpathogenic (Th2) response pattern.

It seems to be safe to conclude that there are numerous distinct regulatory pathways to protect an individual from autoimmune disease. There are regulatory T cells of CD4, and of CD8 phenotype, and there are in addition NK and NK1 T cells, which may have roles in regulation (Sarantopoulos et al. 2004).

5.1
Autoantigen *Retrouvé*: Recognition/Presentation in the Target Organ

The terminal act of an autoimmune disease is initiated when the autoimmune T cell recognizes its specific autoantigenic epitope properly presented within the target tissue. This is less trivial than it may sound. First, as mentioned initially, autoimmune effector T cells do not routinely gain entry into the CNS, an organ that is secluded from the rest of the body by a tight blood–brain barrier (BBB). The only cells that can pass though the resting BBB are a few fully activated T cells (Hickey et al. 1991; Wekerle et al. 1986). Microcinematography suggests that these lymphoblasts interact with the sparse cell adhesion molecules present on the BBB's inner surface to gain access to the CNS parenchyma (Vajkoczy et al. 2001).

The BBB can, however, be rendered more permeable when activated by proinflammatory signals. Following activation, BBB endothelium cells express new sets of cell adhesion molecules, chemokines, and other structures, which, together, allow additional inflammatory cells to enter the CNS. The first class of immune cells to gain access into the CNS are postactivated T cells, which during their stay in peripheral immune tissues assume properties that allow them to migrate through endothelial barriers with particular ease (Flügel et al. 2001). These migratory effector T cells enter the CNS target tissues in masses and interact there with primed microglia cells that present local autoantigen. Only later in the course of a florid autoimmune reaction does the BBB get completely broken and allow the influx of macrophages, unspecific T cells, and permeation of blood molecules.

After successful intrusion into the CNS, the autoimmune effector T cell is confronted with a second problem, the search for a competent antigen-presenting cell. We have also mentioned above that the healthy CNS tissues barely hold any MHC class I or class II proteins, and there are no professional APCs. However, the CNS contains a large number of resident cells, which can be induced to produce and acquire MHC determinants and other structures required to productively present (auto-)antigens. These include microglia cells, and also astrocytes as well as macrophage-like cells surrounding the CNS microvessels (Aloisi et al. 2000). Importantly, none of these facultative APCs produces the myelin autoantigens, which are the targets of autoaggressive T cells in MS and most variants of EAE. These myelin structures must be released from myelin or myelin-forming oligodendrocytes, and taken up by the induced APCs, which process them and present them in a proper, T cell-readable MHC context.

How many effector T cells must invade the CNS in order to produce disease? Traditionally, we assumed that a small population would be sufficient. These T cells, activated following recognition of autoantigen, would secrete soluble factors that then would attract accessory inflammatory cells, macrophages, and activate them to ultimately damage glia and neurons (Steinman 1996). Recently, studies using fluorescent biomarkers—GFP—showed that unexpectedly high numbers of effector T cells indeed go into the CNS, especially in the critical early phase of lesion generation. In T cell line-transferred EAE, for example, literally thousands of effector T cells cross the BBB within a few hours immediately before onset of clinical CNS disease (Flügel et al. 2001).

These studies further demonstrated that many, if not all of these T cells rapidly zigzag through the CNS parenchyma and finally dock on MHC class II-induced APCs and become activated (Fig. 1). Thus, within short periods of time, the infiltrated tissue is flooded with cytokine, chemokines, and other pro-inflammatory molecules released by the T cells, a process that readily explains the rapid onset of clinical EAE.

What is the fate of effector cells within the CNS target tissue? In the best studied EAE models, it appears that very few, if any effector T cells leave the tissue again after a disease episode. Most of them seem to die locally by apoptosis (Pender et al. 1991; Schmied et al. 1993). At least in the EAE models quoted, T cells do not seem to carry information from the CNS back to the peripheral immune system. There may be, however, a different link between the two compartments. Several groups have observed that during intense inflammation the CNS lesions can acquire phenotypically distinguishable dendritic cells, professional APCs (Fischer et al. 2000; Serafini et al. 2000; Suter et al. 2000). Such DCs can be the cytokine induced progeny of resident microglia cells, or, alternatively, arise from infiltrating bone marrow-derived macrophages or, a third possibility, immigrate into the tissue via the blood stream. There is evidence that DCs take up CNS material, process it, and export it to the outside. According to one theory, presentation of various myelin proteins may recruit autoimmune T cells from the naïve immune repertoire. This would explain the phenomenon of determinant spreading, which describes the broadening of an autoimmune T cell clone repertoire during an autoimmune response starting by one specificity and spreading out to additional new epitopes on the initial autoantigen (intramolecular spreading) or even other proteins (intermolecular spreading) (Vanderlugt and Miller 2002).

How does an autoimmune T cell create damage in its target organ? Does it attack directly the target tissues, or does it recruit and arm accessory cells to do the final job? Several observations indicate that cellular helpers are required. For a long time, the prevalent concept had it that a few specific autoimmune T cells are sufficient to trigger all the events underlying autoimmune tissue inflammation. More recently, and as mentioned above, using tracer technologies that allow the real-time identification of autoimmune effector T cells showed, however, that in the early, critical stages of inflammation, a large proportion, i.e., most if not all of the infiltrating T cells are indeed specific effector cells. There is a mass invasion of the target organ by effector cells. Many of these T cells make contacts with local antigen-presenting cells, in the CNS mainly activated microglia cells or perivascular macrophages, and become activated.

Yet there is an impressive body of data showing that effector cells by themselves are not sufficient to produce the pathogenic tissue damage.

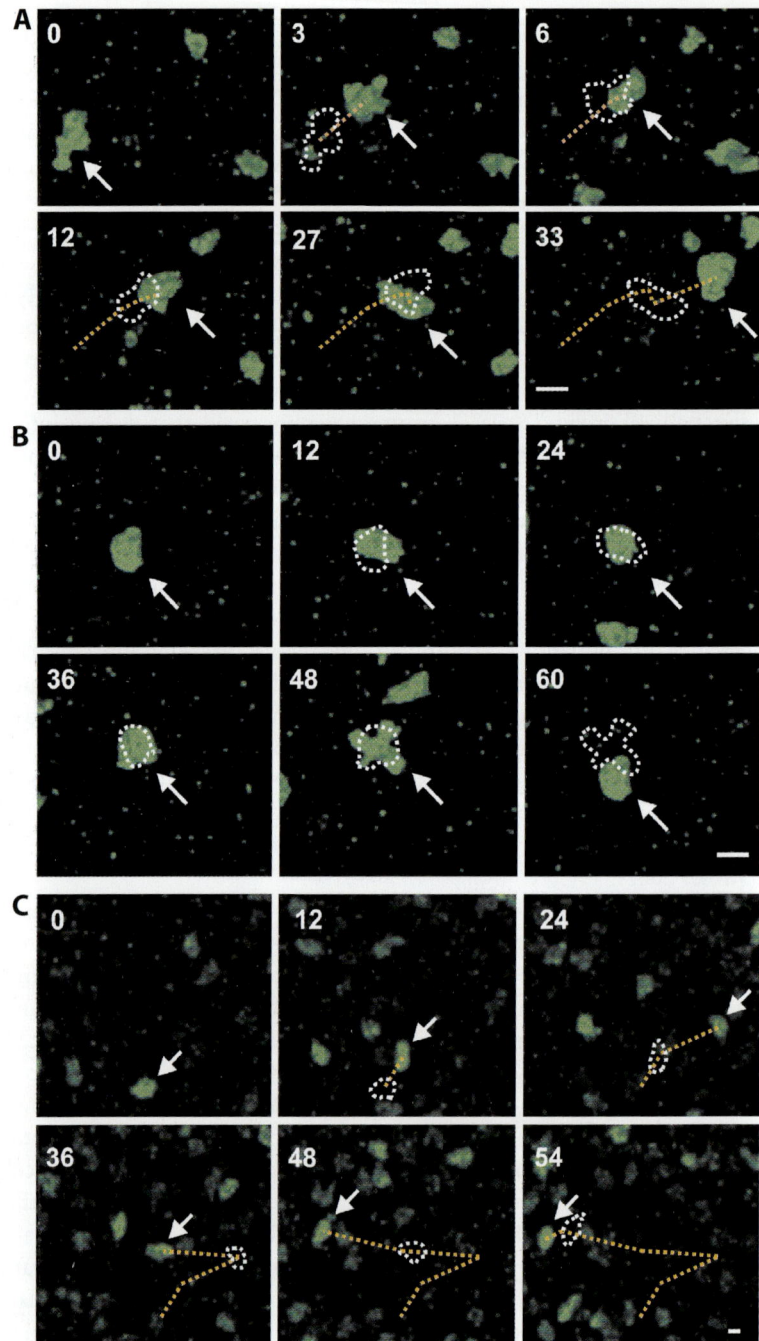

Fig. 1A–C Motility of (auto-)antigen-specific T cells in EAE lesions. **A, B** Two-photon live microscopy of $T_{MBP-GFP}$ cells in acute spinal cord slices. Two types of T cell movements are observed within CNS lesions: motile (**A**) and stationary (**B**) $T_{MBP-GFP}$ cells. *Numbers* indicate time after start of the analysis (minutes). *Dotted lines* indicate the trajectories and the cell shape of the preceding pictures. *Arrows* point to the tracked cells. Representative cells of ten videos from four independent experiments. Bars, 10 µm. **C** Locomotion of $T_{OVA-GFP}$ cells in living spinal cord slices analyzed by two-photon analysis (4 days after co-transfer of T_{MBP} cells and $T_{OVA-GFP}$ cells). A representative cell of six videos from three independent experiments is shown. Bar, 10 µm. (From Kawakami et al. 2005)

Comparing, for example, different T cell line-mediated EAE variants, the degree of clinical severity was remarkably tightly correlated with the number and state of activation of co-invading macrophages (Berger et al. 1997). In the Lewis rat, for example, MBP-specific T cells transfer severe, potentially lethal CNS inflammation; the mature pathological lesion is characterized by a number of activated macrophages that impressively exceeds the number of lymphocytes. In stark contrast is the lesion of EAE-mediated by T cells specific for S100β, a protein produced by astrocytes. When transferred into naïve rats, anti-S100β T cells produce large infiltrates, but unexpectedly mild clinical disease. The inflammatory infiltrates are dominated by T cells, with only a sprinkle of macrophages. It appears that the pathogenic potential of an encephalitogenic T cell correlates with the degree of activation it reaches during the early mass invasion phase. Highly pathogenic T cells are maximally activated and recruit maximal numbers of macrophages, while T cells with modest encephalitogenicity are less activated and attract many fewer macrophages (Kawakami et al. 2004).

The role of macrophages as terminal effector cells is corroborated by depletion experiments. Macrophages can be efficiently depleted in vivo by administration of particulate materials that contain a cellular toxin. These particles are taken up by macrophages, which digest off the lipoid capsules, set free their toxic contents and then succumb to the toxic contents. Using the macrophage depletion approach, several groups showed that in MBP-specific EAE of the Lewis rat, T cells readily gain access to the CNS, but in the absence of macrophages, clinical severity is greatly reduced (Huitinga et al. 1990; Tran et al. 1998; Martiney et al. 1998).

It should also be noted that macrophages are not the only amplifiers of autoimmune T cell attacks. Myelin-specific autoantibodies are additional players, especially in EAE forms involving large-scale demyelination. The autoantibodies in question must bind to a surface structure on the outer membrane of myelin or myelin-forming oligodendrocytes. The only structure that reliably satisfies this criterion is MOG, a glycoprotein that makes about 0.1% of all myelin proteins, but indeed is exclusively positioned on the outside of myelin membranes (Linington et al. 1988; Schluesener et al. 1987). The injection of anti-MOG antibodies into MBP-specific EAE rats greatly aggravates clinical severity, and this is due to the binding of the antibodies to myelin sheaths, resulting in large, confluent demyelinating plaques. More recently, a transgenic knock-in mouse was constructed, whose own germline J(H) locus was replaced by the rearranged immunoglobulin H chain V gene of the classic demyelinating MOG-specific MAb. In this mouse, more than 30% of all B cells produced MOG binding autoantibodies, which substantially enhanced T cell-mediated EAE (Litzenburger et al. 1998).

There is evidence that complement plays a major role in autoantibody-dependent destruction of myelin sheaths. Depletion of complement in vivo reduces anti-MOG demyelination in Lewis rats (Linington et al. 1989), and demyelination is also mitigated by treatment of soluble complement receptor (Piddlesden et al. 1994). While complement may lyse the myelin membrane via the membrane attack complex (Mead et al. 2002), additional toxic mechanisms, including the production of anaphylatoxins and macrophage opsonization cannot be excluded.

6
Conclusion

Immune tolerance of CNS tissues has been often ascribed to T cell ignorance. We were used to assuming that potentially autoimmune T cells have no access to the CNS, which is shielded from the peripheral immune and blood systems by a tight blood–brain barrier. In addition, CNS-specific autoantigens, such as the encephalitogenic protein components of CNS myelin, were considered to be strictly absent from the peripheral immune system, adding another dimension to immune ignorance.

We know now that this immunological separation of nervous and immune systems is more than leaky. T cells, if activated, do gain access to the CNS, and conversely, an ever-increasing number of CNS autoantigens is demonstrated within the immune tissues, central as well peripheral. Further, the peripheral immune repertoire abounds with CNS-specific autoreactive T lymphocytes. These autoimmune T cells are completely innocuous, when remaining in a resting state, but they start to attack the body's own CNS when activated (a proven mechanism), or when escaping counter-regulatory control loops (a hypothetical scenario).

Cui bono? Why is the immune repertoire loaded with potentially perilous T cells? Are these indeed slumbering time bombs, or could they have a positive, beneficial function?

There is evidence that autoreactive T cells participate in tissue regeneration. Besides pro-inflammatory mediators, which are of use in fighting intruded microbial organisms or newly arising tumor cells, T cells are able to produce a respectable range of mediators furthering cell survival and regeneration. Neurotrophins are paramount examples (Kerschensteiner et al. 2003). Thus there is the serious possibility that autoreactive T cell spot areas of degeneration and stem the pathological process by releasing trophic factors (Schwartz 2001).

Detailed insights into the interactions between brain-specific T cells and their target tissues in the CNS will therefore be used from two distinct points of view. Such information will help to identify and neutralize pathogenic, autoaggressive T cells, such as in multiple sclerosis. In addition, beneficial autoreactive T cells can be used as therapeutic tolls to support regeneration in neurodegenerative processes.

References

Aloisi F, Ria F, Adorini L (2000) Regulation of T cell responses by CNS antigen presenting cells: different roles for microglia and astrocytes. Immunol Today 21:141–147

Anderson AC, Nicholson LB, Legge KL, Turchin V, Zaghouani H, Kuchroo VK (2000) High frequency of autoreactive myelin proteolipid protein-specific T cells in the periphery of naive mice: Mechanisms of selection of the self-reactive repertoire. J Exp Med 191:761–770

Antony JM, Van Marle G, Opii W, Butterfield DA, Mallet F, Yong VW, Wallace JL, Deacon RM, Warren K, Power C (2004) Human endogenous retrovirus glycoprotein-mediated induction of redox reactants causes oligodendrocyte death and demyelination. Nature Neurosci 1088–1095

Ben-Nun A, Wekerle H, Cohen IR (1981) Vaccination against autoimmune encephalomyelitis using attenuated cells of a T lymphocyte line reactive against myelin basic protein. Nature 292:60–61

Berger T, Weerth S, Kojima K, Linington C, Wekerle H, Lassmann H (1997) Experimental autoimmune encephalomyelitis: the antigen specificity of T-lymphocytes determines the topography of lesions in the central and peripheral nervous system. Lab Invest 76:355–364

Bernard CCA (1977) Suppressor T cells prevent experimental autoimmune encephalomyelitis in mice. Clin Exp Immunol 29:100–109

Boehm T, Scheu S, Pfeffer K, Bleul CC (2003) Thymic medullary epithelial cell differentiation, thymocyte emigration, and the control of autoimmunity require lympho-epithelial cross talk via LTβR. J Exp Med 198:757–769

Brahic M, Bureau J-F (1997) Multiple sclerosis and retroviruses. Ann Neurol 42:984–985

Brocke S, Gaur A, Piercy C, Gautam AM, Gijbels K, Fathman CG, Steinman L (1993) Induction of relapsing paralysis in experimental autoimmune encephalomyelitis by bacterial superantigen. Nature 365:642–644

Brocke S, Hausmann S, Steinman L, Wucherpfennig KW (1998) Microbial peptides and superantigens in the pathogenesis of autoimmune diseases of the central nervous system. Semin Immunol 10:57–67

Campagnoni AT, Macklin WB (1988) Cellular and molecular aspects of myelin protein gene expression. Mol Neurobiol 2:41–89

Chin RK, Lo JC, Kim O, Blink SE, Christiansen PA, Peterson P, Wang Y, Ware C, Fu Y-X (2003) Lymphotoxin pathway directs thymic *Aire* expression. Nature Immunol 4:1121–1127

Derbinski J, Schulte A, Kyewski B, Klein L (2001) Promiscuous gene expression in medullary thymic epithelial cells mirrors the peripheral self. Nature Immunol 2:1032–1039

Dittel BN, Stefanova I, Germain RN, Janeway CA (1999) Cross-antagonism of a T cell clone expressing two distinct T cells receptors. Immunity 11:289–298

Fischer H-G, Bonifas U, Reichmann G (2000) Phenotype and functions of brain dendritic cells emerging during chronic infection of mice with *Toxoplasma gondii*. J Immunol 164:4826–4834

Flügel A, Berkowicz T, Ritter T, Labeur M, Jenne D, Li Z, Ellwart J, Willem M, Lassmann H, Wekerle H (2001) Migratory activity and functional changes of green fluorescent effector T cells before and during experimental autoimmune encephalomyelitis. Immunity 14:547–560

Freund J, Lipton MM, Thompson GE (1953) Aspermatogenesis in the guinea pig induced by testicular tissue and adjuvants. J Exp Med 97:711–725

Fujinami RS, Oldstone MBA (1985) Amino acid homology between the encephalitogenic site of myelin basic protein (MBP) and virus: mechanism for autoimmunity. Science 230:1043–1046

Furtado GC, Curotto de Lafaille MA, Kutchukhidze N, Lafaille JJ (2002) Interleukin 2 signaling is required for CD4$^+$ regulatory T cell function. J Exp Med 196:851–857

Gaur A, Fathman CG, Steinman L, Brocke S (1993) SEB induced anergy: modulation of immune response to T cell determinants of myoglobin and myelin basic protein. J Immunol 150:3062–3069

Grima B, Zelenika D, Pessac B (1992) A novel transcript overlapping the myelin basic protein gene. J Neurochem 59:2318–2323

Heber-Katz E, Acha-Orbea H (1989) The V-region disease hypothesis: evidence from autoimmune encephalomyelitis. Immunol Today 10:164–169

Hickey WF (2001) Basic principles of immunological surveillance of the normal central nervous system. Glia 36:118–124

Hickey WF, Hsu BL, Kimura H (1991) T lymphocyte entry into the central nervous system. J Neurosci Res 28:254–260

Hinz T, Weidmann E, Kabelitz D (2001) Dual TCR expressing T lymphocytes in health and disease. Int.Arch Allergy Appl Immunol 125:16–20

Hori S, Haury M, Coutinho A, Demengeot J (2002) Specificity requirements for selection and effector functions of CD25$^+$4$^+$ regulatory T cells in anti-myelin basic protein T cell receptor transgenic mice. Proc Natl Acad Sci U S A 99:8213–8218

Huitinga I, Van Rooijen N, De Groot CJA, Uitdehaag BMJ, Dijkstra CD (1990) Suppression of experimental allergic encephalomyelitis in Lewis rats after elimination of macrophages. J Exp Med 172:1025–1033

Ichikawa HT, Williams LP, Segal BM (2002) Activation of APCs through CD40 or Toll-like receptor 9 overcomes tolerance and precipitates autoimmune disease. J Immunol 169:2781–2787

Jiang H, Zhang S-L, Pernis B (1992) Role of CD8$^+$ T cells in murine experimental allergic encephalomyelitis. Science 256:1213–1215

Jiang H, Ware R, Stall A, Flaherty L, Chess L, Pernis B (1995) Murine CD8$^+$ T cells that specifically delete autologous CD4$^+$ T cells expressing Vβ8 TCR: a role of the Qa-1 molecule. Immunity 2:185–194

Jolicoeur C, Hanahan D, Smith KM (1994) T-cell tolerance toward a transgenic β-cell antigen and transcription of endogenous pancreatic genes in thymus. Proc Natl Acad Sci U S A 91:6707–6711

Kawakami N, Lassmann S, Li Z, Odoardi F, Ritter T, Ziemssen T, Klinkert WEF, Ellwart J, Bradl M, Krivacic K, Lassmann H, Ransohoff RM, Volk H-D, Wekerle H, Linington C, Flügel A (2004) The activation status of neuroantigen-specific T cells in the target organ determines the clinical outcome of autoimmune encephalomyelitis. J Exp Med 199:185–197

Kawakami N, Nägerl UV, Odoardi F, Bonhoeffer T, Wekerle H, Flügel A (2005) Live imaging of effector cell trafficking and autoantigen recognition within the unfolding autoimmune encephalomyelitis lesion. J Exp Med 201:1805–1814

Kerschensteiner M, Stadelmann C, Dechant G, Wekerle H, Hohlfeld R (2003) Neurotrophic cross-talk between the nervous and immune systems: implications for neurological diseases. Ann Neurol 53:292–304

Klein L, Klugmann M, Nave K-A, Tuohy VK, Kyewski BA (2000) Shaping of the autoreactive T cell repertoire by a splice variant of self protein expressed in thymic epithelial cells. Nature Med 6:56–61

Koh D-R, Fung-Leung W-P, Ho A, Gray D, Acha-Orbea H, Mak TW (1992) Less mortality but more relapses in experimental allergic encephalomyelitis in CD8$^{-/-}$ mice. Science 256:1210–1213

Kojima K, Berger T, Lassmann H, Hinze-Selch D, Zhang Y, Gehrmann J, Wekerle H, Linington C (1994) Experimental autoimmune panencephalitis and uveoretinitis in the Lewis rat transferred by T lymphocytes specific for the S100β molecule, a calcium binding protein of astroglia. J Exp Med 180:817–829

Kojima K, Lassmann H, Wekerle H, Linington C (1997) The thymus and self tolerance: co-existence of encephalitogenic S-100β specific T cells and their nominal autoantigen, S-100β, in the normal rat thymus. Int Immunol 9:897–904

Lang HLE, Jacobsen H, Ikemizu S, Andersson C, Harlos K, Madsen L, Hjorth P, Sondergaard L, Svejgaard A, Wucherpfennig K, Stuart DI, Bell JI, Jones EY, Fugger L (2002) A functional and structural basis for TCR cross-reactivity in multiple sclerosis. Nature Immunol 3:940–943

Langrish CL, Chen Y, Blumenschein WM, Mattson J, Basham B, Sedgwick JD, McClanahan T, Kastelein RA, Cua DJ (2005) IL-23 drives a pathogenic T cell population that induces autoimmune inflammation. J Exp Med 201:233–240

Lanzavecchia A, Sallusto F (2001) Regulation of T cell immunity by dendritic cells. Cell 106:263–266

Lassmann H, Brück W, Lucchinetti C (2001) Heterogeneity of multiple sclerosis pathogenesis: implications for diagnosis and therapy. Trends Mol Med 7:115–121

Lider O, Reshef T, Béraud E, Ben-Nun A, Cohen IR (1988) Anti-idiotypic network induced by T-cell vaccination against experimental autoimmune encephalomyelitis. Science 239:181–183

Linington C, Webb M, Woodhams PL (1984) A novel myelin-associated glycoprotein defined by a mouse monoclonal antibody. J Neuroimmunol 6:387–396

Linington C, Bradl M, Lassmann H, Brunner C, Vass K (1988) Augmentation of demyelination in rat acute allergic encephalomyelitis by circulating mouse monoclonal antibodies directed against a myelin/oligodendrocyte glycoprotein. Am J Pathol 130:443–454

Linington C, Morgan BP, Scolding NJ, Wilkins P, Piddlesden S, Compston DA (1989) The role of complement in the pathogenesis of experimental allergic encephalomyelitis. Brain 112:895–911

Litzenburger T, Fässler R, Bauer J, Lassmann H, Linington C, Wekerle H, Iglesias A (1998) B lymphocytes producing demyelinating autoantibodies: development and function in gene-targeted transgenic mice. J Exp Med 188:169–180

Litzenburger T, Blüthmann H, Morales P, Pham-Dinh D, Dautigny A, Wekerle H, Iglesias A (2000) Development of MOG autoreactive transgenic B lymphocytes: Receptor editing in vivo following encounter of a self-antigen distinct from MOG. J Immunol 165:5360–5366

Llewelyn M, Cohen J (2003) Superantigens: microbial agents that corrupt immunity. Lancet Infect Dis 2:156–162

Marrack P, Kappler JW (1990) The staphylococcal enterotoxins and their relatives. Science 248:705–710

Martiney JA, Rajan AJ, Charles PC, Cerami A, Ulrich PC, Macphail S, Tracey KJ, Brosnan CF (1998) Prevention and treatment of experimental autoimmune encephalomyelitis by CNI-1493, a macrophage deactivating agent. J Immunol 160:5588–5595

Mathis D, Benoist C (2004) Back to central tolerance. Immunity 20:509–516

Mead RJ, Singhrao SK, Neal JW, Lassmann H, Morgan BP (2002) The membrane attack complex demyelination associated with a of complement causes severe cute axonal injury. J Immunol 168:458–465

Melms A, Schalke BCG, Kirchner T, Müller-Hermelink HK, Albert E, Wekerle H (1988) Thymus in myasthenia gravis: isolation of T-lymphocyte lines specific for the nicotinic acetylcholine receptor from thymuses of myasthenic patients. J Clin Invest 81:902–908

Nemazee D, Hogquist KA (2003) Antigen receptor selection by editing or downregulation of V(D)J recombination. Curr Opin Immunol 15:182–189

Nussenzweig MC (1998) Immune receptor editing: revise and select. Cell 95:875–878

Olivares-Villagómez D, Wang Y, Lafaille JJ (1998) Regulatory CD4$^+$ T cells expressing endogenous T cell receptor chains protect myelin basic protein-specific transgenic mice from spontaneous autoimmune encephalomyelitis. J Exp Med 188:1883–1894

Pender MP, Nguyen KB, McCombe PA, Kerr JFR (1991) Apoptosis in the nervous system in experimental allergic encephalomyelitis. J Neurol Sci 104:81–87

Perron H, Garson JA, Bedin F, Beseme F, Paranhos-Baccala G, Komurian-Pradel F, Mallet J, Tuke PW, Voisset C, Blond JL, Lalande B, Seigneurin JM, Mandr B, The Collaborative Research Group on Multiple Sclerosis (1997) Molecular identification of a novel retrovirus repeatedly isolated from patients with multiple sclerosis. Proc Natl Acad Sci U S A 94:7583–7588

Piddlesden SJ, Storch MK, Hibbs M, Freeman AM, Lassmann H, Morgan BP (1994) Soluble recombinant complement receptor 1 inhibits inflammation and demyelination in antibody-mediated demyelinating experimental allergic encephalomyelitis. J Immunol 152:5477–5484

Posnett DN Yarilina AA (2001) Sleeping with the enemy—endogenous superantigens in humans. Immunity 15:503–506

Pribyl TM, Campagnoni CW, Kampf K, Kashima T, Handley VW, McMahon J, Campagnoni AT (1993) The human myelin basic protein gene is included within a 179-kilobase transcription unit: expression in the immune and central nervous system. Proc Natl Acad Sci U S A 90:10695–10699

Rott O, Wekerle H, Fleischer B (1992) Protection from experimental allergic encephalomyelitis by application of a bacterial superantigen. Int Immunol 4:347–354

Sarantopoulos S, Lu LR, Cantor H (2004) Qa-1 restriction of CD8$^+$ suppressor T cells. J Clin Invest 114:1218–1221

Schiffenbauer J, Johnson HM, Butfiloski EJ, Wegrzyn L, Soos JM (1993) Staphylococcal enterotoxins can reactivate experimental allergic encephalomyelitis. Proc Natl Acad Sci U S A 90:8543–8546

Schlissel MS (2003) Regulating antigen-receptor gene assembly. Nature Rev Immunol 3:890–899

Schluesener HJ, Sobel RA, Linington C, Weiner HL (1987) A monoclonal antibody against a myelin oligodendrocyte glycoprotein induces relapses and demyelination in central nervous system autoimmune disease. J Immunol 139:4016–4021

Schmied M, Breitschopf H, Gold R, Zischler H, Rothe G, Wekerle H, Lassmann H (1993) Apoptosis of T lymphocytes—a mechanism to control inflammation in the brain. Am J Pathol 143:446–452

Schwartz M (2001) Protective autoimmunity as a T-cell response to central nervous system trauma: prospects for therapeutic vaccines. Progr Neurobiol 65:489–496

Segal BM, Shevach EM (1996) IL-12 unmasks latent autoimmune disease in resistant mice. J Exp Med 184:771–775

Serafini B, Columba-Cabezas S, Di Rosa F, Aloisi F (2000) Intracerebral recruitment and maturation of dendritic cells in the onset and progression of experimental autoimmune encephalomyelitis. Am J Pathol 157:1991–2002

Steinman L (1996) A few autoreactive cells in an autoimmune infiltrate control a vast population of nonspecific cells: a tale of smart bombs and the infantry. Proc Natl Acad Sci U S A 93:2253–2256

Su I Tarakhovsky A (2000) B-1 cells: orthodox or conformist? Curr Opin Immunol 12:191–194

Sun D, Qin Y, Chluba J, Epplen JT, Wekerle H (1988) Suppression of experimentally induced autoimmune encephalomyelitis by cytolytic T–T-cell interactions. Nature 332:843–845

Suter T, Malipiero U, Otten L, Ludewig B, Muelethaler-Mottet A, Mach B, Reith W, Fontana A (2000) Dendritic cells and differential use of MHC class II transactivator promoters in the central nervous system in experimental autoimmune encephalitis. Eur J Immunol 30:794–802

Swierkosz JE, Swanborg RH (1977) Immunoregulation of experimental allergic encephalomyelitis: conditions for induction of suppressor cells and analysis of mechanism. J Immunol 119:1501–1506

Tran EH, Hoekstra K, Van Rooijen N, Dijkstra CD, Owens T (1998) Immune invasion of the central nervous system parenchyma and experimental allergic encephalomyelitis, but not leukocyte extravasation from blood, are prevented in macrophage depleted mice. J Immunol 161:3767–3775

Uchida D, Hatakeyama S, Matsushima A, Han HW, Ishido S, Hotta H, Kudoh J, Shimizu N, Doucas V, Kuroda N, Matsumoto M (2004) AIRE functions as an E3 ubiquitin ligase. J Exp Med 199:167–172

Vajkoczy P, Laschinger M, Engelhardt B (2001) α4-Integrin-VCAM binding mediates G protein independent capture of encephalitogenic T cell blasts to CNS white matter microvessels. J Clin Invest 108:557–565

Van de Keere F, Tonegawa S (1998) CD4$^+$ T cells prevent spontaneous experimental autoimmune encephalomyelitis in anti-myelin basic protein T cell receptor transgenic mice. J Exp Med 188:1875–1882

Vanderlugt CL, Miller SD (2002) Epitope spreading in immune mediated diseases: implications for immunotherapy. Nature Rev Immunol 2:85–95

Waldner H, Collins M, Kuchroo VK (2004) Activation of antigen-presenting cells by microbial products breaks self tolerance and induces autoimmune disease. J Clin Invest 113:990–997

Walker LSK, Abbas AK (2002) The enemy within: keeping self-reactive T cells at bay in the periphery. Nature Rev Immunol 2:11–19

Wekerle H, Ketelsen U-P (1977) Intrathymic pathogenesis and dual genetic control of myasthenia gravis. Lancet i:678–680

Wekerle H, Linington C, Lassmann H, Meyermann R (1986) Cellular immune reactivity within the CNS. Trends Neurosci 9:271–277

Wucherpfennig KW, Strominger JL (1995) Molecular mimicry in T cell-mediated autoimmunity: viral peptides activate human T cell clones specific for myelin basic protein. Cell 80:695–705

Zuklys S, Balciunaite G, Agarwal A, Fasler-Kan E, Palmer E, Holländer GA (2000) Normal thymic architecture and negative selection are associated with *Aire* expression, the gene defective in the autoimmune-polyendocrinopathy-candidiasis-ectodermal dystrophy (APECED). J Immunol 165:1976–1983

Naturally Arising Foxp3-Expressing CD25$^+$CD4$^+$ Regulatory T Cells in Self-Tolerance and Autoimmune Disease

S. Sakaguchi (✉) · R. Setoguchi · H. Yagi · T. Nomura

Department of Experimental Pathology, Institute for Frontier Medical Sciences, Kyoto University, 53 Shogoin Kawahara-cho, 606-8507 Sakyo-ku, Kyoto, Japan
shimon@frontier.kyoto-u.ac.jp

1	Introduction	52
2	Self-Tolerance Maintained by Thymus-Produced Natural Treg: Induction of Autoimmune Disease by Their Manipulation at the Cellular and Molecular Level	53
2.1	Induction of Autoimmune Disease in Normal Rodents by Depleting Treg from the Periphery	53
2.2	Thymic Production of Natural Treg and Induction of Autoimmune Disease by Abrogating Their Production	54
2.3	Induction of Autoimmune Disease by Molecular Alteration of Treg Development, Maintenance, or Function	55
2.3.1	Foxp3	55
2.3.2	IL-2/IL-2R	56
2.3.3	CTLA-4	56
2.3.4	CD40 and GITR	57
3	IPEX as an Example of Human Autoimmune Disease Due to a Genetic Defect of Naturally Arising CD25$^+$CD4$^+$ Treg: Its Implications for Immunologic Self-Tolerance and Autoimmune Disease in Humans	57
4	Contribution of Impaired Immunoregulation and Host Genetic Factors to the Development of Autoimmune Disease: A Possible Mechanism of Autoimmune Disease	58
4.1	Altered Balance Between Natural Treg and Self-Reactive T Cells as a Possible Cause of Autoimmune Disease	58
4.2	The Role of Host Genes in Determining the Phenotype of Autoimmune Disease	59
4.3	A Hypothesis on the Cause and Mechanism of Autoimmune Disease	60
5	Conclusion and Perspective	62
	References	62

Abstract Naturally arising CD25$^+$CD4$^+$ regulatory T cells, which express the transcription factor Foxp3, play key roles in the maintenance of immunologic self-tolerance and negative control of a variety of physiological and pathological immune responses. The majority of them are produced by the normal thymus as a functionally mature T cell subpopulation specialized for suppressive function. Their generation is in part genetically and developmentally controlled. Genetically determined or environmentally induced abnormality in CD25$^+$CD4$^+$ regulatory T cell development, maintenance, and function can be a cause of autoimmune disease in humans.

Abbreviations

APC	Antigen-presenting cell
ATx	Adult thymectomy
IBD	Inflammatory bowel disease
IPEX	Immune dysfunction polyendocrinopathy enteropathy X-linked syndrome
NTx	Neonatal thymectomy
TCR	T cell receptor
T1D	Type 1 diabetes mellitus
Treg	Regulatory T cells

1
Introduction

Although the cause of autoimmune diseases is largely obscure at present, it is well established that T cells are the key mediators of many autoimmune diseases as the effectors of cell-mediated immunity and helper T cells for autoantibody formation [1]. It has also been well demonstrated that T cells that are reactive with normal self-antigens and hence potentially pathogenic are present in normal individuals [2, 3]. Fundamental questions for understanding the cause and mechanism of autoimmune disease are, therefore, what specificities and potencies of self-reactive T cells can be produced by the thymus, how their activation and expansion is physiologically controlled in the periphery, and what conditions are required for their activation and expansion to cause autoimmune disease. In addition, given that both genetic and environmental factors contribute to the pathogenetic process of common autoimmune diseases, such as type 1 diabetes (T1D) and rheumatoid arthritis, one can ask how genetic and environmental factors affect the control of thymic production and peripheral activation/expansion of self-reactive T cells.

There is accumulating evidence that, in addition to clonal deletion or inactivation of self-reactive T cells, T cell-mediated dominant control is another important mechanism of immunologic self-tolerance (see [4–7] for review). The normal immune system harbors naturally arising regulatory T cells (Treg) that engage in suppressing the activation and expansion of pathogenic self-reactive T cells in the periphery, thereby preventing autoimmune disease. Impaired thymic development of natural Treg or their abnormality in number or function in the periphery indeed leads to the spontaneous occurrence of various organ-specific autoimmune diseases in otherwise normal rodents and also in humans [7]. Based on recent findings, we shall discuss in this article a possible mechanism of autoimmune disease due to impaired immunoregulation mediated by natural Treg.

2
Self-Tolerance Maintained by Thymus-Produced Natural Treg: Induction of Autoimmune Disease by Their Manipulation at the Cellular and Molecular Level

As evidence for the crucial role of natural Treg in the maintenance of natural self-tolerance, autoimmune diseases immunopathologically resembling their human counterparts can be produced in normal rodents by removing natural Treg from the periphery, abrogating their thymic production, or altering their survival or function at the molecular level.

2.1
Induction of Autoimmune Disease in Normal Rodents by Depleting Treg from the Periphery

Several lines of investigations suggested that T cells capable of preventing the development of autoimmune disease are present in normal animals [7]. For example, autoimmune disease spontaneously develops in mice that have received thymectomy in a critical neonatal period (day 2–4 after birth, see below) or in rats that are subjected to thymectomy in adults and several subsequent doses of X-irradiation; the development of autoimmune disease in these animals can be prevented by inoculation of T cells, especially CD4$^+$ T cells from histocompatible normal mice or rats [8, 9]. Based on these findings, attempts were made to produce autoimmune disease by removing a purported autoimmune-suppressive population from normal animals, directly and not indirectly, by neonatal thymectomy (NTx) or Tx plus X-irradiation. Transfer of spleen cell suspensions depleted of particular T cell subpopulations to histocompatible T cell-deficient mice or rats elicits autoimmune disease in otherwise normal animals. Several differentiation antigens such as CD5, CD45RC, RT6.1, or CD25 can identify Treg cells with varying degrees of accuracy [10–15]. CD25-expressing cells constitute only 5%–10% of CD4$^+$ T cells in normal naïve mice and the transfer of CD25$^+$ T cell-depleted populations to syngeneic mice reliably induces autoimmunity such as autoimmune gastritis, thyroiditis, diabetes/insulitis, adrenalitis, sialadenitis, oophoritis, or orchitis. Importantly, co-transfer of $CD25^+CD4^+$ T cells prevents such autoimmune disease induction [15]. A similar protocol of cell transfer, especially to T/B cell-deficient SCID mice also elicited colitis [6]. Autoimmune/inflammatory diseases thus produced are clinically and immunopathologically similar to their human counterparts, such as autoimmune gastritis/pernicious anemia, premature ovarian failure with autoimmune oophoritis, Hashimoto's thyroiditis, adrenalitis/Addison disease, insulitis/T1D, and inflammatory bowel disease (IBD). Thus, depletion or reduction of naturally arising $CD25^+CD4^+$ Treg leads to spontaneous triggering of pathogenic autoimmune responses, and also heightened immune responses to non-self-antigens including invading or co-habiting microbes as shown in IBD, which is presumably due to excessive immune responses to commensal bacteria in the intestine.

2.2
Thymic Production of Natural Treg and Induction of Autoimmune Disease by Abrogating Their Production

Similar autoimmune diseases also develop when mature $CD4^+CD8^-$ thymocyte suspensions, 5% of which are $CD25^+$, are transferred to athymic nude mice after removing $CD25^+$ cells; reconstitution of the removed population prevents the autoimmunity [16]. This indicates that the normal thymus is continuously producing both Treg and pathogenic self-reactive T cells, releasing both to the periphery, irrespective of thymic expression of some peripheral self-antigens targeted in autoimmune disease [17].

$CD25^+CD4^+$ $CD8^-$ Treg in the thymus and the periphery appear to form a cell lineage continuity. They share many immunologic characteristics, including autoimmune-preventive activity, a cell surface phenotype that indicates their antigen-primed state, in vitro hyporesponsiveness to antigenic stimulation, potent in vitro suppressive activity, and expression of *Foxp3*, a gene highly specific for natural Treg (see below) [7, 16]. Furthermore, NTx around day 3 after birth produces organ-specific autoimmune diseases similar to those produced in nude mice by the transfer of $CD25^+$ cell-depleted spleen cells or thymocytes; and inoculation of $CD25^+CD4^+$ T cells from non-Tx mice prevents the autoimmune development in NTx mice [18]. $CD25^+CD4^+$ T cells become detectable in the periphery of normal mice from around day 3 after birth [18]. These findings collectively indicate that thymic production of natural Treg is developmentally programmed, and that abrogation of their thymic generation from the beginning of their ontogeny, for example by NTx, leads to the paucity of Treg in the periphery, causing autoimmune disease.

2.3
Induction of Autoimmune Disease by Molecular Alteration of Treg Development, Maintenance, or Function

Several molecules expressed in natural Treg, in particular the transcription factor Foxp3, IL-2/IL-2 receptor, and CTLA-4, are closely associated with their generation, maintenance, and function. Their molecular defects indeed lead to the development of autoimmune/inflammatory disease.

2.3.1
Foxp3

Foxp3 was found as the defective gene in the Scurfy strain of mice, which is an X-linked recessive mutant with lethality in hemizygous males within a month after birth, exhibiting hyperactivation of $CD4^+$ T cells, and overproduction of proinflammatory cytokines [19]. *Foxp3* encodes Scurfin, a new member of the forkhead/winged-helix family of transcription factors [20]. Mutations of the human gene *FOXP3*, the ortholog of the murine *Foxp3*, were subsequently found to be the cause of IPEX (immune dysregulation, polyendocrinopathy, enteropathy, X-linked syndrome), which is an X-linked immunodeficiency syndrome associated with autoimmune disease in multiple endocrine organs (such as T1D and thyroiditis), IBD, allergic dermatitis, and fatal infections ([21], see below).

Foxp3 plays a specific role in the development and function of natural $CD25^+CD4^+$ Treg [22–24]. For example, $CD25^+CD4^+$ peripheral T cells and $CD25^+CD4^+CD8^-$ thymocytes express *Foxp3* mRNA, whereas other thymocytes/T cells and B cells do not. Importantly, activation of $CD25^-CD4^+$ T cells, Th1 or Th2 cells fails to induce *Foxp3* expression [22, 23]. Furthermore, retroviral transduction of *Foxp3* to $CD25^-CD4^+$ T cells can convert them to $CD25^+CD4^+$ Treg-like cells both phenotypically and functionally [22, 24]. *Foxp3*-transduced $CD25^-CD4^+$ T cells are able to suppress proliferation of other T cells in vitro and the development of autoimmune disease and IBD in vivo [22].

Analyses of *Foxp3*-transgenic or -deficient mice also revealed an indispensable role of *Foxp3* for the development of $CD25^+CD4^+$ Treg [23, 24]. The number of $CD25^+CD4^+$ T cells increased in *Foxp3*-transgenic mice; furthermore, $CD25^-CD4^+$ T cells and $CD8^+$ T cells in these transgenic mice also expressed high levels of *Foxp3* and exhibited in vitro suppressive activity [24]. *Foxp3*-deficient mice, on the other hand, showed hyperactivation of T cells, as observed in Scurfy mice. In bone marrow (BM) chimera mice with a mixture of BM cells from wild type and *Foxp3*-deficient mice, *Foxp3*-deficient BM cells failed to give rise to $CD25^+CD4^+$ T cells, while *Foxp3*-intact BM cells generated them [23]. Scurfy mice, whose Scurfin protein lacks the fork-head domain, harbor few $CD25^+CD4^+$ Treg, and inoculation of $CD25^+CD4^+$ T cells prevented severe autoimmunity in Scurfy mice [23].

Thus, *Foxp3/FOXP3* appears to be a master control gene for the development and function of natural $CD25^+CD4^+$ Treg. Disruption of the *Foxp3* gene abrogates the development of Treg, leading to hyperactivation of T cells reactive with self-antigens, commensal bacteria in the intestine, or innocuous environmental substances, thus causing autoimmune polyendocrinopathy, IBD, and allergy, respectively.

2.3.2
IL-2/IL-2R

A number of findings indicate that IL-2 is an essential cytokine for peripheral survival, activation, and thymic generation of natural Treg and that CD25 (the IL-2R α chain) is not a mere marker for natural Treg but an indispensable molecule for high-affinity IL-2 binding to IL-2R. First, administration of neutralizing anti-IL-2 monoclonal antibody (mAb) to normal naïve mice for a limited period selectively reduces the number of $CD25^+CD4^+$ T cells in the thymus and periphery, resulting in the development of organ-specific autoimmune diseases similar to those produced by depletion of $CD25^+CD4^+$ T cells [25]. The IL-2-neutralization inhibits in vivo physiological proliferation of $CD25^+CD4^+$ T cells that are presumably responding to normal self-antigens [25]. Second, IL-2, IL-2Rα (CD25), or IL-2Rβ (CD122) deficiency all produces similar fatal lymphoproliferative inflammatory disease with autoimmune components (e.g., IBD, lymphoproliferation, and lymphocytic infiltration into multiple organs), generally called IL-2 deficiency syndrome [26]. Notably, the number of $CD25^+CD4^+$ T cells is selectively reduced in the thymus and periphery of IL-2-deficient mice, irrespective of the normal number, composition, and function of other $CD4^+$ and $CD8^+$ T cells [27, 28]. The syndrome can be prevented by inoculation of IL-2-replete spleen cells or thymocytes [28–31]. While transfer of IL-2-deficient BM cells produces multi-organ inflammation in RAG-deficient mice, co-transfer of normal BM cells inhibits the inflammation by giving rise to $CD25^+CD4^+$ Treg [31]. Third, IL-2 is also required for in vivo and in vitro functional activation of Treg and for sustaining their CD25 expression [32].

2.3.3
CTLA-4

An intriguing feature of natural $CD4^+$ Treg is that they constitutively express CTLA-4, whereas naïve T cells express the molecule only following T cell activation [33–35]. Although there is substantial evidence for CTLA-4-transduced negative signaling to activated effector T cells, the following findings support the possible contribution of CTLA-4 to Treg cell-mediated suppression as well. First, administration of anti-CTLA-4 mAb to normal young naïve mice over a limited period elicited autoimmune disease similar to the one produced by depletion of $CD25^+CD4^+$ Treg, without reducing their number [35]. Likewise, anti-CTLA-4 mAb treatment abolished the protective activity of $CD25^+CD4^+$ Treg in a murine IBD model [34]. Second, a lethal lymphoproliferative and autoimmune syndrome that spontaneously develops in CTLA-4-deficient mice is not T cell autonomous but can be inhibited by wild-type T cells [36]. Third, blockade of CTLA-4 by Fab fragments of anti-CTLA-4 mAb abrogated in vitro $CD25^+CD4^+$ Treg cell-mediated suppression in the setting where Treg were prepared from normal mice (hence constitutively expressing CTLA-4) and responder T cells were from CTLA-4-deficient mice [35, 37]. The precise molecular mechanism by which CTLA-4 plays a part in Treg-mediated regulation remains to be determined, especially as to whether the molecule transduces a co-stimulatory signal to Treg or it may directly mediate suppression.

2.3.4
CD40 and GITR

In addition to Foxp3, IL-2/IL-2R, CTLA-4, there are other molecules, such as CD40 and GITR, that control the development and function of natural Treg. Molecular alteration in their expression or function leads to the development of autoimmune diseases similar to those produced by Treg depletion [38, 39].

3
IPEX as an Example of Human Autoimmune Disease Due to a Genetic Defect of Naturally Arising $CD25^+CD4^+$ Treg: Its Implications for Immunologic Self-Tolerance and Autoimmune Disease in Humans

$CD25^+CD4^+$ Treg found in rodents are present in humans as well and share similar immunological characteristics [40]. Based on the fact that the development of natural Treg is in part developmentally controlled, it has been suspected that certain autoimmune diseases in humans are due to defects of $CD25^+CD4^+$ natural Treg in maintaining self-tolerance. In this regard, IPEX is so far the clearest example that abnormality in naturally arising Treg is a primary cause of human autoimmune disease and for that matter IBD and allergy. Although IPEX is a rare disease, it has important implications for the mechanism of immunologic self-tolerance as well as the etiology and the pathogenetic mechanisms of autoimmune and other immunological diseases.

First, this is the best illustration that the mechanism of dominant self-tolerance is physiologically operating in humans. Because of random inactivation of the X-chromosome (lyonization) in individual Treg, some hemizygous females may have *FOXP3*-defective Treg and *FOXP3*-normal ones as a mosaic, but they are completely normal, as are female Scurfy mice, and do not show intermediate disease phenotypes [41]. This indicates that the residual normal Treg dominantly control self-reactive T cells in such hemizygous females.

Second, human autoimmune disease can occur as a result of a solely intrinsic defect of the T-cell immune system. IPEX patients generally develop autoimmune disease within several months after birth and sometimes already at the time of birth [21]. This indicates that autoimmune disease has started to develop in utero in some patients, indicating that autoimmune disease can be triggered without requiring participation of plausible autoimmune-causing environmental agents that might affect the target organs or tissue

Third, defects of a single gene are able to cause autoimmune diseases in multiple organs and tissues by affecting Treg-mediated dominant control of self-reactive T cells. This is illustrated by the clinical findings that IPEX patients frequently develop not only T1D and thyroiditis but also various other autoimmune diseases, including hemolytic anemia, thrombocytopenic purpura, and arthritis [21].

Furthermore, Foxp3 abnormality can have a more dominant effect in the pathogenesis of various autoimmune diseases than other polymorphic genes known to influence the genetic susceptibility to autoimmune disease. For example, T1D develops in more than 80% of IPEX patients, including even those bearing diabetes-protective HLA haplotypes [42].

4
Contribution of Impaired Immunoregulation and Host Genetic Factors to the Development of Autoimmune Disease: A Possible Mechanism of Autoimmune Disease

4.1
Altered Balance Between Natural Treg and Self-Reactive T Cells as a Possible Cause of Autoimmune Disease

The above findings in rodents and humans indicate that, in general, any genetic abnormality or environmental insult can be a cause or a predisposing factor of autoimmune disease if it affects the development, maintenance, and function of natural Treg and tipped the balance between natural Treg and self-reactive T cells toward the dominance of the latter [43].

As examples of such genetic causes, defects of the Foxp3, CTLA-4, CD40, IL-2, CD25, or CD122 genes elicit severe autoimmune diseases in rodents and humans presumably through impairing the generation or function of natural $CD25^+CD4^+$ Treg, as discussed above. This also suggests that the polymorphisms of these genes may contribute to determining the genetic susceptibility to autoimmune disease by affecting Treg development or function. For example, the polymorphism of the IL-2 and CTLA-4 genes, which are known to associate with genetic susceptibility to T1D in NOD mice and humans [44, 45], may affect natural Treg-mediated mechanism of self-tolerance, as neutralizing anti-IL-2 antibody or blocking anti-CTLA-4 antibody exacerbate T1D in NOD mice, in part, by affecting Treg survival and activation (see above).

As environmental causes of autoimmune disease, a physical, chemical, or biological agent can cause autoimmune disease when it reduces natural $CD25^+CD4^+$ Treg in the periphery or affects their thymic production or function [7]: for example, administration of cyclosporin A (CsA), infection with mouse T lymphotropic virus (MTLV), or low-dose fractionated X irradiations [46–49]. These autoimmune inductions can be attributed to specific immunological properties of natural $CD25^+CD4^+$ Treg. For example, natural $CD25^+CD4^+$ Treg recognizing self-antigens are continuously proliferating in the periphery and hence are more radiosensitive than other T cells [25, 50]. Inhibition of IL-2 production, for example by CsA, may reduce natural Treg in the periphery by affecting their thymic production or peripheral survival. In addition, the early period in life seems to be more susceptible to such environmental insults because it is relatively easy to deplete a small number of natural Treg in the periphery or because self-reactive T cells produced by the thymus can more easily expand owing to the paucity of Treg in the periphery [18], as illustrated by neonatal CsA treatment and MTLV infection in mice [46, 47]. It is noteworthy in this regard that in utero infection with rubella virus later causes T1D and other autoimmune endocrinopathies (such as thyroid autoimmunity) at high incidences [51, 52]. Infection with rubella virus at a particular stage of intrauterine life might affect developing natural Treg and thereby trigger autoimmunity as the virus infects T cells and impairs proliferation of various tissue cells, including T cells.

4.2
The Role of Host Genes in Determining the Phenotype of Autoimmune Disease

When autoimmune responses are triggered by reduction or dysfunction of natural Treg, it is of note that their deficiency or dysfunction by itself cannot determine which organs or tissues are targeted by the responses [52, 53]. The genetic makeup of the host mainly determines the phenotype of the autoimmunity triggered by altered T cell regulation. For example, NTx predominantly produces autoimmune oophoritis in the A strain, autoimmune gastritis in the BALB/c but not DBA/2 strain (which shares the H-2^d MHC haplotype), and no apparent organ-specific autoimmunity in the C57BL/6 strain [53]. Administration of neutralizing anti-IL-2 mAb produced gastritis in BALB/c mice, exacerbated T1D in NOD mice [25], and produced de novo autoimmune peripheral neuritis in NOD mice [25]. ATx and subsequent fractionated X irradiations predominantly induces thyroiditis in PVG/c rats with the RT1^c MHC haplotype, and T1D in MHC congenic PVG-RT1^u rats [54]. Thus, MHC and non-MHC genes contribute to determining the phenotype of autoimmune disease triggered upon reduction or dysfunction of natural Treg. Polymorphisms of these genes may affect the formation of a self-reactive repertoire of effector as well as regulatory T cells through thymic positive or negative selection, or peripheral activation of each T cell population, or both.

4.3
A Hypothesis on the Cause and Mechanism of Autoimmune Disease

The findings discussed above lead to formulation of a possible mechanism of autoimmune disease. That is, the development of many, if not all, autoimmune diseases, especially organ-specific ones, may be determined by two elements: one is the degree of deficiency or dysfunction of natural Treg, or the balance between natural Treg and self-reactive T cells, and the other the host genes, including MHC and non-MHC genes, which determine the phenotype of the autoimmune disease including the specificity and intensity of the autoimmune responses triggered by abnormal Treg cell-mediated control. This possible pathogenetic mechanism of autoimmune disease has the following implications. First, unless the abnormality of Treg is present, host genes per se are unable to cause autoimmune disease; for example, mothers of IPEX patients are completely healthy even if they share phenotype-determining genes with their affected children [41]. Second, the degree of the abnormality of Treg is able to influence the manifestation of the genetically predetermined phenotype. In general, the longer and/or the more severe the reduction or dysfunction of $CD25^+CD4^+$ Treg is, the higher the incidence is of the genetically predisposed particular autoimmune diseases and the wider the spectrum of autoimmune diseases is in a genetically determined hierarchical pattern. In the BALB/c strain, for example, the order of incidence in the hierarchy is: autoimmune gastritis, oophoritis, thyroiditis, adrenalitis, insulitis/T1D, and others [15]. In IPEX, a high incidence of T1D and its early onset (within 1 year in the majority of cases [21], see above) could be attributed to so severe a deficiency or dysfunction of natural Treg. Notably, thorough depletion of natural Treg from the normal immune system can induce novel autoimmune diseases that have been postulated to be of autoimmune etiology in humans, but with little evidence. For example, autoimmune neuritis or autoimmune myocarditis, resembling human CIDP (chronic inflammatory demyelinating polyneuropathy) or giant cell myocarditis, respectively, can be induced in NOD and BALB/c mice, respectively ([25], Ono et al., unpublished data). Third, this possible mechanism of autoimmune disease implies that a single causative agent or a single genetic abnormality affecting the Treg-mediated control, or the balance between Treg and self-reactive effector T cells, may lead to the occurrence of different autoimmune diseases, frequently more than one, in a single individual, as in IPEX. On the other hand, different causative agents affecting this control may produce the same autoimmune disease through a common mechanism in individuals with similar polymorphisms of the phenotype-determining genes (e.g., BALB/c mice predominantly develop autoimmune gastritis following CsA treatment, MTLV infection, fractionated X irradiation, or genetical alteration of Treg cell ontogeny). In this respect, many, if not all, autoimmune diseases may have a common mechanism, and not necessarily a specific etiology for each autoimmune disease [43]. It remains to be determined whether the mechanism of autoimmune development in IPEX and congenital rubella syndrome, both of which develop T1D and thyroiditis, share a common mechanism.

It is not our assertion, however, that every autoimmune disease is due to abnormality in Treg-mediated immunoregulation. It is plausible that genetic anomalies or environmental insults may primarily activate autoimmune effector T cells, not Treg, to the degree that they can overcome normal Treg cell-mediated downregulation. For example, strong stimulation of potentially self-reactive T cells with self-antigens emulsified in complete Freund's adjuvant activates them to cause autoimmune tissue damage. Such autoimmune responses are, however, generally self-limiting and the tissue damage appears to resolve eventually if the animals can survive the acute phase of autoimmunity. Furthermore, in such an antigen-induced autoimmune disease, depletion of natural Treg can render a genetically resistant strain of mice susceptible and make the disease more chronic, indicating that the repertoire and strength of natural Treg can contribute to the genetic susceptibility to antigen-induced autoimmune disease [55].

5
Conclusion and Perspective

There is now substantial evidence in animals and humans that naturally arising Treg play crucial roles in the maintenance of immunologic self-tolerance and their abnormality can be a cause of autoimmune disease. Further study of Treg, especially the molecular basis of their generation, activation, and function, will contribute to our understanding of the cause and mechanism of autoimmune disease. Furthermore, in addition to the present method of treating autoimmune disease by physically destroying autoimmune effector T cells as much and as specifically as possible, use of Treg may be a future strategy for the treatment and prevention of autoimmune disease through reestablishing dominant self-tolerance.

Acknowledgements The authors thank Dr. Zoltan Fehervari for critical reading of the manuscript. This work was supported by grants-in-aid from the Ministry of Education, Science, Sports and Culture, the Ministry of Human Welfare, and the Science and Technology Agency of Japan.

References

1. Walker LS, Abbas AK (2002) The enemy within: keeping self-reactive T cells at bay in the periphery. Nat Rev Immunol 2:11–19
2. Wekerle H, Bradl M, Linington C, Kaab G, Kojima K (1996) The shaping of the brain-specific T lymphocyte repertoire in the thymus. Immunol Rev 149:231–243
3. Danke NA, Koelle DM, Yee C, Beheray S, Kwok WW (2004) Autoreactive T cells in healthy individuals. J Immunol 172:5967–5972
4. Sakaguchi S (2000) Regulatory T cells: key controllers of immunologic self-tolerance. Cell 101:455–458
5. Shevach EM (2000) Regulatory T cells in autoimmmunity. Annu Rev Immunol 18:423–449
6. Maloy KJ, Powrie F (2001) Regulatory T cells in the control of immune pathology. Nat Immunol 2:816–822
7. Sakaguchi S (2004) Naturally arising CD4+ regulatory t cells for immunologic self-tolerance and negative control of immune responses. Annu Rev Immunol 22:531–562
8. Sakaguchi S, Takahashi T, Nishizuka Y (1982) Study on cellular events in post-thymectomy autoimmune oophoritis in mice. II. Requirement of Lyt-1 cells in normal female mice for the prevention of oophoritis. J Exp Med 156:1577–1586
9. Penhale WJ, Farmer A, McKenna RP, Irvine WJ (1973) Spontaneous thyroiditis in thymectomized and irradiated Wistar rats. Clin Exp Immunol 15:225–236
10. Sakaguchi S, Fukuma K, Kuribayashi K, Masuda T (1985) Organ-specific autoimmune diseases induced in mice by elimination of T cell subset. I. Evidence for the active participation of T cells in natural self-tolerance; deficit of a T cell subset as a possible cause of autoimmune disease. J Exp Med 161:72–87

11. Sugihara S, Izumi Y, Yoshioka T, Yagi H, Tsujimura T, Tarutani O, Kohno Y, Murakami S, Hamaoka T, Fujiwara H (1988) Autoimmune thyroiditis induced in mice depleted of particular T cell subsets. I. Requirement of Lyt-1 dull L3T4 bright normal T cells for the induction of thyroiditis. J Immunol 141:105–113
12. Smith H, Lou YH, Lacy P, Tung KS (1992) Tolerance mechanism in experimental ovarian and gastric autoimmune diseases. J Immunol 149:2212–2218
13. Powrie F, Mason D (1990) OX-22high CD4+ T cells induce wasting disease with multiple organ pathology: prevention by the OX-22low subset. J Exp Med 172:1701–1708
14. McKeever U, Mordes JP, Greiner DL, Appel MC, Rozing J, Handler ES, Rossini AA (1990) Adoptive transfer of autoimmune diabetes and thyroiditis to athymic rats. Proc Natl Acad Sci U S A 87:7618–7622
15. Sakaguchi S, Sakaguchi N, Asano M, Itoh M, Toda M (1995) Immunologic self-tolerance maintained by activated T cells expressing IL-2 receptor alpha-chains (CD25). Breakdown of a single mechanism of self-tolerance causes various autoimmune diseases. J Immunol 155:1151–1164
16. Itoh M, Takahashi T, Sakaguchi N, Kuniyasu Y, Shimizu J, Otsuka F, Sakaguchi S (1999) Thymus and autoimmunity: production of CD25+CD4+ naturally anergic and suppressive T cells as a key function of the thymus in maintaining immunologic self-tolerance. J Immunol 162:5317–5326
17. Kyewski B, Derbinski J (2004) Self-representation in the thymus: an extended view. Nat Rev Immunol 4:688–698
18. Asano M, Toda M, Sakaguchi N, Sakaguchi S (1996) Autoimmune disease as a consequence of developmental abnormality of a T cell subpopulation. J Exp Med 184:387–396
19. Godfrey VL, Wilkinson JE, Russell LB (1991) X-linked lymphoreticular disease in the scurfy (sf) mutant mouse. Am J Pathol 138:1379–1387
20. Brunkow ME, Jeffery EW, Hjerrild KA, Paeper B, Clark LB, Yasayko SA, Wilkinson JE, Galas D, Ziegler SF, Ramsdell F (2001) Disruption of a new forkhead/winged-helix protein, scurfin, results in the fatal lymphoproliferative disorder of the scurfy mouse. Nat Genet 27:68–73
21. Gambineri E, Torgerson TR, Ochs HD (2003) Immune dysregulation, polyendocrinopathy, enteropathy, and X-linked inheritance (IPEX), a syndrome of systemic autoimmunity caused by mutations of FOXP3, a critical regulator of T-cell homeostasis. Curr Opin Rheumatol 15:430–435
22. Hori S, Nomura T, Sakaguchi S (2003) Control of regulatory T cell development by the transcription factor Foxp3. Science 299:1057–1061
23. Fontenot JD, Gavin MA, Rudensky AY (2003) Foxp3 programs the development and function of CD4+CD25+ regulatory T cells. Nat Immunol 4:330–336
24. Khattri R, Cox T, Yasayko SA, Ramsdell F (2003) An essential role for Scurfin in CD4+CD25+ T regulatory cells. Nat Immunol 4:337–342
25. Setoguchi R, Hori S, Takahashi T, Sakaguchi S (2005) Homeostatic maintenance of natural Foxp3(+) CD25(+) CD4(+) regulatory T cells by interleukin (IL)-2 and induction of autoimmune disease by IL-2 neutralization. J Exp Med 201:723–735
26. Horak I, Lohler J, Ma A, Smith KA (1995) Interleukin-2 deficient mice: a new model to study autoimmunity and self-tolerance. Immunol Rev 148:35–44

27. Papiernik M, de Moraes ML, Pontoux C, Vasseur F, Penit C (1998) Regulatory CD4 T cells: expression of IL-2R alpha chain, resistance to clonal deletion and IL-2 dependency. Int Immunol 10:371–378
28. Wolf M, Schimpl A, Hunig T (2001) Control of T cell hyperactivation in IL-2-deficient mice by CD4(+)CD25(-) and CD4(+)CD25(+) T cells: evidence for two distinct regulatory mechanisms. Eur J Immunol 31:1637–1645
29. Furtado GC, Curotto de Lafaille MA, Kutchukhidze N, Lafaille JJ (2002) Interleukin 2 signaling is required for CD4(+) regulatory T cell function. J Exp Med 196:851–857
30. Malek TR, Yu A, Vincek V, Scibelli P, Kong L (2002) CD4 regulatory T cells prevent lethal autoimmunity in IL-2Rbeta-deficient mice. Implications for the nonredundant function of IL-2. Immunity 17:167–178
31. Almeida AR, Legrand N, Papiernik M, Freitas AA (2002) Homeostasis of peripheral CD4+ T cells: IL-2R alpha and IL-2 shape a population of regulatory cells that controls CD4+ T cell numbers. J Immunol 169:4850–4860
32. Thornton AM, Donovan EE, Piccirillo CA, Shevach EM (2004) Cutting edge: IL-2 is critically required for the in vitro activation of CD4+CD25+ T cell suppressor function. J Immunol 172:6519–6523
33. Salomon B, Lenschow DJ, Rhee L, Ashourian N, Singh B, Sharpe A, Bluestone JA (2000) B7/CD28 costimulation is essential for the homeostasis of the CD4+CD25+ immunoregulatory T cells that control autoimmune diabetes. Immunity 12:431–440
34. Read S, Malmstrom V, Powrie F (2000) Cytotoxic T lymphocyte-associated antigen 4 plays an essential role in the function of CD25(+)CD4(+) regulatory cells that control intestinal inflammation. J Exp Med 192:295–302
35. Takahashi T, Tagami T, Yamazaki S, Uede T, Shimizu J, Sakaguchi N, Mak TW, Sakaguchi S (2000) Immunologic self-tolerance maintained by CD25(+)CD4(+) regulatory T cells constitutively expressing cytotoxic T lymphocyte-associated antigen 4. J Exp Med 192:303–310
36. Bachmann MF, Kohler G, Ecabert B, Mak TW, Kopf M (1999) Cutting edge: lymphoproliferative disease in the absence of CTLA-4 is not T cell autonomous. J Immunol 163:1128–1131
37. Tang Q, Boden EK, Henriksen KJ, Bour-Jordan H, Bi M, Bluestone JA (2004) Distinct roles of CTLA-4 and TGF-beta in CD4+CD25+ regulatory T cell function. Eur J Immunol 34:2996–3005
38. Kumanogoh A, Wang X, Lee I, Watanabe C, Kamanaka M, Shi W, Yoshida K, Sato T, Habu S, Itoh M, Sakaguchi N, Sakaguchi S, Kikutani H (2001) Increased T cell autoreactivity in the absence of CD40–CD40 ligand interactions: a role of CD40 in regulatory T cell development. J Immunol 166:353–360
39. Shimizu J, Yamazaki S, Takahashi T, Ishida Y, Sakaguchi S (2002) Stimulation of CD25(+)CD4(+) regulatory T cells through GITR breaks immunological self-tolerance. Nat Immunol 3:135–142
40. Baecher-Allan C, Hafler DA (2004) Suppressor T cells in human diseases. J Exp Med 200:273–276
41. Tommasini A, Ferrari S, Moratto D, Badolato R, Boniotto M, Pirulli D, Notarangelo LD, Andolina M (2002) X-chromosome inactivation analysis in a female carrier of FOXP3 mutation. Clin Exp Immunol 130:127–130

42. Owen CJ, Jennings CE, Imrie H, Lachaux A, Bridges NA, Cheetham TD, Pearce SH (2003) Mutational analysis of the FOXP3 gene and evidence for genetic heterogeneity in the immunodysregulation, polyendocrinopathy, enteropathy syndrome. J Clin Endocrinol Metab 88:6034–6039
43. Sakaguchi S, Sakaguchi N (1994) Thymus, T cells, and autoimmunity: various causes but a common mechanism of autoimmune disease. In: Autoimmunity: physiology and diseases. Wiley-Liss, Hoboken NJ, pp 203–227
44. Ueda H, Howson JM, Esposito L, Heward J, Snook H, Chamberlain G, Rainbow DB, Hunter KM, Smith AN, Di Genova G, Herr MH, Dahlman I, Payne F, Smyth D, Lowe C, Twells RC, Howlett S, Healy B, Nutland S, Rance HE, Everett V, Smink LJ, Lam AC, Cordell HJ, Walker NM, Bordin C, Hulme J, Motzo C, Cucca F, Hess JF, Metzker ML, Rogers J, Gregory S, Allahabadia A, Nithiyananthan R, Tuomilehto-Wolf E, Tuomilehto J, Bingley P, Gillespie KM, Undlien DE, Ronningen KS, Guja C, Ionescu-Tirgoviste C, Savage DA, Maxwell AP, Carson DJ, Patterson CC, Franklyn JA, Clayton DG, Peterson LB, Wicker LS, Todd JA, Gough SC (2003) Association of the T-cell regulatory gene CTLA4 with susceptibility to autoimmune disease. Nature 423:506–511
45. Encinas JA, Wicker LS, Peterson LB, Mukasa A, Teuscher C, Sobel R, Weiner HL, Seidman CE, Seidman JG, Kuchroo VK (1999) QTL influencing autoimmune diabetes and encephalomyelitis map to a 0.15-cM region containing Il2. Nat Genet 21:158–160
46. Sakaguchi S, Sakaguchi N (1989) Organ-specific autoimmune disease induced in mice by elimination of T cell subsets. V. Neonatal administration of cyclosporin A causes autoimmune disease. J Immunol 142:471–480
47. Morse SS, Sakaguchi N, Sakaguchi S (1999) Virus and autoimmunity: induction of autoimmune disease in mice by mouse T lymphotropic virus (MTLV) destroying CD4+ T cells. J Immunol 162:5309–5316
48. Sakaguchi N, Miyai K, Sakaguchi S (1994) Ionizing radiation and autoimmunity. Induction of autoimmune disease in mice by high dose fractionated total lymphoid irradiation and its prevention by inoculating normal T cells. J Immunol 152:2586–2595
49. Sakaguchi S, Ermak TH, Toda M, Berg LJ, Ho W, Fazekas de St Groth B, Peterson PA, Sakaguchi N, Davis MM (1994) Induction of autoimmune disease in mice by germline alteration of the T cell receptor gene expression. J Immunol 152:1471–1484
50. Fisson S, Darrasse-Jeze G, Litvinova E, Septier F, Klatzmann D, Liblau R, Salomon BL (2003) Continuous activation of autoreactive CD4+ CD25+ regulatory T cells in the steady state. J Exp Med 198:737–746
51. Ginsberg-Fellner F, Witt ME, Fedun B, Taub F, Dobersen MJ, McEvoy RC, Cooper LZ, Notkins AL, Rubinstein P (1985) Diabetes mellitus and autoimmunity in patients with the congenital rubella syndrome. Rev Infect Dis 7 [Suppl 1]: S170–S176
52. Sakaguchi S (2000) Animal models of autoimmunity and their relevance to human diseases. Curr Opin Immunol 12:684–690
53. Sakaguchi S, Sakaguchi N (2000) Role of genetic factors in organ-specific autoimmune diseases induced by manipulating the thymus or T cells, and not self-antigens. Rev Immunogenet 2:147–153

54. Fowell D, Mason D (1993) Evidence that the T cell repertoire of normal rats contains cells with the potential to cause diabetes. Characterization of the CD4+ T cell subset that inhibits this autoimmune potential. J Exp Med 177:627–636
55. Reddy J, Illes Z, Zhang X, Encinas J, Pyrdol J, Nicholson L, Sobel RA, Wucherpfennig KW, Kuchroo VK (2004) Myelin proteolipid protein-specific CD4+CD25+ regulatory cells mediate genetic resistance to experimental autoimmune encephalomyelitis. Proc Natl Acad Sci U S A 101:15434–15439

Sex Hormones and SLE: Influencing the Fate of Autoreactive B Cells

J. F. G. Cohen-Solal[1] · V. Jeganathan[1] · C. M. Grimaldi[1] · E. Peeva[2] · B. Diamond[1] (✉)

[1]Department of Medicine, Columbia University Medical Center, 1130 St. Nicholas Avenue, Audobon III Bldg 9th Fl., New York, NY 10032, USA
bd2137@columbia.edu

[2]Department of Microbiology and Immunology, Albert Einstein College of Medicine, Bronx, NY 10461, USA

1	Introduction	68
1.1	Estrogen, Prolactin, and the Immune System	70
1.1.1	Estrogen	70
1.1.2	Prolactin	72
2	Estrogen, Prolactin, and B Cell Fate in the R4A Model	74
2.1	Estrogen	74
2.2	Prolactin	78
3	Clinical Relevance	79
4	Conclusion	80
	References	81

Abstract The prevalence of systemic lupus erythematosus (SLE) is far higher in females than in males and numerous investigations to understand this gender bias have been conducted. While it is plausible that some sex-linked genes may contribute to the genetic predisposition for the disease, other likely culprits are the sex hormones estrogen and prolactin. In this chapter we review studies that have addressed the influence of sex hormones in SLE activity and discuss the recent data established in a BALB/c mouse transgenic for the heavy chain of an anti-DNA antibody. These mice are prone to develop lupus following exposure to exogenous sex hormones. We describe how estrogen and prolactin influence B cell maturation and selection, permitting B cells to mature to immunocompetence. Finally, we discuss the relevance and implications of these data for human disease.

1
Introduction

Systemic lupus erythematosus (SLE) is a polygenic autoimmune disease. The disease is characterized by a breakdown of B cell tolerance, which results in the development of tissue-specific and non-tissue-specific autoantibodies that mediate a variety of pathologic outcomes. The common targets of many of the autoantibodies are ubiquitous nuclear antigens: single- or double-stranded DNA, chromatin, nuclear proteins such as Ro/SS-A or U1RNP. The most common clinical manifestations include glomerulonephritis, arthritis, vasculitis, cerebritis, pericarditis, cytopenias, and serositis [1]. It is now apparent that the predisposition to producing autoantibodies is genetically determined, and that many genes and genetic loci can contribute to this predisposition. The production of autoantibodies can precede clinical disease by several years [2]. Recently, it has become clear that target organ vulnerability to autoimmune attack is also genetically determined [3]. Thus, some individuals will experience more tissue destruction than others, despite harboring the same autoreactivity.

Susceptibility to SLE is influenced by nongenetic factors also, and there is compelling evidence that sex hormones can exacerbate disease, in at least some individuals.

SLE is nine times more common in women than men [4]. It has a characteristic age of onset after menarche and before menopause. Outside the period of female reproductive activity, the onset of disease is uncommon and without sex preference [5, 6]. These observations suggest that endogenous sex hormones may play a role in the development of the disease, with estrogen acting to trigger disease and androgen to reduce disease susceptibility. Consistent with this hypothesis, some women with SLE have low levels of plasma androgen [7] and abnormal patterns of estradiol metabolism, leading to increased estrogenic activity [8].

Because endogenous estrogen may promote SLE disease, clinical studies have been conducted to question the safety of exogenous estrogen therapies, hormone replacement therapy (HRT), and oral contraception (OCP). Early studies described a link between estrogen and disease flares [9-14], but later studies failed to show a correlation [15-20]. Two large retrospective surveys suggested that the use of exogenous estrogen increases the risk of developing SLE: HRT with a relative risk of 2.1 [21] and OCP with a relative risk of 1.9 [22]. The recent Safety of Estrogens in Lupus Erythematosus: National Assessment trial demonstrated that HRT increases the number of mild and moderate flares, while OCP does not. Why there should be discordance between HRT and OCP is not resolved [23]. One possible explanation is the heterogeneity of the genetic background of SLE patients, which might influence the response to estrogen. This would flatten the statistics of large cohorts and might explain the inconsistent results obtained for small cohorts. The discrepant studies on the effects of estrogen have highlighted the need for additional research to determine the molecular pathways affected by estrogens and potential genetic links between estrogen susceptibility and the onset and exacerbation of disease.

Murine models that spontaneously develop a syndrome resembling human SLE have been exploited to question the potential effects of estrogen. Data obtained with the lupus-prone NZB/W F1 mice clearly demonstrate that estrogen can modulate disease. Female mice treated with 17β-estradiol manifest an earlier onset of lupus and an earlier mortality [24]. Similar results have been established for lupus-prone MRL/lpr mice [25–27]. Conversely, when female mice are ovariectomized and treated with testosterone [24, 28] or simply treated with an antiestrogenic drug such as tamoxifen [29] or ICI-182,780 [27] or fed with an antiestrogenic diet [30], they exhibit a prolonged lifespan.

SLE severity has also been linked to elevated prolactin levels. Approximately 15%–20% of patients have elevated prolactin levels [31]. Few have pituitary adenomas; therefore, the etiology of the prolactin elevation is unclear [32]. In NZB/W F1 mice, increasing prolactin levels results in earlier onset of disease and earlier mortality [33, 34].

We have begun to dissect the role of estrogen and prolactin in the fate of autoreactive B cells using a nonspontaneous mouse model of autoantibody production, the R4A transgenic mouse. This mouse is transgenic for the γ2b heavy chain of the R4A anti-DNA antibody. In BALB/c mice, approximately 5%–10% of the B cells express the transgene; the remaining B cells express a full endogenous heavy chain repertoire. All B cells express an endogenous light chain [35–37]. The association of some light chains with the R4A heavy chain generates an antibody with no binding to DNA. Other light chains confer low-affinity DNA binding and still others confer high-affinity DNA binding. The B cells making antibodies with no or low affinity for DNA mature to immunocompetence, but those B cells making high-affinity anti-DNA antibodies are subject to tolerance induction.

Female BALB/c R4A mice are not spontaneously autoimmune. After administration of exogenous estrogen, they develop elevated titers of high-affinity anti-dsDNA antibodies composed of the R4A heavy chain and a number of different light chains, and display kidney deposition of these antibodies [38]. Exogenous estrogen is a sufficient factor for the development of an SLE serology in this model. A doubling of serum prolactin in BALB/c R4A transgenic mice also leads to autoantibody production, demonstrating that prolactin as well as estrogen can alter B cell repertoire selection, and B cell activation [39]. This model, therefore, provides the opportunity to observe how estrogen and prolactin alter B cell selection and maturation and allow autoreactive R4A B cells to survive and mature to antibody secreting cells.

In this chapter, we will review the mechanisms by which estrogen and prolactin appear to contribute to autoantibody production. Based on the R4A model, we will describe the mechanisms responsible for the estrogen- or prolactin-dependant breakdown of B cell tolerance. We will discuss the clinical relevance of these observations for SLE patients. It is highly probable that both hormones may also affect target organ sensitivity to autoantibody attack. This question will not be addressed in this review, but remains an important topic for future study.

1.1
Estrogen, Prolactin, and the Immune System

1.1.1
Estrogen

Estrogens are steroid hormones synthesized from a cholesterol backbone and produced predominantly in the ovary in response to follicle-stimulating hormone (FSH); 17β-estradiol is the most abundant estrogenic compound in the circulation. Metabolic precursors of estrogen include progesterone, dehydroepiandrosterone, and testosterone. Some catabolites of 17β-estradiol such as 16-hydroxyestrone display high estrogenic activity. Many SLE patients have high levels of 16-hydroxyestrone and low levels of androgen [8]. Among the many effects of estrogen is increased prolactin secretion.

Two types of estrogen receptor, estrogen receptor α (ERα) and estrogen receptor β (ERβ) mediate the effects of estrogen. They are expressed not only in reproductive tissues but also in multiple other cell types, including cells of the immune system, such as monocytes and macrophages [40], NK cells [41], B and T lymphocytes [34] [42]. These receptors are targets for both endogenous and exogenous estrogens and for pharmacological estrogen receptor modulators. The classic signaling pathway for estrogen is ligand-dependent receptor activation with activated estrogen receptors acting as transcription factors [43]. There are differences in the structure and cellular distribution of ERα and β that suggest different biological roles for the two receptors. In addition, there appears to be membrane-associated estrogen receptors, which are expressed by T lymphocytes [44] and macrophages [45] but not B lymphocytes [46]. These receptors are involved in nongenomic rapid responses to estrogen. It is not clear whether these receptors are an alternative splice variant of ERα/β [47] or the recently described membrane G-protein-coupled estrogen receptor GPR30 [48].

Estrogens affect both B and T lymphopoiesis. B cell development in the bone marrow is inhibited by 17β-estradiol and during pregnancy B cell lymphopoiesis is reduced [49]. In estrogen-treated mice, lymphoid-restricted progenitors are selectively depleted [50]. Estrogen induces thymic atrophy with a reduction of T cell lymphopoiesis; this atrophy is mainly attributable to the effects of ERα engagement. While all T cell subsets are reduced, there is a disproportionate loss of CD4$^+$CD8$^+$ double-positive cells [51]. The CD4$^+$ to CD8$^+$ T cell ratio is altered with an increase of CD8$^+$ T cells [52]. Furthermore, a reversible thymic atrophy is observed during pregnancy.

It has been reported that pregnancy is associated with a bias toward the production of Th2 cytokines by T cells. C57Bl/6 mice are usually resistant to *Leishmania* infection due to a strong Th1 response, but during pregnancy female C57BL/6 mice become susceptible to *Leishmania*. This susceptibility correlates with a switch from a Th1 to a Th2 pattern of cytokine secretion by splenocytes with decreased secretion of IFNγ and increased secretion of IL4, IL5, and IL10 [53]. While a shift to a Th2 bias has been attributed to estrogen, estrogen can also enhance a Th1 response. The IFNγ promoter possesses an estrogen response element that allows estrogen to directly stimulate IFNγ secretion through a mechanism that requires ERα expression in hematopoietic cells [54, 55].

Estrogen also affects monocyte differentiation. Estrogen treatment increases FasL expression in the human monocytic cell line U937 through estrogen response elements present in the FasL promoter [40]. Estrogen also induces apoptosis in monocytes, which is dependent on ERβ engagement. In addition, 17β-estradiol increases TNFα synthesis and decreases IL-10 synthesis in PMA-differentiated U937 cells [56]. Tamoxifen, a pure ERβ antagonist and partial ERα agonist, and ICI-182,780, an antagonist of both ERα and β, completely abolish induction of TNFα [56]. In contrast, transcription and protein synthesis of CD16 (FcγRIII), an activation receptor, are significantly increased in the absence of estrogen. In estrogen-deprived macrophages, the higher level of CD16, is responsible upon cross-linking for the secretion of significantly more TNFα, IL-1β, and IL-6 [57]. Thus, the cytokine profile induced by the presence or absence of estrogen is complex and dependent on the combination of activating factors.

To determine the action of estrogen on autoimmune pathologies, several studies have been performed with peripheral blood mononuclear cells (PBMCs) from healthy donors and SLE patients. PBMCs of healthy donors stimulated in vitro with pokeweed mitogen and treated with 17β-estradiol show enhanced immunoglobulin secretion. This increase in immunoglobulin production is dose-dependant for concentrations of 17β-estradiol ranging from 10^{-10} to 10^{-8} M (eq 0.03–3 ng/ml), and is also observed in PBMCs of

SLE patients with an accompanying enhancement of anti-dsDNA IgG production [58]. Treatment of PBMCs from SLE patients with 17β-estradiol at 10^{-8}M also causes a decrease in both apoptosis and TNFα production and an increase in IL-10 production, mostly due to estrogen's effects on monocytes [59]. This is in contrast to the effect of estrogen on PBMCs of healthy donors.

As highlighted in Table 1, data obtained with mouse models of SLE display a strong link between response to estrogen and a female bias in disease susceptibility and conversely the absence of response to estrogen in the absence of female susceptibility [60–67].

The studies with MRL/lpr mice illustrate an estrogen paradox that also appears to exist in human disease [68]. In experimental autoimmune encephalomyelitis (EAE), estrogen ameliorates disease manifestations, while in lupus estrogen worsens disease. In human disease, estrogen ameliorates rheumatoid arthritis while potentially leading to exacerbations in SLE. This may reflect the fact that estrogen alters not only the induction of autoreactivity, but also effector mechanisms of target organ injury.

1.1.2
Prolactin

Prolactin functions as the lactogenic master hormone but is also an immunomodulator that affects apoptosis, activation, and proliferation of immune cells. Prolactin (PRL) is a peptide hormone secreted by the anterior pituitary and by cells of the immune system. It binds to surface receptors of the cytokine superfamily (PRLR), which are expressed in the breast and the uterus in the female and in the prostate in the male, and are also found on lymphohematopoietic cells. [69]

Prolactin induces the dimerization of PRLRs, which trigger the activation of the Janus Kinase/Stat pathway [70] or the MAPK pathway [71]. The prolactin-PRLR system is regulated at the translational level by the expression of a nonactivatable PRLR isoform, which serves as a decoy receptor, [72] and at the post-translational level by prolactin phosphorylation, which is necessary for agonist activity [73, 74].

Prolactin promotes lymphocyte development enhancing pro-B cell generation [75] as well as CD4,CD8 double-negative thymocyte maturation into double-positive cells [76, 77]. As PRL- and PRLR-deficient mice display normal hematopoiesis, prolactin appears to play an adjunct role [78, 79]. In vitro, prolactin supports splenocyte stimulation by mitogen but alone does not induce proliferation [80]. A major effect of prolactin may be upregulation of anti-apoptotic factors such as Bcl-2 and downregulation of pro-apoptotic factors such as Bax [81]. Prolactin also influences both Th1 and Th2 cytokine

Table 1 SLE-prone mice models: gender bias and sensibility to estrogens

Mice	Mean survival (weeks)		Sensibility to sex hormones	Autoantibodies	Lupus symptoms
	Female	Male			
NZB	63	67	None	Anti-erythrocyte Anti-ssDNA Anti-dsDNA	Hemolytic anemia, Mild glomerulonephritis
(NZB × NZW) F1	35	58	Estrogen accelerates Androgen protects	Anti-dsDNA	Severe glomerulonephritis
(SWR × NZW) F1	29	64	Estrogen accelerates	Anti-ssDNA Anti-dsDNA	Severe glomerulonephritis
MRL/lpr	20	22	Dichotomous effect of estrogen: Accelerate B cell symptoms Protect from T cell symptoms	Anti-ssDNA Anti-Sm	Severe glomerulonephritis, Synovitis, Polyarthritis, Lymphadenopathy
MRL/+	73	98	Estrogen slightly accelerates	Anti-Sm	Late onset, Glomerulonephritis
BXSB/MP	68	20	None	Anti-erythrocyte Anti-ssDNA Anti-dsDNA	Severe glomerulonephritis, Hemolytic anemia, Vasculitis, Lymphadenopathy
Motheaten	3.2	3.2	Not tested	Anti-ssDNA Anti-dsDNA	Severe glomerulonephritis, Pneumonitis, Alopecia

production: prolactin-mediated upregulation of IL-6 and IFNγ and downregulation of IL-2 have been reported [82–84].

Roughly 15%–20% of lupus patients of both sexes have hyperprolactinemia [31], the etiology of which is unknown. Studies of PBMCs from lupus patients have revealed that they produce more prolactin than PBMCs of healthy donors. In vitro, prolactin stimulates production of IgM, IgG, and anti-dsDNA antibodies [85, 86] as well as IFNγ [82] from PBMCs of lupus patients. In lupus-prone mice, an excess of prolactin is associated with accelerated onset of the disease and early mortality [33, 34, 39]. In MRL-lpr/fas lupus prone mice, lactation correlates with postpartum arthritic flares [87]. Conversely, treatment of NZB/NZW F1 mice with bromocriptine (which inhibits prolactin secretion) causes a decrease in serum anti-DNA antibody titer and improves survival [88].

2
Estrogen, Prolactin, and B Cell Fate in the R4A Model

2.1
Estrogen

The breakdown of tolerance of autoreactive B cells is central to the development of SLE. Because R4A transgenic mice are not spontaneously autoimmune and do not develop elevated titers of anti-DNA antibody until they are given exogenous estrogen, the model opens a window to the cellular and molecular basis of the actions of estrogen.

The development of B cells is controlled by multiple checkpoints, which are set in order to ensure competency of B cell receptor signaling and to eliminate autoreactivity (Fig. 1). The first checkpoints are in the bone marrow, at the pro-B cell to pre-B transition. The newly synthesized mu heavy chains associate with surrogate light chains to form a pre-B cell receptor (pre-BCR). Afterwards the mu heavy chain combines with a kappa or lambda light chain to form the BCR. The cells that are able to form a functional pre-BCR and BCR continue differentiating due to a "tonic signal" that appears to be antigen-independent [89]. Some of the newly expressed BCRs display autoreactivity [90] and are purged from the pool by one of three mechanisms: deletion by apoptosis [91, 92], functional inactivation called anergy [93], and receptor editing, which replaces the autoreactive BCR with a nonautoreactive BCR [94, 95].

Immature B cells are subject to negative selection in the bone marrow upon BCR ligation. Alternatively, they mature to become T1 transitional cells [97] that migrate from the bone marrow to the spleen [98]. T1 B cells continue

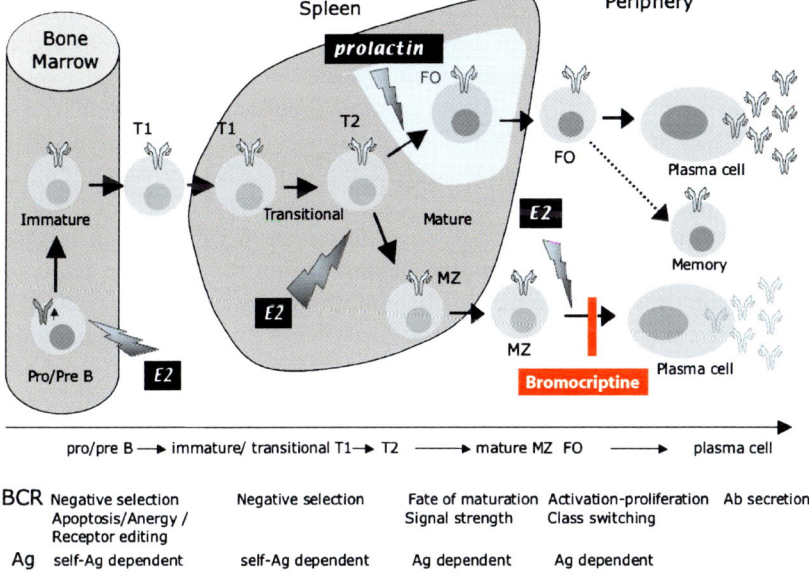

Fig. 1 Influence of sex hormones on BALB/c R4A tg B cells development. (*E2* 17-β-estradiol, *MZ B cells* marginal zone B cells, *FO B cells* follicular B cells)

their development in the spleen, where they are targets for a second round of negative selection in the periarteriolar lymphoid sheath [99]. Surviving T1 B cells enter the primary follicle and become T2 cells. There is some controversy whether BCR engagement of T2 B cells can also mediate negative selection or whether it constitutes a survival factor that permits the B cell to mature to immunocompetence [100, 101]. Clearly, T1 and T2 cells differ as T1 B cells express Fas and are readily susceptible to Fas L-induced apoptosis; T2 B cells repress Fas, express Bcl-2 and/or BAFF receptor, and are less susceptible to apoptosis [101, 102]. Some investigators believe the T2 stage of development is followed by a T3 stage [103]. The functional differences between these stages are not well defined.

Late T2 cells mature into marginal zone (MZ) B cells or follicular B cells. Engagement of the BCR signal appears necessary to drive this differentiation. It appears that late transitional B cells are subject to positive selection by BCR ligation, with antigen presented by follicular dendritic cells [101, 104]. Strong to intermediate BCR signaling promotes the maturation into follicular B cells and weaker signaling into MZ B cells. This emerging concept is supported by studies of mice with deletions of molecules involved in the BCR signaling pathway [99, 105, 106] and is generally a well-accepted concept despite some contradictory data [107]. Follicular B cells are conventional B2 cells that respond to T-dependent antigen stimulation. They can form short-lived plasma cells, which reside in the red pulp in the spleen. With help from CD4 T cells, follicular B cells can also constitute a germinal center response, proliferate, and undergo somatic hypermutation, affinity maturation, and isotype class switching. These T cell-dependent, high-affinity B cells surviving germinal center selection give rise to memory B cells and long-lived plasma cells [108]. MZ B cells are predominantly responsible for the rapid secretion of IgM against T independent blood-borne pathogens, but they also can undergo heavy chain class switching, and perhaps limited somatic mutation [109]. MZ B cells are a major source of circulating low-affinity autoantibodies. Immune complexes composed of antibodies secreted by MZ-derived plasmocytes are believed to be presented to follicular B cells by follicular dendritic cells; thus, MZ B cells participate indirectly in T-dependant B cell responses [110].

In the BALB/c R4A transgenic female mice, most of the B cells express an endogenous mu chain, while 5%–10% express the transgene encoded γ2b heavy chain [96]. The transgenic heavy chain can pair with a variety of light chains to produce BCRs with affinities for dsDNA ranging from nondetectable to high [35–37]. Three distinct DNA-reactive B cell populations have been described: one that secretes low-affinity anti-DNA antibody and two that produce high-affinity anti-DNA antibody. The population with low-affinity for DNA is not tolerized and matures in peripheral lymphoid organs [36]. One population of high-affinity autoreactive B cells expresses a germ line encoded light chain and is deleted at the immature B cell stage. Its existence has been identified in BALB/c mice transgenic for both R4A and Bcl-2 [37] and in R4A transgenic NZB/W mice [35]. In these strains, these high-affinity autoreactive B cells mature to immunocompetence. R4A transgenic mice harbor a second population of high-affinity autoreactive B cells that is anergic and displays somatically mutated light chains, suggesting that their autoreactivity developed after encounter with antigen and germinal center maturation. These B cells can be identified as they secrete anti-DNA antibodies after LPS stimulation [111]. Thus, R4A BALB/c mice possess well-characterized populations of autoreactive B cells that make it valuable for studying the effects of sex hormones on B cell development.

To study the effects of estrogen, R4A mice were treated with implants of 17β-estradiol that release hormone to achieve a constant serum concentration of 75–100 pg/ml (about 10^{-9} M) for 2 months. This concentration corresponds to the highest physiological level reached during the estrus cycle.

Female BALB/c R4A mice given 17β-estradiol display the expected alteration in lymphopoiesis with a decreased number of bone marrow B220$^+$ cells [49]. They have enhanced titers of anti-DNA antibodies encoded by the R4A transgene. The analysis of the kidney by immunohistochemistry reveals the deposition of IgG2b in the glomeruli. Hybridomas generated from estradiol-treated mice demonstrate that naïve B cells with a transgene encoded heavy chain and a germline encoded light chain are rescued by hormone treatment [112]. Analysis of estradiol-treated mice also shows that the number of transitional B cells is decreased, reflecting decreased lymphopoiesis and that the ratio of T1:T2 cells is shifted toward more T2 cells. The population of mature B cells is increased and the percentage of MZ B cells is doubled [113]. These data are summarized in Fig 1.

High-affinity DNA-reactive B cells expressing the R4A heavy chain differentiate into MZ B cells. The maturation of these B cells is T cell-independent, as the phenomenon occurs in mice with CD4 T cell depletion [38]. There is, however, no secretion of anti-DNA antibodies in CD4 T cell-depleted mice, suggesting that autoreactive B cell activation may require CD40 ligation (Diamond and Grimaldi, unpublished data).

A detailed analysis of B cell maturation in estradiol-treated mice demonstrates that DNA-reactive B cells are usually eliminated at the T2 stage. When they are induced to mature by estradiol, they acquire a MZ phenotype. Furthermore, the high-affinity DNA-reactive B cells appear to out-compete the low-affinity DNA-reactive B cells. Thus, 17β-estradiol permits the survival of potentially pathogenic B cells and diminishes the survival of autoreactive B cells presumed to play a protective role in the elimination of apoptotic debris.

Estradiol exerts a direct effect on B cells as B cells express both estrogen receptors, ERα and ERβ. The analysis of the gene expression profile of splenic B cells from mice treated with estrogen or placebo demonstrates that estrogen upregulates molecules of the apoptotic pathway (Bcl-2) and molecules of the BCR signaling pathway (SHP1 and CD22) [38]. Bcl-2, an anti-apoptotic molecule, has been shown to be upregulated in B220$^+$ cells as they traverse negative selection [114]. The Bcl-2 promoter possesses an estrogen response element, and is upregulated by the direct action of estrogen [115]. Transfection of B cell lines with a constitutively activated mutant ERα upregulates Bcl-2, confirming a direct effect of estradiol on Bcl-2 expression. Similarly, the constitutively activated ERα also upregulates CD22 and SHP-1 in B cells [38]. CD22 is a cell surface receptor that possesses two immunoreceptor tyrosine-based inhibitory motifs (ITIM). Once phosphorylated, these ITIM motifs recruit SHP1, a protein tyrosine phosphatase, which dephosphorylates protein tyrosine kinases and inhibits BCR signaling. A 20% increase in expression of CD22 and SHP1 in transfected B cell is sufficient to reduce the calcium response induced by BCR cross-linking [38]. This observation substantiates the hypothesis that a slight variation in the strength of BCR signaling can

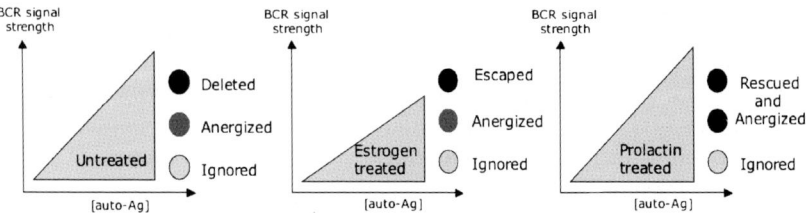

Fig. 2 The strength of the BCR signal determines susceptibility to autoreactivity. DNA reactive B cells are normally deleted, anergized or ignored. Estrogen treatment reduces the BCR signaling strength to a level that is insufficient to delete potentially high-affinity DNA reactive B cells. Prolactin treatment rescue the high-affinity DNA reactive B cells without alteration of the signaling strength of the BCR, by increasing B cell co-stimulation

alter B cell fate and can result from the direct effect of estrogen. The overall model for estrogen effects on B cell development begins with a weaker BCR signal in estrogen-treated mice, leading to the rescued autoreactive B cells from apoptosis and the maturation of transitional B cells into MZ B cells [116] (illustrated in Fig. 2). The capacity of estrogen to rescue immature B cells from BCR-induced apoptosis has been confirmed in vitro using splenic B cells from estrogen-treated and placebo-treated BALB/c R4A mice [38].

Tamoxifen is a partial estrogen agonist, partial estrogen antagonist. When given to R4A transgenic mice together with estradiol, it antagonizes the secretion of anti-DNA antibodies [116]. While Bcl-2 remains upregulated, there is no upregulation of either CD22 or SHP-1. The DNA-reactive B cells do not mature to acquire an MZ phenotype. Thus, the stronger BCR signal that exists in the absence of upregulation of CD22 and SHP-1 appears to mediate tolerance induction.

2.2
Prolactin

When prolactin was given to BALB/c R4A mice, there was an expansion of transgene-expressing B cells and a rise in titer of anti-DNA antibodies. The autoreactive B cells matured as follicular B cells, although they expressed the same light chains as MZ B cells rescued from deletion by estradiol. The mechanism for B cell rescue appears to be upregulation of CD40 on B cells and CD40L on T cells, leading to the protection of transitional B cells normally destined for deletion [117].

Estrogen and prolactin have a reciprocal relationship; estrogen increases prolactin secretion by the pituitary and prolactin decreases estrogen secretion [69]. Female BALB/c R4A transgenic mice were treated with 17β-estradiol with or without bromocriptine, a specific inhibitor of prolactin secretion [118]. The analysis of peripheral B cells of both groups revealed the same number of transgene-expressing B cells. The bromocriptine-induced reduction in prolactin does not negate the estrogen-dependent rescue of autoreactive B cells, but B cells from bromocriptine-treated mice do not spontaneously secrete autoantibodies. B cells of estrogen and bromocriptine-treated mice did not secrete anti-DNA antibodies in response to IL-4 and anti-CD40 antibody in vitro, but they did respond to LPS stimulation [117]. These results demonstrate that estrogen allows the rescue of high-affinity DNA-reactive B cells from negative selection through a prolactin-independent pathway, but prolactin is implicated in the activation of those B cells.

Several studies of mice with deletions of molecules belonging to the BCR signal transduction pathway have demonstrated that a slight variation in the strength of the signal can dramatically compromise B cell maturation and promote autoimmune diseases [119–121]. BALB/c R4A transgenic mice have an estrogen or prolactin inducible lupus-like serology, while C57B1/6 R4A are not responsive to exogenous estrogen or prolactin (Peeva, unpublished data). Why BALB/c mice lose B cell tolerance while C57B1/6 mice do not is not known. It would appear that any component of the BCR-signaling pathway or co-stimulatory pathway that might be regulated by estrogen or prolactin could be decisive for the escape from the negative selection. The analysis of polymorphisms of these molecules in humans will be a major focus for research.

3
Clinical Relevance

A major goal of many studies of lupus is to identify genes directly or indirectly incriminated in the breakdown of B cell tolerance and to determine genes that lead to enhanced disease severity that are regulated by estrogen. The gender bias in SLE may not be explained solely by the contribution of estrogen but we believe that some women with SLE, like BALB/c mice, have an enhanced susceptibility to estrogen. The identification of estrogen or prolactin-inducible genes will help to characterize the subpopulation of patients that may have a disease exacerbated by hormones.

Bcl-2, CD22, SHP1, ERα, prolactin, and prolactin receptor are all molecules of interest in studies of hormonal effects on B cell development. One study concluded there was no linkage of a bcl-2 polymorphism with SLE in a large cohort of 378 Mexican patients and 112 Swedish simplex families [122]. Four polymorphisms, a SNP (–394) C→T and a micro-deletion polymorphism (–195) Δ CTGA in the promoter region, a missense SNP (541) G→C in exon 1 (which changes the amino acid sequence G171A), and a SNP (903) C→T in exon 2 have been described for the human *shp1* gene [123], but no studies have been published demonstrating a linkage with SLE. Several polymorphisms have been described for the murine CD22 [124], and one study suggested that a polymorphism of human CD22 associates with SLE. Liu has proposed that ERα gene polymorphisms may be important in lupus nephritis patients in the Chinese population. The PpXx ERα genotype may be associated with susceptibility to SLE in males [125]. Moreover, the frequency of the *ppXx* genotype was greater in childhood onset SLE than in controls (pc = 0.0009) or adults (pc = 0.027) in Korean patients [126]. Recently, a study on 260 patients with SLE from northern Sweden has confirmed the association of p (T→C) and x (A→G) polymorphisms with a milder form of SLE characterized by skin manifestations, later onset, and less organ damage [127]. A SNP (–1149) G→T in the promoter of the prolactin gene has been characterized. One disease association study of a cohort of SLE patients demonstrated an increased frequency of the prolactin *–1149 G* allele compared with control subjects [128], but another failed to replicate this observation [129]. It may be that identifying patients with a hormonally modulated disease needs to be accomplished before critical genetic polymorphisms can be identified.

4
Conclusion

It is clear that both estrogen and prolactin exert immunomodulatory effects, including effects on both immature and mature B cells. Their impact on lupus onset and disease exacerbation is well established in mouse models. The BALB/c R4A transgenic mice are prone to develop lupus-like symptoms only upon hormone exposure. The breakdown of tolerance induced by estrogen correlates with the upregulation of molecules from both B cell apoptotic pathways and the BCR signalosome leading to survival of autoreactive cells and maturation to a MZ phenotype. This maturation and activation of autoantibody-secreting cells is due to an altered strength of BCR signaling. The absence of disease in C57Bl/6 R4A transgenic mice treated with estrogen emphasizes the role of genetic background in the breakdown of B cell tolerance and perhaps explains the controversial situation observed in the human disease. Moreover, the data suggest that only a subset of SLE patients is likely to have estrogen-exacerbated disease and invites us to pursue research on potential estrogen-responsive genomic factors that are B cell-specific and to expand the study to other cell types influencing B cell development such as stromal cells, monocytes, dendritic cells, and T cells, which are known to be responsive to estrogen.

Prolactin also alters B cell selection, but does so by rescuing transitional B cells through a CD40–CD40 ligand interaction. Whether it acts directly on B cells, like estrogen, or indirectly, is not yet established. Like estrogen, prolactin's ability to break B cell tolerance is dependent on genetic background. These studies suggest that pathways affected by these hormones may constitute therapeutic targets for diminishing the predisposition to autoantibody formation, and that effective therapies that focus on the targets may expand the time of disease remission.

References

1. Boumpas DT, Austin HA 3rd, Fessler BJ, Balow JE, Klippel JH, Lockshin MD (1995) Systemic lupus erythematosus: emerging concepts. Part 1. Renal, neuropsychiatric, cardiovascular, pulmonary, and hematologic disease. Ann Intern Med 122:940–950
2. Arbuckle MR, McClain MT, Rubertone MV, Scofield RH, Dennis GJ, James JA, Harley JB (2003) Development of autoantibodies before the clinical onset of systemic lupus erythematosus. N Engl J Med 349:1526–1533
3. Wakeland EK, Liu K, Graham RR, Behrens TW (2001) Delineating the genetic basis of systemic lupus erythematosus. Immunity 15:397–408
4. Cervera R, Khamashta MA, Font J, Sebastiani GD, Gil A, Lavilla P, Domenech I, Aydintug AO, Jedryka-Goral A, de Ramon E et al (1993) Systemic lupus erythematosus: clinical and immunologic patterns of disease expression in a cohort of 1,000 patients. The European Working Party on Systemic Lupus Erythematosus. Medicine (Baltimore) 72:113–124
5. Tucker LB, Menon S, Schaller JG, Isenberg DA (1995) Adult- and childhood-onset systemic lupus erythematosus: a comparison of onset, clinical features, serology, and outcome. Br J Rheumatol.34:866–872
6. Font J, Pallares L, Cervera R, Lopez-Soto A, Navarro M, Bosch X, Ingelmo M (1991) Systemic lupus erythematosus in the elderly: clinical and immunological characteristics. Ann Rheum Dis 50:702–705
7. Lahita RG, Bradlow HL, Ginzler E, Pang S, New M (1987) Low plasma androgens in women with systemic lupus erythematosus. Arthritis Rheum 30:241–248
8. Lahita RG, Bradlow HL, Kunkel HG, Fishman J (1979) Alterations of estrogen metabolism in systemic lupus erythematosus. Arthritis Rheum 22:1195–1198
9. Pimstone BL (1968) S.L.E. cells after oral contraceptives. Lancet 25:1153
10. Chapel TA, Burns RE (1971) Oral contraceptives and exacerbation of lupus erythematosus. Am J Obstet Gynecol 110:366–369
11. Travers RL, Hughes GR (1978) Oral contraceptive therapy and systemic lupus erythematosus. J Rheumatol 5:448–451

12. Garovich M, Agudelo C, Pisko E (1980) Oral contraceptives and systemic lupus erythematosus. Arthritis Rheum 23:1396–1398
13. Furukawa F, Tachibana T, Imamura S, Tamura T (1991) Oral contraceptive-induced lupus erythematosus in a Japanese woman. J Dermatol 18:56–58
14. Barrett C, Neylon N, Snaith ML (1986) Oestrogen-induced systemic lupus erythematosus. Br J Rheumatol 25:300–301
15. Jungers P, Liote F, Dehaine V, Dougados M, Viriot J, Pelissier C, Kuttenn F (1990) Hormonal contraception and lupus (in French; review). Ann Med Interne (Paris) 141:253–256
16. Julkunen HA (1991) Oral contraceptives in systemic lupus erythematosus: side-effects and influence on the activity of SLE. Scand J Rheumatol 20:427–433
17. Buyon JP, Belmont HM, Kalunian KC (1995) Postmenopausal hormone therapy and systemic lupus erythematosus. Ann Intern Med 123:961
18. Arden NK, Lloyd ME, Spector TD, Hughes GR (1994) Safety of hormone replacement therapy (HRT) in systemic lupus erythematosus (SLE). Lupus 3:11–13
19. Kreidstein S, Urowitz MB, Gladman DD, Gough J (1997) Hormone replacement therapy in systemic lupus erythematosus. J Rheumatol 24:2149–2152
20. Mok CC, Lau CS, Ho CT, Lee KW, Mok MY, Wong RW (1998) Safety of hormonal replacement therapy in postmenopausal patients with systemic lupus erythematosus. Scand J Rheumatol 27:342–346
21. Sanchez-Guerrero J, Liang MH, Karlson EW, Hunter DJ, Colditz GA (1995) Postmenopausal estrogen therapy and the risk for developing systemic lupus erythematosus. Ann Intern Med 122:430–433
22. Sanchez-Guerrero J, Karlson EW, Liang MH, Hunter DJ, Speizer FE, Colditz GA (1997) Use of oral contraceptives and the risk of developing systemic lupus erythematosus. Arthritis Rheum 40:804–808
23. Buyon JP, Petri M, Kim M, Kalunian K, Grossman J, Hahn B, Merrill J, Sammaritano L, Lockshin M, Alarcon G, Manzi S, Belmont H, Sigler L, Dooley M, VonFeldt J, McCune W, Friedman A, Diamond B, Mackay M, Cronin M (2003) Estrogen/cyclic progesterone replacement is associated with an increased rate of mild/moderate but not severe flares in SLE patients in the SELENA trial (abstract). Arthritis Rheum 48:3659–660
24. Roubinian JR, Talal N, Greenspan JS, Goodman JR, Siiteri PK (1978) Effect of castration and sex hormone treatment on survival, anti-nucleic acid antibodies, and glomerulonephritis in NZB/NZW F1 mice. J Exp Med 147:1568–1583
25. Carlsten H, Tarkowski A, Holmdahl R, Nilsson LA (1990) Oestrogen is a potent disease accelerator in SLE-prone MRL lpr/lpr mice. Clin Exp Immunol 80:467–473
26. Carlsten H, Nilsson N, Jonsson R, Backman K, Holmdahl R, Tarkowski A (1992) Estrogen accelerates immune complex glomerulonephritis but ameliorates T cell-mediated vasculitis and sialadenitis in autoimmune MRL lpr/lpr mice. Cell Immunol 144:190–202
27. Dhaher YY, Greenstein BD, Khamashta MA, Hughes GR (2001) Effects of oestradiol and the oestrogen antagonist Ici 182,780 on the delayed type hypersensitivity (DTH) index and on serum levels of IgM and IgG in ovariectomised Balb/C and MRL/Mp-Lpr/Lpr mice, a model of systemic lupus erythematosus (SLE). Autoimmunity 33:237–243
28. Roubinian JR, Talal N, Greenspan JS, Goodman JR, Siiteri PK (1979) Delayed androgen treatment prolongs survival in murine lupus. J Clin Invest 63:902–911

29. Sthoeger ZM, Zinger H, Mozes E (2003) Beneficial effects of the anti-oestrogen tamoxifen on systemic lupus erythematosus of (NZBxNZW)F1 female mice are associated with specific reduction of IgG3 autoantibodies. Ann Rheum Dis 62:341–346
30. Auborn KJ, Qi M, Yan XJ, Teichberg S, Chen D, Madaio MP, Chiorazzi N (2003) Lifespan is prolonged in autoimmune-prone (NZB/NZW) F1 mice fed a diet supplemented with indole-3-carbinol. J Nutr 133:3610–3613
31. Allen SH, Sharp GC, Wang G, Conley C, Takeda Y, Conroy SE, Walker SE (1996) Prolactin levels and antinuclear antibody profiles in women tested for connective tissue disease. Lupus 5:30–37
32. Funauchi M, Ikoma S, Enomoto H, Sugiyama M, Ohno M, Hamada K, Kanamaru A (1998) Prolactin modulates the disease activity of systemic lupus erythematosus accompanied by prolactinoma. Clin Exp Rheumatol 16:479–482
33. McMurray R, Keisler D, Izui S, Walker SE (1994) Hyperprolactinemia in male NZB/NZW (B/W) F1 mice: accelerated autoimmune disease with normal circulating testosterone. Clin Immunol Immunopathol 71:338–343
34. McMurray R, Keisler D, Kanuckel K, Izui S, Walker SE (1991) Prolactin influences autoimmune disease activity in the female B/W mouse. J Immunol 147:3780–3787
35. Spatz L, Saenko V, Iliev A, Jones L, Geskin L, Diamond B (1997) Light chain usage in anti-double-stranded DNA B cell subsets: role in cell fate determination. J Exp Med 185:1317–1326
36. Bynoe MS, Spatz L, Diamond B (1999) Characterization of anti-DNA B cells that escape negative selection. Eur J Immunol 29:1304–1313
37. Kuo P, Bynoe MS, Wang C, Diamond B (1999) Bcl-2 leads to expression of anti-DNA B cells but no nephritis: a model for a clinical subset. Eur J Immunol 29:3168–3178
38. Grimaldi CM, Cleary J, Dagtas AS, Moussai D, Diamond B (2002) Estrogen alters thresholds for B cell apoptosis and activation. J Clin Invest 109:1625–1633
39. Peeva E, Michael D, Cleary J, Rice J, Chen X, Diamond B (2003) Prolactin modulates the naive B cell repertoire. J Clin Invest 111:275–283
40. Mor G, Sapi E, Abrahams VM, Rutherford T, Song J, Hao XY, Muzaffar S, Kohen F (2003) Interaction of the estrogen receptors with the Fas ligand promoter in human monocytes. J Immunol 170:114–122
41. Curran EM, Berghaus LJ, Vernetti NJ, Saporita AJ, Lubahn DB, Estes DM (2001) Natural killer cells express estrogen receptor-alpha and estrogen receptor-beta and can respond to estrogen via a non-estrogen receptor-alpha-mediated pathway. Cell Immunol 214:12–20
42. Tornwall J, Carey AB, Fox RI, Fox HS (1999) Estrogen in autoimmunity: expression of estrogen receptors in thymic and autoimmune T cells. J Gend Specif Med 2:33–40
43. Gruber CJ, Tschugguel W, Schneeberger C, Huber JC (2002) Production and actions of estrogens. N Engl J Med 346:340–352
44. Benten WP, Lieberherr M, Giese G, Wunderlich F (1998) Estradiol binding to cell surface raises cytosolic free calcium in T cells. FEBS Lett 422:349–353
45. Benten WP, Stephan C, Lieberherr M, Wunderlich F (2001) Estradiol signaling via sequestrable surface receptors. Endocrinology 142:1669–1677
46. Benten WP, Stephan C, Wunderlich F (2002) B cells express intracellular but not surface receptors for testosterone and estradiol. Steroids 67:647–654

47. Razandi M, Pedram A, Greene GL, Levin ER (1999) Cell membrane and nuclear estrogen receptors (ERs) originate from a single transcript: studies of ERalpha and ERbeta expressed in Chinese hamster ovary cells. Mol Endocrinol 13:307–319
48. Revankar CM, Cimino DF, Sklar LA, Arterburn JB, Prossnitz ER (2005) A transmembrane intracellular estrogen receptor mediates rapid cell signaling. Science 307:1625–1630
49. Medina KL, Smithson G, Kincade PW (1993) Suppression of B lymphopoiesis during normal pregnancy. J Exp Med 178:1507–1515
50. Medina KL, Garrett KP, Thompson LF, Rossi MI, Payne KJ, Kincade PW (2001) Identification of very early lymphoid precursors in bone marrow and their regulation by estrogen. Nat Immunol 2:718–724
51. Rijhsinghani AG, Thompson K, Bhatia SK, Waldschmidt TJ (1996) Estrogen blocks early T cell development in the thymus. Am J Reprod Immunol 36:269–277
52. Erlandsson MC, Gomori E, Taube M, Carlsten H (2000) Effects of raloxifene, a selective estrogen receptor modulator, on thymus, T cell reactivity, and inflammation in mice. Cell Immunol 205:103–109
53. Krishnan L, Guilbert LJ, Russell AS, Wegmann TG, Mosmann TR, Belosevic M (1996) Pregnancy impairs resistance of C57BL/6 mice to Leishmania major infection and causes decreased antigen-specific IFN-gamma response and increased production of T helper 2 cytokines. J Immunol 156:644–652
54. Fox HS, Bond BL, Parslow TG (1991) Estrogen regulates the IFN-gamma promoter. J Immunol 146:4362–4367
55. Maret A, Coudert JD, Garidou L, Foucras G, Gourdy P, Krust A, Dupont S, Chambon P, Druet P, Bayard F, Guery JC (2003) Estradiol enhances primary antigen-specific CD4 T cell responses and Th1 development in vivo. Essential role of estrogen receptor alpha expression in hematopoietic cells. Eur J Immunol 33:512–521
56. Carruba G, D'Agostino P, Miele M, Calabro M, Barbera C, Bella GD, Milano S, Ferlazzo V, Caruso R, Rosa ML, Cocciadiferro L, Campisi I, Castagnetta L, Cillari E (2003) Estrogen regulates cytokine production and apoptosis in PMA-differentiated, macrophage-like U937 cells. J Cell Biochem 90:187–196
57. Kramer PR, Kramer SF, Guan G (2004) 17 beta-estradiol regulates cytokine release through modulation of CD16 expression in monocytes and monocyte-derived macrophages. Arthritis Rheum 50:1967–1975
58. Kanda N, Tamaki K (1999) Estrogen enhances immunoglobulin production by human PBMCs. J Allergy Clin Immunol 103:282–288
59. Evans MJ, MacLaughlin S, Marvin RD, Abdou NI (1997) Estrogen decreases in vitro apoptosis of peripheral blood mononuclear cells from women with normal menstrual cycles and decreases TNF-alpha production in SLE but not in normal cultures. Clin Immunol Immunopathol 82:258–262
60. Andrews BS, Eisenberg RA, Theofilopoulos AN, Izui S, Wilson CB, McConahey PJ, Murphy ED, Roths JB, Dixon FJ (1978) Spontaneous murine lupus-like syndromes. Clinical and immunopathological manifestations in several strains. J Exp Med 148:1198–1215
61. Theofilopoulos AN, Dixon FJ (1985) Murine models of systemic lupus erythematosus. Adv Immunol 37:269–390
62. Cohen PL, Eisenberg RA (1991) Lpr and gld: single gene models of systemic autoimmunity and lymphoproliferative disease. Annu Rev Immunol 9:243–269

63. Carlsten H, Tarkowski A, Holmdahl R, Nilsson LA (1990) Oestrogen is a potent disease accelerator in SLE-prone MRL lpr/lpr mice. Clin Exp Immunol 80:467–473
64. Yu CC, Tsui HW, Ngan BY, Shulman MJ, Wu GE, Tsui FW (1996) B and T cells are not required for the viable motheaten phenotype. J Exp Med 183:371–380
65. Westhoff CM, Whittier A, Kathol S, McHugh J, Zajicek C, Shultz LD, Wylie DE (1997) DNA-binding antibodies from viable motheaten mutant mice: implications for B cell tolerance. J Immunol 159:3024–3033
66. Shultz LD, Coman DR, Bailey CL, Beamer WG, Sidman CL (1984) "Viable motheaten," a new allele at the motheaten locus. I. Pathology. Am J Pathol 116:179–192
67. Stoll ML, Gavalchin J (2000) Systemic lupus erythematosus-messages from experimental models. Rheumatology (Oxford) 39:18–27
68. Carlsten H, Nilsson N, Jonsson R, Backman K, Holmdahl R, Tarkowski A (1992) Estrogen accelerates immune complex glomerulonephritis but ameliorates T cell-mediated vasculitis and sialadenitis in autoimmune MRL lpr/lpr mice. Cell Immunol 144:190–202
69. Peeva E, Venkatesh J, Michael D, Diamond B (2004) Prolactin as a modulator of B cell function: implications for SLE. Biomed Pharmacother 58:310–319
70. Yu-Lee LY (1997) Molecular actions of prolactin in the immune system. Proc Soc Exp Biol Med 215:35–52
71. Clevenger CV, Kline JB (2001) Prolactin receptor signal transduction. Lupus 10:706–718
72. Kelly PA, Djiane J, Banville D, Ali S, Edery M, Rozakis M (1991) The growth hormone/prolactin receptor gene family. Oxf Surv Eukaryot Genes 7:29–50
73. Wu W, Coss D, Lorenson MY, Kuo CB, Xu X, Walker AM (2003) Different biological effects of unmodified prolactin and a molecular mimic of phosphorylated prolactin involve different signaling pathways. Biochemistry 42:7561–7570
74. Yang L, Kuo CB, Liu Y, Coss D, Xu X, Chen C, Oster-Granite ML, Walker AM (2001) Administration of unmodified prolactin (U-PRL) and a molecular mimic of phosphorylated prolactin (PP-PRL) during rat pregnancy provides evidence that the U-PRL:PP-PRL ratio is crucial to the normal development of pup tissues. J Endocrinol 168:227–238
75. Morales P, Carretero MV, Geronimo H, Copin SG, Gaspar ML, Marcos MA, Martin-Perez J.(1999) Influence of prolactin on the differentiation of mouse B-lymphoid precursors. Cell Growth Differ 10:583–590
76. Moreno J, Varas A, Vicente A, Zapata AG (1998) Role of prolactin in the recovered T-cell development of early partially decapitated chicken embryo. Dev Immunol 5:183–195
77. Carreno PC, Sacedon R, Jimenez E, Vicente A, Zapata AG (2005) Prolactin affects both survival and differentiation of T-cell progenitors. J Neuroimmunol 160:135–145
78. Steger RW, Chandrashekar V, Zhao W, Bartke A, Horseman ND (1998) Neuroendocrine and reproductive functions in male mice with targeted disruption of the prolactin gene. Endocrinology 139:3691–3695
79. Bouchard B, Ormandy CJ, Di Santo JP, Kelly PA (1999) Immune system development and function in prolactin receptor-deficient mice. J Immunol 163:576–182
80. Sandi C, Cambronero JC, Borrell J, Guaza C (1992) Mutually antagonistic effects of corticosterone and prolactin on rat lymphocyte proliferation. Neuroendocrinology 56:574–581

81. Krumenacker JS, Buckley DJ, Leff MA, McCormack JT, de Jong G, Gout PW, Reed JC, Miyashita T, Magnuson NS, Buckley AR (1998) Prolactin-regulated apoptosis of Nb2 lymphoma cells: pim-1, bcl-2, and bax expression. Endocrine 9:163–170
82. Cesario TC, Yousefi S, Carandang G, Sadati N, Le J, Vaziri N.(1994) Enhanced yields of gamma interferon in prolactin treated human peripheral blood mononuclear cells. Proc Soc Exp Biol Med 205:89–95
83. Vidaller A, Llorente L, Larrea F, Mendez JP, Alcocer-Varela J, Alarcon-Segovia D (1986) T-cell dysregulation in patients with hyperprolactinemia: effect of bromocriptine treatment. Clin Immunol Immunopathol 38:337–343
84. Jara LJ, Irigoyen L, Ortiz MJ, Zazueta B, Bravo G, Espinoza LR (1998) Prolactin and interleukin-6 in neuropsychiatric lupus erythematosus. Clin Rheumatol 17:110–114
85. Gutierrez MA, Molina JF, Jara LJ, Garcia C, Gutierrez-Urena S, Cuellar ML, Gharavi A, Espinoza LR (1996) Prolactin-induced immunoglobulin and autoantibody production by peripheral blood mononuclear cells from systemic lupus erythematosus and normal individuals. Int Arch Allergy Immunol 109:229–235
86. Jacobi AM, Rohde W, Volk HD, Dorner T, Burmester GR, Hiepe F (2001) Prolactin enhances the in vitro production of IgG in peripheral blood mononuclear cells from patients with systemic lupus erythematosus but not from healthy controls. Ann Rheum Dis 60:242–247
87. Ratkay LG, Weinberg J, Waterfield JD (2000) The effect of lactation in the postpartum arthritis of MRL-lpr/fasmice. Rheumatology (Oxford) 39:646–651
88. Walker SE (2001) Bromocriptine treatment of systemic lupus erythematosus. Lupus 10:762–728
89. Monroe JG (2004) Ligand-independent tonic signaling in B-cell receptor function. Curr Opin Immunol 16:288–295
90. Wardemann H, Yurasov S, Schaefer A, Young JW, Meffre E, Nussenzweig MC (2003) Predominant autoantibody production by early human B cell precursors. Science 301:1374–1377
91. Nemazee DA, Burki K (1989) Clonal deletion of B lymphocytes in a transgenic mouse bearing anti-MHC class I antibody genes. Nature 337:562–566
92. Chen C, Nagy Z, Prak EL, Weigert M (1995) Immunoglobulin heavy chain gene replacement: a mechanism of receptor editing. Immunity 3:747–755
93. Fulcher DA, Basten A (1994) Reduced life span of anergic self-reactive B cells in a double-transgenic model. J Exp Med 179:125–134
94. Tiegs SL, Russell DM, Nemazee D (1993) Receptor editing in self-reactive bone marrow B cells. J Exp Med 177:1009–1020
95. Gay D, Saunders T, Camper S, Weigert M (1993) Receptor editing: an approach by autoreactive B cells to escape tolerance. J Exp Med 177:999–1008
96. Offen D, Spatz L, Escowitz H, Factor S, Diamond B (1992) Induction of tolerance to an IgG autoantibody. Proc Natl Acad Sci U S A 89:8332–8336
97. Hardy RR, Hayakawa K (1991) developmental switch in B lymphopoiesis. Proc Natl Acad Sci U S A 88:11550–11554
98. Carsetti R, Kohler G, Lamers MC (1995) Transitional B cells are the target of negative selection in the B cell compartment. J Exp Med 181:2129–2140

99. Loder F, Mutschler B, Ray RJ, Paige CJ, Sideras P, Torres R, Lamers MC, Carsetti R (1999) B cell development in the spleen takes place in discrete steps and is determined by the quality of B cell receptor-derived signals. J Exp Med 190:75–89
100. Allman D, Lindsley RC, DeMuth W, Rudd K, Shinton SA, Hardy RR (2001) Resolution of three nonproliferative immature splenic B cell subsets reveals multiple selection points during peripheral B cell maturation. J Immunol 167:6834–6840
101. Su TT, Rawlings DJ (2002) Transitional B lymphocyte subsets operate as distinct checkpoints in murine splenic B cell development. J Immunol 168:2101–2110
102. Petro JB, Gerstein RM, Lowe J, Carter RS, Shinners N, Khan WN (2003) Transitional type 1 and 2 B lymphocyte subsets are differentially responsive to antigen receptor signaling. J Biol Chem 277:48009–48019
103. Hardy RR, Li YS, Allman D, Asano M, Gui M, Hayakawa K (2000) B-cell commitment, development and selection, Immunol Rev 175:23–32
104. Su TT, Guo B, Kawakami Y, Sommer K, Chae K, Humphries LA, Kato RM, Kang S, Patrone L, Wall R, Teitell M, Leitges M, Kawakami T, Rawlings DJ (2002) PKC-beta controls I kappa B kinase lipid raft recruitment and activation in response to BCR signaling. Nat Immunol 3:780–786
105. Martin F, Kearney JF (2000) Selection from newly formed to marginal zone B cells depends on the rate of clonal production, CD19, and btk. Immunity 12:39–49
106. Cariappa A, Tang M, Parng C, Nebelitskiy E, Carroll M, Georgopoulos K, Pillai S (2001) The follicular versus marginal zone B lymphocyte cell fate decision is regulated by Aiolos, Btk, and CD21. Immunity 14:603–615
107. Anzelon AN, Wu H, Rickert RC (2003) Pten inactivation alters peripheral B lymphocyte fate and reconstitutes CD19 function. Nat Immunol 4:287–294
108. McHeyzer-Williams LJ, McHeyzer-Williams MG (2005) Antigen-specific memory B cell development. Annu Rev Immunol 23:487–513
109. Song H, Cerny J (2003) Functional heterogeneity of marginal zone B cells revealed by their ability to generate both early antibody-forming cells and germinal centers with hypermutation and memory in response to a T-dependent antigen. J Exp Med 198:1923–1935
110. Ferguson AR, Youd ME, Corley RB (2004) Marginal zone B cells transport and deposit IgM-containing immune complexes onto follicular dendritic cells. Int Immunol 16:1411–1422
111. Iliev A, Spatz L, Ray S, Diamond B (1994) Lack of allelic exclusion permits autoreactive B cells to escape deletion. J Immunol 153:3551–3556
112. Bynoe MS, Grimaldi CM, Diamond B (2000) Estrogen up-regulates Bcl-2 and blocks tolerance induction of naive B cells. Proc Natl Acad Sci U S A 97:2703–2708
113. Grimaldi CM, Michael DJ, Diamond B (2001) Cutting edge: expansion and activation of a population of autoreactive marginal zone B cells in a model of estrogen-induced lupus. J Immunol 167:1886–1890
114. Hande S, Notidis E, Manser T (1998) Bcl-2 obstructs negative selection of autoreactive, hypermutated antibody V regions during memory B cell development. Immunity 8:189–198
115. Perillo B, Sasso A, Abbondanza C, Palumbo G (2000) 17beta-estradiol inhibits apoptosis in MCF-7 cells, inducing bcl-2 expression via two estrogen-responsive elements present in the coding sequence. Mol Cell Biol 20:2890–2901

116. Grimaldi CM, Hicks R, Diamond B (2005) B cell selection and susceptibility to autoimmunity. J Immunol 174:1775–1781
117. Peeva E, Grimaldi C, Spatz L, Diamond B (2002) Bromocriptine restores tolerance in estrogen-treated mice. J Clin Invest 106:1373–1379
118. Neidhart M (1997) Bromocriptine has little direct effect on murine lymphocytes, the immunomodulatory effect being mediated by the suppression of prolactin secretion. Biomed Pharmacother 151:118–125
119. Cornall RJ, Cyster JG, Hibbs ML, Dunn AR, Otipoby KL, Clark EA, Goodnow CC (1998) Polygenic autoimmune traits: Lyn, CD22, and SHP-1 are limiting elements of a biochemical pathway regulating BCR signaling and selection. Immunity 8:497–508
120. Nishimura H, Nose M, Hiai H, Minato N, Honjo T (1999) Development of lupus-like autoimmune diseases by disruption of the PD-1 gene encoding an ITIM motif-carrying immunoreceptor. Immunity 11:141–151
121. Bolland S, Ravetch JV (2000) Spontaneous autoimmune disease in Fc(gamma)RIIB-deficient mice results from strain-specific epistasis. Immunity 13:277–285
122. Johansson C, Castillejo-Lopez C, Johanneson B, Svenungsson E, Gunnarsson I, Frostegard J, Sturfelt G, Truedsson L, Lofstrom B, Alcocer-Varela J, Lundberg I, Gyllensten UB, Alarcon-Segovia D, Alarcon-Riquelme ME (2000) Association analysis with microsatellite and SNP markers does not support the involvement of BCL-2 in systemic lupus erythematosus in Mexican and Swedish patients and their families. Genes Immun 1:380–385
123. Cao H, Hegele RA (2002) Identification of polymorphisms in the human SHP1 gene. J Hum Genet 47:445–447
124. Lajaunias F, Ibnou-Zekri N, Fossati Jimack L, Chicheportiche Y, Parkhouse RM, Mary C, Reininger L, Brighouse G, Izui S (1999) Polymorphisms in the Cd22 gene of inbred mouse strains. Immunogenetics 49:991–995
125. Liu ZH, Cheng ZH, Gong RJ, Liu H, Liu D, Li LS (2002) Sex differences in estrogen receptor gene polymorphism and its association with lupus nephritis in Chinese. Nephron 90:174–180
126. Lee YJ, Shin KS, Kang SW, Lee CK, Yoo B, Cha HS, Koh EM, Yoon SJ, Lee J (2004) Association of the oestrogen receptor alpha gene polymorphisms with disease onset in systemic lupus erythematosus. Ann Rheum Dis 63:1244–1249
127. Johansson M, Arlestig L, Moller B, Smedby T, Rantapaa-Dahlqvist S (2005) Estrogen receptor alpha gene polymorphisms in systemic lupus erythematosus. Ann Rheum Dis 64:1611–1617
128. Stevens A, Ray D, Alansari A, Hajeer A, Thomson W, Donn R, Ollier WE, Worthington J, Davis JR (2001) Characterization of a prolactin gene polymorphism and its associations with systemic lupus erythematosus. Arthritis Rheum 44:2358–2366
129. Mellai M, Giordano M, D'Alfonso S, Marchini M, Scorza R, Giovanna Danieli M, Leone M, Ferro I, Liguori M, Trojano M, Ballerini C, Massacesi L, Cannoni S, Bomprezzi R, Momigliano-Richiardi P (2003) Prolactin and prolactin receptor gene polymorphisms in multiple sclerosis and systemic lupus erythematosus. Hum Immunol 64:274–284

Innate (Over)immunity and Adaptive Autoimmune Disease

M. Recher[1,2] (✉) · K. S. Lang[2]

[1]University Hospital Bruderholz, Institute of Internal Medicine,
4101 Bruderholz, Switzerland
mike.recher@ksbh.ch

[2]Institute for Experimental Immunology, University Hospital Zürich,
Schmelzbergstrasse 12, 8091 Zürich, Switzerland

1	Introduction	89
2	Autoimmunity and/or Infection	90
3	Innate Regulators of Autoreactive T Cell Priming	93
4	Regulatory T Cells and Their Relation to Toll-Like Receptor Signals	95
5	Lack of (Auto)immunity After Innate Overactivation: A Role for Interferons and the Nervous System	96
6	Autoreactivity and Conversion to Autoimmune Disease	97
7	Conclusion	99
References		100

Abstract Autoimmune disease is characterized by clinical symptoms mediated by adaptive (T cell and B cell) immune reactions towards autoantigen-expressing tissue. Here we discuss that autoimmune disease is often preceded by autoreactivity, meaning the priming of autoantigen-specific immune cells without relevant tissue damage. Recent experimental evidence has demonstrated that both the induction of autoreactivity and the conversion into autoimmune disease is controlled by the activation of the nonspecific innate immune system. Also, the "inflammatory status" of the target organ critically influences the onset of overt autoimmune disease.

1 Introduction

Autoimmune diseases in humans are chronic syndromes characterized by typical, often relapsing, clinical symptoms combined with diagnostic results of adaptive humoral (autoantibodies) or cellular (autoreactive T cells) responses directed against autoantigen-expressing tissues. Important human autoimmune diseases include autoimmune diabetes mellitus, rheumatoid arthritis, multiple sclerosis, and myasthenia gravis. Remarkably, autoimmunity often associates with, or is triggered by virus infections and is associated with certain MHC alleles [1]. Endocrine organs such as the adrenal gland (Morbus Addison), the thyroid gland (Hashimoto thyroiditis, Graves disease) and endocrine cells in the stomach are often involved in autoimmunity [2]. Since there barely exists an organ where autoimmunity has not been reported, the frequent involvement of endocrine organs may reflect relatively easy diagnosis or special pathogenetic features. This review will focus on mechanisms involved in the activation and effector function of autoreactive T cells and attempts to explain some clinical observations in a novel way to suggest new therapeutic strategies.

2
Autoimmunity and/or Infection

The thymus negatively selects T cells with autoantigen-specific surface receptors. This negative selection process requires the presence of peripheral autoantigen in the thymus. Although this review will not focus on the thymic selection process, it is noteworthy that the transcription factor AIRE has been proposed to assure thymic expression of peripheral antigens [3]. AIRE was identified as the mutated gene in humans with Autoimmune Polyendocrinopathy-Candidiasis-Ectodermal Dystrophy (APECED), a familiar polyendocrine autoimmune disease [4]. To study central tolerance and peripheral autoimmunity, several T cell receptor transgenic mice specific for relevant extralymphatic peripheral autoantigens have been developed during the past decade [5]. Interestingly, central tolerance appeared to be more the exception than the rule. These findings implicate that naïve autoantigen-specific T cells are probably common, much more than widely believed. However, most T cell receptor transgenic autoimmune mouse models fail to induce disease spontaneously, at least during the relatively short lifespan of a laboratory mouse [5]. Thus, while accepting the importance of the presence of the final adaptive effector cells in mediating clinical disease, it seems even more essential to understand the pathways that initially led to their induction, i.e., why, where, and how are these autoreactive B and T cells primed? Several explanations have been offered:

1. Molecular mimicry, meaning that an infectious agent shares a protein-epitope with a self-protein within the peripheral target tissue [6]. Cross-

reactivity has been proposed to be involved in the association of infection with beta hemolytic streptococci and rheumatic fever, B3 Coxsackievirus and myocarditis, various viruses and multiple sclerosis, *Borrelia burgdorferi* and Lyme arthritis and B4 Coxsackie virus, rubella virus or CMV and diabetes type I. Since epitope binding occurs in a MHC-restricted manner, molecular mimicry may also explain the associations with MHC alleles [7]. However, confirmation of molecular mimicry involvement in autoimmunity requires more than simple associations. The endogenous as well as the foreign epitopes must be identified and the induction of cross-reactive T cells during disease should be confirmed. In a best case scenario, deletion of either epitope should result in absence or reduction of autoimmunity in an animal model [8]. Based on these criteria, molecular mimicry has not been demonstrated convincingly. Nevertheless, molecular mimicry may sometimes still contribute to autoimmunity in some cases [9–11].

2. A more common first step in the autoimmune disease pathway involves organ damage and release of so far immunologically ignored autoantigen and its presentation by antigen-presenting cells (APCs) in draining lymph nodes and the spleen. For example, ischemic myocardial infarction leads to the increase of myocardial proteins measurable in blood and may induce autoimmune myo/epi/pericarditis some weeks later (Dressler syndrome). Similarly, mechanical eye injury may lead to autoimmune destruction of the other undamaged eye [12, 13]. In infection-associated autoimmunity, cytopathic virus (e.g., B3 Coxsackie virus) replication may cause myocardial apoptosis and release of heart muscle proteins. T cells against both the virus and against autoantigen are primed in local lymph nodes and the spleen and are recruited to the heart [14]. Depending on the virus, molecular mimicry may in addition enhance autoimmune attack. Once started, autoimmunity destroys additional heart muscle tissue and autoantigen is again released, which maintains the process and may involve additional epitopes (epitope spreading).

Despite these complexities, autoantigen-specific T cells usually seem to ignore the peripheral antigen in the absence of an organ pathology or inflammation. This view was supported from experiments in a mouse diabetes model where a viral antigen (lymphocytic choriomeningitis virus (LCMV) -glycoprotein GP or LCMV-nucleoprotein NP) is expressed solely in the pancreatic islets due to expression control by the rat insulin promoter (RIP-GP and RIP-NP mice) [15, 16]. If these mice are crossed with mice in which all (transgenic) T cells recognize the same viral antigen, no activation of T cells is induced (Ignorance) (Fig. 1). In contrast, if the RIP-GP or RIP-NP mice are systemically

RIP-GP model

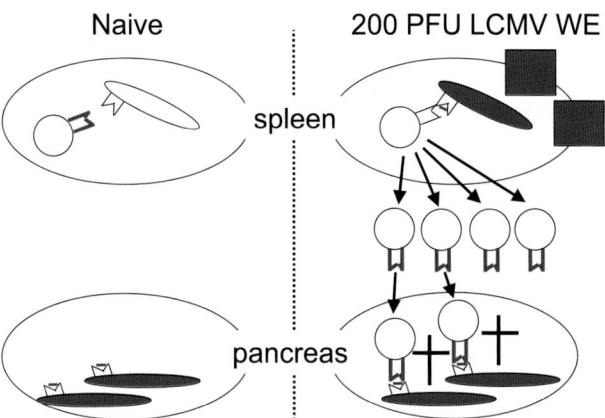

Fig. 1 RIP-GP mice express the LCMV glycoprotein under the rat insulin promoter. These mice express the LCMV antigen specifically in the pancreatic islets. T cells specific for the LCMV glycoprotein exist but are not activated since the antigen is not expressed by antigen-presenting cells (APCs) in the spleen (*left*). If these mice are infected with LCMV, virus replicates in the spleen, LCMV glycoprotein is presented by splenic APCs followed by an activation of CD8$^+$ T cells. These effector cells then home to the pancreas where they encounter LCMV antigen on islets cells. This leads to the destruction of beta islets cells and to overt diabetes (*right*)

infected with LCMV, the T cells proliferate, migrate within the pancreas, and induce diabetes within days (RIP-GP) or weeks (RIP-NP). When researchers aimed to induce myasthenia-like autoimmune disease by injection of acetylcholine receptor autoantigen, the response was low. Only repeated autoantigen injection in combination of so-called adjuvans could induce autoimmunity [17]. Adjuvans as an essential part in inducing autoimmunity were later shown to activate the innate immune system, including macrophages and dendritic cells [18]. From this point of view, autoimmunity develops similarly to an adaptive immune response against pathogens. There, the so-called danger hypothesis postulates that adaptive immune responses (e.g., against a virus) are enhanced in the presence of additional pathogen-related signals [19, 20]. For example, immunization with LCMV antigen-peptide alone is insufficient to activate adaptive cellular immune responses. However, if the same antigen is delivered in the form of a virus-like particle or virus-derived signals, the immune response is greatly enhanced [21–23]. Interestingly, T cell receptor transgenic mice specific for basic myelin protein developed multiple sclerosis-like disease in a conventional mouse facility while remaining healthy under specific pathogen-free (SPF) housing conditions [5, 24]. Thus, additional inflammatory signals, even if their origin is unrelated to the autoantigen-expressing tissue, may accelerate and support the induction of autoimmune disease.

3
Innate Regulators of Autoreactive T Cell Priming

During the last few years, so-called danger signals have been characterized molecularly. They, amongst others, include bacterial and viral oligonucleotides, bacterial and fungal cell wall components such as lipopolysaccharides (LPS), or bacterial proteins derived from flagellae [25, 26]. They all have in common that they are ligands for specific pattern-recognition receptors called toll-like receptors (TLRs) on innate antigen-presenting cells [25]. The TLR family is built of ten members, each specifically recognizing a different pattern. For example, TLR4 recognizes LPS and TLR9 is engaged by DNA oligonucleotides. Intracellular TLR signaling involves different adaptor molecules such as MyD88 or TRIF and commonly results in the activation of the transcription factor NF-kappa B [27]. Consequences of toll-like receptor triggering are the release of interferons and other cytokines as well as the expression of co-stimulatory molecules. In an autoimmune myocarditis model, only autoantigen-presenting dendritic cells, additionally and specifically activated by toll-like receptor stimulation, induced myocarditis and heart failure. Dendritic cells carrying autoantigen without TLR engagement failed to induce autoimmunity [28]. Thus, be it immune or autoimmune responses, the activation of these antigen-presenting cells by toll-like receptor engagement leads to an enhanced activation of adaptive immune responses. Ligands of toll-like receptors are not restricted to pathogen-related products. "Stressed" cells are another source of potent innate immunity [29, 30]. This activation has been reported to be partially mediated by so-called heat shock proteins (HSPs) [29]. Upregulated during cellular damage, HSPs are potent activators of toll-like receptors. In the RIP-GP model, autoimmune diabetes could be induced more easily by administration of endogenous heat shock protein in addition to virus peptide [31]. However, LPS contamination of HsP preparations may be at least partly responsible for some of the observed effects [32]. A recent report has identified uric acid released from damaged cells as another source of innate immune activation [33]. The underlying mechanisms of innate immunity triggering adaptive autoimmune responses include enhanced expression of the aforementioned co-stimulatory molecules by toll-like receptor-triggered

APCs. Among these co-stimulatory molecules, the B7 group built of CD80 and CD86, both binding to the T cell activating CD28 protein, has been characterized most extensively [34, 35]. In addition, co-stimulatory interactions of Ox40-OX40L and ICOS-B7H-2 have been demonstrated to facilitate T cell priming both in vitro and in vivo [36, 37]. Balancing these activating co-stimulatory receptors, there exist negative signals that inhibit the priming of both autoreactive or pathogen-specific T cells (Table 1). These are provided for example by PD-1 or CTLA4 [38, 39]. PD-1 or CTLA4-expressing, antigen-presenting naïve DCs lead to the tolerization/anergy of specific T cells [40]. In contrast, DCs lacking PD-1 or CTLA4 lead to the activation of the same T cells.

Table 1

Mechanism	Proteins involved	Enhancement (+) or suppression (−) of autoimmune disease	Selected references
Thymic selection			
Expression of autoantigens	AIRE	−	3, 4
Initial priming			
Co-stimulation	CD80, CD86, OX40	+	34–36
Tolerance	PD-1, CTLA-4	−	38–40
Regulatory T cells	FoxP3, IL10, TGF-beta, CTLA-4	−	42, 46
Homing			
Retention of T cells	S1P, IP10	−	67–69
Reduced homing in peripheral organs	CXCR3	+	66
Effector function in target organ			
T cell intrinsic anergy	Cbl-b	−	74
Enhancement of peripheral antigen presentation	TNF, IFNγ, IFNα	+	71, 72, 77
Apoptosis	FASL	−	76

4
Regulatory T Cells and Their Relation to Toll-Like Receptor Signals

Another control mechanism of autoreactive T cell priming has been proposed to be mediated by so-called naturally arising regulatory T cells. These T cells develop in the thymus, are mostly but not exclusively CD25$^+$, and are functionally characterized by expression of the transcription factor FoxP3 [41, 42]. Upon T cell receptor triggering, so-called T regulatory cells seem to suppress the activation of CD4$^+$ and CD8$^+$ T cells both in vitro and in vivo assays. The mechanism of suppression is still debated but seems to be partly contact-dependent, although cytokines such as IL-10, IL-4, and TGFβ may play an additional important role. The contact-dependent suppression involves CTLA4, whose expression is tightly regulated by FoxP3 [41]. Recent evidence has revealed that regulatory T cells paradoxically require the cytokine IL-2, which was known for some time to accelerate T cell activation [43, 44]. Together with the fact that CD25 functions as an IL-2 receptor chain, it might be suggested that regulation is achieved by simply depriving T cells from IL-2. However, IL-2 knock-out mice lack regulatory T cells and die of severe autoimmunity, while their T cell response upon various immunizations is, at least initially, quite normal [45]. In contrast, in vivo neutralization of IL-2 results in autoimmune disease by selective reduction of FOXP3-expressing CD25$^+$CD4$^+$ T cells [46]. Depletion of regulatory T cells clearly lowers the threshold of autoreactive T cell priming. However, simple administration of antigen in the absence of regulatory T cells is only associated with autoreactive T cell activation when co-stimulation (e.g., via CD28) is present [47]. Thus, different levels exist that assure peripheral ignorance/nonresponsiveness of autoreactive T cells. These include regulatory T cells or signals derived from TLR engagement. All may influence the upregulation of co-stimulatory or downregulation of co-inhibitory molecules on dendritic cells and other antigen-presenting cells. TLR-triggered APCs are also capable of overcoming the control by regulatory T cells. For example, activated antigen-presenting DCs with upregulated co-stimulatory molecules fail to initiate T cell priming as long as CD25$^+$ T cells are present [47, 48]. However, the same regulatory T cells no longer inhibit T cell priming when DCs produce cytokines such as IL-6 following TLR engagement [48]. Also, regulatory T cells themselves express TLRs [49]. Thus, T cell priming only occurs if APC activation via TLR-mediated signals exceeds a certain threshold, a mechanism which may hinder the formation of adaptive autoimmunity. In mouse studies, deliberate induction of regulatory T cells has been successfully used to limit autoimmune diabetes, allergic encephalitis, and myasthenia gravis in vivo [50–52]. Taken together, while the phenomenon of regulation is undisputed, some details of the mechanisms at work remain elusive.

5
Lack of (Auto)immunity After Innate Overactivation: A Role for Interferons and the Nervous System

As discussed, autoimmune responses are induced similarly to an immune response against pathogens. Both involve an early phase of innate immune activation followed by the activation of adaptive T and B cell responses. It is noteworthy that innate immunity may be overactivated to a state resulting in suppression rather than priming of T cells. Interestingly, some clinically acute infections such as measles virus infection show a phenotype of early severe inflammatory disease and immunosuppression later. Measles patients frequently suffer from superinfectious bacterial pneumonia and often fail to react with a delayed type hypersensitivity (DTH) reaction to intradermal tuberculin protein, a classical type IV immune response according to Coombs [53]. In mice, measles virus leads to intense activation of macrophages and dendritic cells that finally results in an overactivated state associated with increased apoptosis and failure to prime T cell responses [54, 55]. Consistently, an infection with LCMV-Clone 13 causes DC apoptosis, which partly explains the lack of a functional T cell response in vivo [56, 57]. Notably, the apoptotic pathways in both virus models required type I interferon signaling [55]. A similar immunosuppressive activity has been observed following Listeria monocytogenes infection in vivo, which was demonstrated to be lethal only if type I interferon signaling was functional [58, 59]. In the presence of type I interferon signaling, splenocyte apoptosis following *Listeria* infection was enhanced. Thus, besides the widely known antiviral activity, type I interferons display important immunosuppressive capacities. Another clinical example of such induced immunosuppression is cerebral ischemic stroke, where superinfection and sepsis are leading causes of death. In a murine stroke model, bacterial pneumonia was rapidly observed in almost 100% of cases [60]. This could be prevented by the administration of the beta-blocker propanolol correlating with decreased splenocyte apoptosis. These results are consistent with those from the *Listeria* infection model described above [60]. Propanolol counteracts the signals derived from the sympathetic nerve and its transmitter noradrenalin. The same counteracting is physiologically done by the vagus nerve and its main transmitter acetylcholine. Acetylcholine administration renders APCs more resistant to inducing experimental sepsis in vivo [61]. In light of these recent findings, a possible psychosomatic contribution in induction and progress of autoimmune responses may be worth re-evaluating [62, 63]. Intriguingly, nicotine acts as an acetylcholine agonist and has been demonstrated to suppress lethal sepsis, provocatively implicating a "smoke or die" regimen for patients with severe systemic inflammatory syndromes [64]. Taken together, innate immunity typically results in two rather opposing consequences: mostly, adaptive immune responses are favored. However, in case of inappropriate innate overimmunity, immunosuppression is induced, meaning that adaptive immune responses are greatly suppressed. This may partly explain why severe burn injuries or acute pancreatitis are not regularly followed by autoimmune disease, despite the potential systemic release of autoantigens by tissue destruction. Rather, vigorous innate immune activation during such states is linked to an immunosuppression with a great risk of superinfection, sepsis, and death.

6
Autoreactivity and Conversion to Autoimmune Disease

Once autoantigen becomes systemically released, innate immunity is induced and adaptive responses therefore primed, the described criteria of autoreactivity are fulfilled. Autoreactivity describes a state where adaptive autoimmune responses (T cells and/or autoantibodies) are measurable; however, overt disease is still absent. This state can be observed in patients where autoreactive T cells are detectable years before onset of disease. Also, detection of autoantibodies is often possible in "healthy" persons without any further signs of autoimmune disease. In general, this may reflect a quality or quantity of the autoimmune responses below a threshold required for initiation of disease [65]. Furthermore, the conversion of autoreactivity into overt autoimmune disease requires additional immunological and inflammatory processes. First, autoreactive T cells have to be recruited to the peripheral target organ. Here, expression and function of chemokines and their respective receptors play an important role. For example, effector T cells express the chemokine CXCR3, which results in migration toward an IP-10 gradient. Interestingly, islets of NOD mice that spontaneously develop diabetes with age have been reported to express increased age-related amounts of IP-10. LCMV-infected CXCR3-deficient RIP-GP mice develop delayed autoimmune diabetes associated with a decreased lymphocyte infiltration in autoantigen-expressing islets [66]. FTY, a novel drug binding to sphingosine receptors retains activated lymphocytes within lymphoid organs and reduces peripheral organ infiltration, thereby delaying or preventing diabetes in the LCMV RIP-GP model [67, 68]. Strikingly, prediabetic mice that already showed islet T cell infiltrations could be "cured" by a systemic virus infection [69]. This correlated with the fact that upon viral infection, IP10 expression became upregulated in lymph nodes, including the pancreatic lymph node. Islet T cells therefore migrated toward the lymph node away from the islets, where they were eventually eliminated by activation induced cell death [69]. In contrast, islet expression of several immune activating molecules has been shown to favor immune cell accumulations in the peripheral target organ and to accelerate disease [70–72]. Nevertheless, autoimmune responses are complex since the encounter of autoreactive T cells and autoantigen-expressing cells may not always accelerate autoimmune disease. For example, T cell transgenic mice specific for pancreatic islet antigen on the NOD mouse background rapidly induced insulitis; however, the mice rarely progressed to overt diabetes. Diabetes induction was even less than in nontransgenic control mice [5]. One possible mechanism explaining this disease-delaying state might arise is T cell intrinsic anergy or deletion, a common finding following immunizations with high or persistent antigen immunizations [73]. The ubiquitin ligase cbl-b has been demonstrated to critically promote T cell anergy and to reduce the transition of autoreactivity and autoimmune disease [65, 74]. Another mechanism of peripheral tolerance depends on the peripheral target organ itself. This proposal is based on the fact that some tumors have been demonstrated to express FAS ligand, which may hinder tumor destruction due to apoptosis of attacking FAS-expressing T cells [75]. The same was observed in autoimmune uveitis, where the eye tissue constitutively expresses FAS ligand [76]. Another important parameter of the peripheral target organ was identified in RIP-GP mice. When RIP-GP mice were immunized with LCMV peptide in an optimized prime-boost strategy, up to 90% of all CD8$^+$ T cells in the blood were specific for the islet antigen. However, the mice still remained healthy. Recent experiments revealed that one limiting factor is islet MHC class I expression [77]. Only high MHC class I expression on islet cells allowed specific

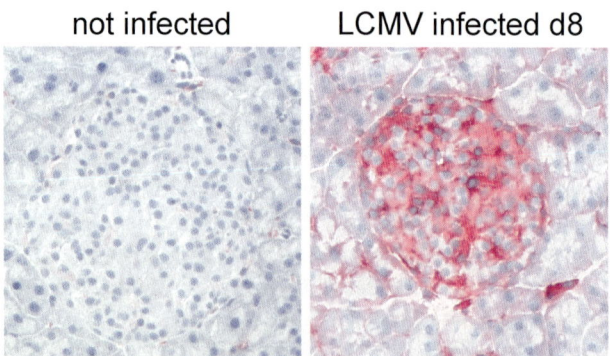

Fig. 2 In naïve C57BL/6 mice (*left*) or C57BL/6 mice 8 days after infection with 200 plaque forming units (PFU) LCMV-WE (*right*), MHC I expression on pancreatic islets is shown by immunohistology

T cells to cause diabetes. MHC class I expression on pancreatic islets depended on intact TLR signaling and signals driven by systemic type I interferons [77]. Remarkably, endocrine pancreatic islet cells were far more susceptible to up-regulation of MHC class I following systemic release of interferon alpha when compared to the exocrine pancreas (Fig. 2). Thus, a state of autoreactivity could be converted into overt autoimmune disease by nonspecific activation of innate immunity. This might explain why several virus infections are related to autoimmune diseases and that disease relapse is often observed in association with generalized virus infection. While viruses may rarely share epitopes with autoantigens (molecular mimicry), most viruses probably activate TLRs and change the immune status (e.g., MHC class I expression) of the autoantigen-expressing peripheral target organ.

7
Conclusion

Autoimmune disease depends on three general criteria (Table 1). First, autoreactive T cells have to be primed before they, second, are recruited to the peripheral autoantigen-expressing target organ. Thirdly, these T cells have to be able to destroy the autoantigen-presenting tissue. In all these steps, innate immunity is a limiting factor leading to autoimmune disease (Table 1). This happens in analogy to an immune response against a pathogen, where adaptive responses depend on innate resistance mechanisms.

The innate triggering of T cell priming can be classified into three groups. First, triggering of TLRs enhances the probability of T cell priming. Second, co-stimulation results in either positive or negative effects on T cell priming. Third, regulatory T cells generally influence T cell responses, especially in the absence of TLR signals. In addition, the autonomous nervous system may balance innate immune activation. While most early autoimmune research has focused on autoimmune B and T cells so far, it has recently become clear that innate immunity is a superposed regulator of autoimmunity. This has also been underscored by the successful introduction of TNFα antagonists in clinical autoimmunity trials [78]. Other clinical targets could be antagonists of TLRs or modulators of the interferon signaling cascade. The suppressive activities of regulatory T cells represents another means to ameliorate autoimmune diseases [51]. It remains to be established how to differentiate innate immunity and related autoimmune disease from innate overactivation and related immunosuppression. Though counterintuitive, also innate overactivation may have the potential to ameliorate autoimmune disease, while bearing the risk of superinfection.

Acknowledgements The authors thank Prof. H. Hengartner, Prof. R.M. Zinkernagel, Dr. H.C. Probst, and Dr. A. Bergthaler for discussions and critical reading of the manuscript.

References

1. Sonderstrup G, McDevitt HO (2001) DR, DQ, and you: MHC alleles and autoimmunity. J Clin Invest 107:795–796
2. Anderson MS (2002) Autoimmune endocrine disease. Curr Opin Immunol 14:760–764
3. Liston A, Lesage S, Wilson J, Peltonen L, Goodnow CC (2003) Aire regulates negative selection of organ-specific T cells. Nat Immunol 4:350–354
4. Bjorses P, Aaltonen J, Horelli-Kuitunen N, Yaspo ML, Peltonen L (1998) Gene defect behind APECED a new clue to autoimmunity. Hum Mol Genet 7:1547–1553
5. Lafaille JJ (2004) T-cell receptor transgenic mice in the study of autoimmune diseases. J Autoimmunol 22:95–106
6. Kukreja A, Maclaren NK (2000) Current cases in which epitope mimicry is considered as a component cause of autoimmune disease: immune-mediated (type 1) diabetes. Cell Mol Life Sci 57:534–541
7. Stratmann T, Martin-Orozco N, Mallet-Designe V, Poirot L, McGavern D, Losyev G, Dobbs CM, Oldstone MB, Yoshida K, Kikutani H et al (2003) Susceptible MHC alleles, not background genes, select an autoimmune T cell reactivity. J Clin Invest 112:902–914
8. Benoist C, Mathis D (2001) Autoimmunity provoked by infection: how good is the case for T cell epitope mimicry? Nat Immunol 22:797–801
9. McClain MT, Heinlen LD, Dennis GJ, Roebuck J, Harley JB, James JA (2005) Early events in lupus humoral autoimmunity suggest initiation through molecular mimicry. Nat Med 11:85–89
10. Olson JK, Ludovic Croxford J, Miller SD (2004) Innate and adaptive immune requirements for induction of autoimmune demyelinating disease by molecular mimicry. Mol Immunol 40:1103–1108
11. Olson JK, Eagar TN, Miller SD (2002) Functional activation of myelin-specific T cells by virus-induced molecular mimicry. J Immunol 169:2719–2726
12. Gregoratos G (1990) Pericardial involvement in acute myocardial infarction. Cardiol Clin 8:601–608
13. Gregerson DS (2002) Peripheral expression of ocular antigens in regulation and therapy of ocular autoimmunity. Int Rev Immunol 21:101–121
14. Fairweather D, Kaya Z, Shellam GR, Lawson CM, Rose NR (2001) From infection to autoimmunity. J Autoimmun 16:175–186
15. Ohashi PS, Oehen S, Aichele P, Pircher H, Odermatt B, Herrera P, Higuchi Y, Buerki K, Hengartner H, Zinkernagel RM (1993) Induction of diabetes is influenced by the infectious virus and local expression of MHC class I and tumor necrosis factor-alpha. J Immunol 150:5185–5194

16. Von Herrath MG, Dockter J, Oldstone MB (1994) How virus induces a rapid or slow onset insulin-dependent diabetes mellitus in a transgenic model. Immunity 1:231–242
17. Fuchs S, Nevo D, Tarrab-Hazdai R, Yaar I (1976) Strain differences in the autoimmune response of mice to acetylcholine receptors. Nature 263:329–330
18. O'Neill LA (2004) TLRs: Professor Mechnikov, sit on your hat. Trends Immunol 25:687–693
19. Janeway CA Jr (1992) The immune system evolved to discriminate infectious nonself from noninfectious self. Immunol Today 13:11–16
20. Gallucci S, Matzinger P (2001) Danger signals: SOS to the immune system. Curr Opin Immunol 13:114–119
21. Bachmann MF, Lutz MB, Layton GT, Harris SJ, Fehr T, Rescigno M, Ricciardi-Castagnoli P (1996) Dendritic cells process exogenous viral proteins and virus-like particles for class I presentation to CD8+ cytotoxic T lymphocytes. Eur J Immunol 26:2595–2600
22. Gilbert SC (2001) Virus-like particles as vaccine adjuvants. Mol Biotechnol 19:169–177
23. Kovacsovics-Bankowski M, Clark K, Benacerraf B, Rock KL (1993) Efficient major histocompatibility complex class I presentation of exogenous antigen upon phagocytosis by macrophages. Proc Natl Acad Sci U S A 90:4942–4946
24. Lafaille JJ, Nagashima K, Katsuki M, Tonegawa S (1994) High incidence of spontaneous autoimmune encephalomyelitis in immunodeficient anti-myelin basic protein T cell receptor transgenic mice. Cell 78:399–408
25. Akira S, Hemmi H (2003) Recognition of pathogen-associated molecular patterns by TLR family. Immunol Lett 85:85–95
26. Beutler B (2004) Innate immunity: an overview. Mol Immunol 40:845–859
27. Akira S, Takeda K (2004) Toll-like receptor signalling. Nat Rev Immunol 4:499–511
28. Eriksson U, Ricci R, Hunziker L, Kurrer MO, Oudit GY, Watts TH, Sonderegger I, Bachmaier K, Kopf M, Penninger JM (2003) Dendritic cell-induced autoimmune heart failure requires cooperation between adaptive and innate immunity. Nat Med 9:1484–1490
29. Basu S, Binder RJ, Suto R, Anderson KM, Srivastava PK (2000) Necrotic but not apoptotic cell death releases heat shock proteins, which deliver a partial maturation signal to dendritic cells and activate the NF-kappa B pathway. Int Immunol 12:1539–1546
30. Shi Y, Rock KL (2002) Cell death releases endogenous adjuvants that selectively enhance immune surveillance of particulate antigens. Eur J Immunol 32:155–162
31. Millar DG, Garza KM, Odermatt B, Elford AR, Ono N, Li Z, Ohashi PS (2003) Hsp70 promotes antigen-presenting cell function and converts T-cell tolerance to autoimmunity in vivo. Nat Med 9:1469–1476
32. Gao B, Tsan MF (2003) Endotoxin contamination in recombinant human heat shock protein 70 (Hsp70) preparation is responsible for the induction of tumor necrosis factor alpha release by murine macrophages. J Biol Chem 278:174–179
33. Shi Y, Evans JE, Rock KL (2003) Molecular identification of a danger signal that alerts the immune system to dying cells. Nature 425:516–521

34. McAdam AJ, Schweitzer AN, Sharpe AH (1998) The role of B7 co-stimulation in activation and differentiation of CD4+ and CD8+ T cells. Immunol Rev 165:231–247
35. Greenwald RJ, Freeman GJ, Sharpe AH (2004) The B7 family revisited. Annu Rev Immunol 23:515–548
36. Coyle AJ, Gutierrez-Ramos JC (2004) The role of ICOS and other costimulatory molecules in allergy and asthma. Springer Semin Immunopathol 25:349–359
37. Croft M (2003) Costimulation of T cells by OX40, 4-1BB, and CD27. Cytokine Growth Factor Rev 14:265–273
38. Okazaki T, Iwai Y, Honjo T (2002) New regulatory co-receptors: inducible co-stimulator and PD-1. Curr Opin Immunol 14:779–782
39. Nishimura H, Nose M, Hiai H, Minato N, Honjo T (1999) Development of lupus-like autoimmune diseases by disruption of the PD-1 gene encoding an ITIM motif-carrying immunoreceptor. Immunity 11:141–151
40. Probst HC (2005) Resting dendritic cells induce peripheral CD8+ T cell tolerance through PD-1 and CTLA-4. Nat Immunol 6:280–286
41. Sakaguchi S (2004) Naturally arising CD4+ regulatory t cells for immunologic self-tolerance and negative control of immune responses. Annu Rev Immunol 22:531–562
42. Shevach EM (2000) Regulatory T cells in autoimmmunity. Annu Rev Immunol 18:423–449
43. Nelson BH (2004) IL-2, regulatory T cells, and tolerance. J Immunol 172:3983–3988
44. Malek TR, Bayer AL (2004) Tolerance, not immunity, crucially depends on IL-2. Nat Rev Immunol 4:665–674
45. Kundig TM, Schorle H, Bachmann MF, Hengartner H, Zinkernagel RM, Horak I (1993) Immune responses in interleukin-2-deficient mice. Science 262:1059–1061
46. Setoguchi R, Hori S, Takahashi T, Sakaguchi S (2005) Homeostatic maintenance of natural Foxp3+ CD25+ CD4+ regulatory T cells by interleukin (IL)-2 and induction of autoimmune disease by IL-2 neutralization. J Exp Med 201:723–735
47. Pasare C, Medzhitov R (2004) Toll-dependent control mechanisms of CD4 T cell activation. Immunity 21:733–741
48. Pasare C, Medzhitov R (2003) Toll pathway-dependent blockade of CD4+CD25+ T cell-mediated suppression by dendritic cells. Science 299:1033–1036
49. Caramalho I, Lopes-Carvalho T, Ostler D, Zelenay S, Haury M, Demengeot J (2003) Regulatory T cells selectively express toll-like receptors and are activated by lipopolysaccharide. J Exp Med 197:403–411
50. Homann D, Holz A, Bot A, Coon B, Wolfe T, Petersen J, Dyrberg TP, Grusby MJ, von Herrath MG (1999) Autoreactive CD4+ T cells protect from autoimmune diabetes via bystander suppression using the IL-4/Stat6 pathway. Immunity 11:463–472
51. Homann D, von Herrath M (2004) Regulatory T cells and type 1 diabetes. Clin Immunol 112:202–209
52. Sela M, Mozes E (2004) Therapeutic vaccines in autoimmunity. Proc Natl Acad Sci U S A 101 [Suppl 2]:14586–14592
53. Rall GF (2003) Measles virus 1998–2002: progress and controversy. Annu Rev Microbiol 57:343–367
54. Hahm B, Arbour N, Oldstone MB (2004) Measles virus interacts with human SLAM receptor on dendritic cells to cause immunosuppression. Virology 323:292–302

55. Hahm B, Trifilo MJ, Zuniga EI, Oldstone MB (2005) Viruses evade the immune system through type i interferon-mediated STAT2-dependent, but STAT1-independent, signaling. Immunity 22:247–257
56. Sevilla N, McGavern DB, Teng C, Kunz S, Oldstone MB (2004) Viral targeting of hematopoietic progenitors and inhibition of DC maturation as a dual strategy for immune subversion. J Clin Invest 113:737–745
57. Moskophidis D, Lechner F, Pircher H, Zinkernagel RM (1993) Virus persistence in acutely infected immunocompetent mice by exhaustion of antiviral cytotoxic effector T cells. Nature 362:758–761
58. O'Connell RM, Saha SK, Vaidya SA, Bruhn KW, Miranda GA, Zarnegar B, Perry AK, Nguyen BO, Lane TF, Taniguchi T et al (2004) Type I interferon production enhances susceptibility to Listeria monocytogenes infection. J Exp Med 200:437–445
59. Auerbuch V, Brockstedt DG, Meyer-Morse N, O'Riordan M, Portnoy DA (2004) Mice lacking the type I interferon receptor are resistant to Listeria monocytogenes. J Exp Med 200:527–533
60. Prass K, Meisel C, Hoflich C, Braun J, Halle E, Wolf T, Ruscher K, Victorov IV, Priller J, Dirnagl U et al (2003) Stroke-induced immunodeficiency promotes spontaneous bacterial infections and is mediated by sympathetic activation reversal by poststroke T helper cell type 1-like immunostimulation. J Exp Med 198:725–736
61. Wang H, Yu M, Ochani M, Amella CA, Tanovic M, Susarla S, Li JH, Yang H, Ulloa L, Al-Abed Y et al (2003) Nicotinic acetylcholine receptor alpha7 subunit is an essential regulator of inflammation. Nature 421:384–388
62. Tracey KJ, Czura CJ, Ivanova S (2001) Mind over immunity. FASEB J 15:1575–1576
63. Libert C (2003) Inflammation: a nervous connection. Nature 421:328–329
64. Matthay MA, Ware LB (2004) Can nicotine treat sepsis? Nat Med 10:1161–1162
65. Gronski MA, Boulter JM, Moskophidis D, Nguyen LT, Holmberg K, Elford AR, Deenick EK, Kim HO, Penninger JM, Odermatt B et al (2004) TCR affinity and negative regulation limit autoimmunity. Nat Med 10:1234–1239
66. Frigerio S, Junt T, Lu B, Gerard C, Zumsteg U, Hollander GA, Piali L (2002) Beta cells are responsible for CXCR3-mediated T-cell infiltration in insulitis. Nat Med 8:1414–1420
67. Pinschewer DD, Ochsenbein AF, Odermatt B, Brinkmann V, Hengartner H, Zinkernagel RM (2000) FTY720 immunosuppression impairs effector T cell peripheral homing without affecting induction, expansion, and memory. J Immunol 164:5761–5770
68. Mandala S, Hajdu R, Bergstrom J, Quackenbush E, Xie J, Milligan J, Thornton R, Shei GJ, Card D, Keohane C et al (2002) Alteration of lymphocyte trafficking by sphingosine-1-phosphate receptor agonists. Science 296:346–349
69. Christen U, Benke D, Wolfe T, Rodrigo E, Rhode A, Hughes AC, Oldstone MB, von Herrath MG (2004) Cure of prediabetic mice by viral infections involves lymphocyte recruitment along an IP-10 gradient. J Clin Invest 113:74–84
70. Holz A, Brett K, Oldstone MB (2001) Constitutive beta cell expression of IL-12 does not perturb self-tolerance but intensifies established autoimmune diabetes. J Clin Invest 108:1749–1758

71. Von Herrath MG, Guerder S, Lewicki H, Flavell RA, Oldstone MB (1995) Coexpression of B7-1 and viral ("self") transgenes in pancreatic beta cells can break peripheral ignorance and lead to spontaneous autoimmune diabetes. Immunity 3:727–738
72. Sarvetnick N, Shizuru J, Liggitt D, Martin L, McIntyre B, Gregory A, Parslow T, Stewart T (1990) Loss of pancreatic islet tolerance induced by beta-cell expression of interferon-gamma. Nature 346:844–847
73. Aichele P, Brduscha-Riem K, Zinkernagel RM, Hengartner H, Pircher H (1995) T cell priming versus T cell tolerance induced by synthetic peptides. J Exp Med 182:261–266
74. Jeon MS, Atfield A, Venuprasad K, Krawczyk C, Sarao R, Elly C, Yang C, Arya S, Bachmaier K, Su L et al (2004) Essential role of the E3 ubiquitin ligase Cbl-b in T cell anergy induction. Immunity 21:167–177
75. Hahne M, Rimoldi D, Schroter M, Romero P, Schreier M, French LE, Schneider P, Bornand T, Fontana A, Lienard D et al (1996) Melanoma cell expression of Fas(Apo-1/CD95) ligand: implications for tumor immune escape. Science 274:1363–1366
76. Griffith TS, Brunner T, Fletcher SM, Green DR, Ferguson TA (1995) Fas ligand-induced apoptosis as a mechanism of immune privilege. Science 270:1189–1192
77. Lang KS, Recher M, Junt T, Navarini AA, Harris NL, Freigang S, Odermatt B, Conrad C, Ittner LM, Bauer S et al (2005) Toll-like receptor engagement converts T-cell autoreactivity into overt autoimmune disease. Nat Med 11:138–145
78. Braun J, Sieper J (2003) Overview of the use of the anti-TNF agent infliximab in chronic inflammatory diseases. Expert Opin Biol Ther 3:141–168

Can Unresolved Infection Precipitate Autoimmune Disease?

D. J. B. Marks[1] · N. A. Mitchison[2] (✉) · A. W. Segal[1] · J. Sieper[3]

[1]Centre for Molecular Medicine, University College London, 5 University Street, London WC1E 6JJ, UK

[2]Department of Immunology, Windeyer Institute of Medical Science, University College London, 46 Cleveland Street, London W1T 4JF, UK
n.mitchison@ucl.ac.uk

[3]Department of Rheumatology, Charite Berlin, Campus Benjamin Franklin, Hindenburgdamm 30, 12200 Berlin, Germany

1	Introduction	106
2	**Crohn's Disease**	107
2.1	Infections Unlikely to Cause Crohn's Disease	108
2.2	Defective Neutrophil Function Drives the Disease	109
3	**Ankylosing Spondylitis and the Other Spondyloarthritides**	112
3.1	Absence of Persistent Microbial Antigen	112
3.2	The Triggering Infection	113
3.3	Antibiotics Inhibit Triggering	114
4	**Regulatory Mechanisms in Autoimmunity**	115
4.1	Downregulation Occurs Within Dendritic Cell Clusters	116
4.2	Arenas Where Downregulation May Operate	117
4.3	Fear of Autoimmunity Can Hold Up Vaccine Development	118
	References	118

Abstract Autoimmune diseases are frequently postulated to arise as post-infectious phenomena. Here we survey the evidence supporting these theories, with particular emphasis on Crohn's disease and ankylosing spondylitis. Direct proof that infection establishes persistent autoimmunity remains lacking, although it may provoke a prolonged inflammatory response when occurring on a susceptible immunological background. The argument of infective causality is by no means trivial, since it carries important consequences for the safety of vaccine development.

1
Introduction

We argue here that the risk of unresolved infection precipitating autoimmune disease is very low. The relevant information can be summarized as follows. First, there exists a group of "autoimmune" diseases, so designated because they fulfil (1) a set of generally accepted positive criteria, and (2) the negative criterion that reasonable efforts have failed to find an infectious causal agent. The group includes RA (rheumatoid arthritis), T1D (type 1 diabetes mellitus), MS (multiple sclerosis), and less frequent diseases such as MG (myasthenia gravis) and Graves' disease (thyroid autoimmunity). The positive criteria include presence of autoantibody and self-reactive T cells, immune pathology, MHC associations, and an animal model. Second, another group of diseases exists in which it is postulated that an infectious trigger establishes an autonomous, persistent immunopathology (damage caused by the immune system rather than the infectious agent on its own). This group includes ReA (reactive arthritis) and its related spondylarthropathies such as AS (ankylosing spondylitis), chronic rheumatic fever, Crohn's disease, Coxsackie virus-associated myocarditis, HSK (herpes simplex keratitis), antibiotic-resistant Lyme disease, and a number of tropical diseases [7, 97]. The question posed here concerns this latter group, and in particular whether the pathogen continues to drive the immunopathology in the later phase when the acute infection has subsided. Table 1 lists the evidence bearing on autoimmunity in these diseases.

We conclude from this survey that substantial efforts have so far failed to demonstrate that these infections can lead to self-sustaining autoimmunity. The main problem has been that although the disease typically lasts for years after the acute event, antigen derived from the infective agent, or the pathogen itself, remains detectable. Improved methods, notably PCR, have undermined the case for autoimmunity: Chagas' cardiac myopathy, for instance, has been subjected cogently to this critique [63]. Strikingly, in a mouse model of B3 coxsackievirus-associated myocarditis, $CD4^+$ T cells themselves provide a source of the virus (M. Hesse et al., unpublished data), and in T1D the epidemiology has not convincingly demonstrated association with B4 coxsackievirus infection [50]. The main exception is AS, which we argue here may well represent a true instance of infection precipitating autoimmunity.

A discussion follows of two particularly informative diseases: Crohn's disease and AS. We present here a view of the chronic inflammatory diseases centred on immune dysregulation. Entering the two diseases in Table 1 as contradictory marks a difference, but does not exclude a connection between

Table 1 Where disease may have instigated autoimmunity

Disease	Autoimmunity target	Autoimmunity? Yes	Autoimmunity? No/Not proven
Chagas'	Heart, gut	[62, 71, 92]	[63, 110]
Herpes simplex keratitis	Cornea	[122]	[30, 115]
Malaria	Red blood cell	[28] (protective)	
Onchocerciasis	Eye	[82]	
Onchocerciasis	Skin (SOWDA)	[47, 49]	[23]
B3 coxsackievirus-associated cardiac	Heart	[98, 103]	M. Hesse et al., unpublished data
Rheumatic fever	Heart	[53]	
B4 coxsackievirus-associated T1D	Pancreas	[114]	[46, 50]
Spondyloarthropathy	Joints	Discussed in this chapter	
Crohn's disease	Gut		Discussed in this chapter
Lyme disease (antibiotic resistant)	Joints		T. Kamradt, personal communication

the two. We argue that the neutrophil defect identified as causal in Crohn's disease can on occasion (depending on a genetic factor) allow enteric bacteria to trigger the autoimmunity of AS. We then show how recent advances in understanding immune downregulation have blurred the boundary between self and non-self, and how they strengthen the view that autoimmunity springs from immune dysregulation. Finally, we point out how misplaced fear of autoimmunity can hinder vaccine development.

2
Crohn's Disease

The central problem in Crohn's disease concerns the nature of the stimulus driving the chronic inflammation. We question the primary pathogenic role for infection and favour an alternative mechanism based on impaired neutrophil recruitment.

2.1
Infections Unlikely to Cause Crohn's Disease

The suggestion that *Mycobacterium avium paratuberculosis* (MAP) represents the primary aetiological agent in Crohn's disease was made in the first description of the syndrome [27]. In ruminants, MAP causes a granulomatous ileocolitis known as Johne's disease [19]. Many regard this as the animal equivalent of Crohn's disease, although others point to significant differences between the two diseases [112].

Conventional histochemistry fails to reveal mycobacteria in human Crohn's tissues. However, specialized culture can yield cell-wall-deficient organisms termed spheroplasts [21]. These subsequently develop Ziehl-Neelsen-positive cell walls and contain a MAP genome. Inoculation of animals with these isolates elicits variable phenotypes: mice generate hepatic and splenic granulomata, whilst many other species exhibit no detectable response. Most impressively, goats develop a granulomatous ileitis following oral inoculation.

Case–control studies have examined the human disease specificity of MAP, principally by comparing detection rates of the *IS900* DNA insertion element in patients and controls. The results have proved highly variable, not least due to methodological differences between studies [94]. Of note, a significant proportion of individuals without overt Crohn's disease also carry MAP within the bowel wall and circulating leukocytes, although organisms isolated from Crohn's patients appear to exhibit greater viability [87].

Conclusive evidence for MAP pathogenicity in humans is lacking. A frequently cited case report describes a 7-year-old boy who presented with granulomatous cervical lymphadenopathy, positive for MAP DNA, who 5 years later developed terminal ileitis consistent with Crohn's disease [55]. Whilst this story is interesting, it warrants the proviso that the histological finding of caseating granulomata in the lymph node implicates *Mycobacterium scrofulaceum* (untested) as the causative pathogen. Subsequent inflammatory bowel disease could have arisen coincidentally. Furthermore, under the hypothesis that MAP drives the inflammation of Crohn's disease, anti-mycobacterial treatment should give a cure. Preliminary clinical studies have provided mixed data but no strong evidence that this is the case [36, 52, 105]. The results of a double-blind, randomized controlled trial currently in progress should resolve this issue.

Although MAP may persist abnormally in Crohn's disease, the case for causality remains weak. Any hypothesis invoking MAP as the primary aetiology needs to explain why carriage in healthy individuals does not lead to disease, accepting that *Mycobacterium tuberculosis* induces pathology only in a minority of those infected. This requires the postulation of a susceptible immunological background. The clinical utility of infliximab, an inhibitor of TNF-α, argues against this in that it ameliorates bowel inflammation whilst permitting reactivation of latent mycobacteria [86]. Additionally, the failure to detect MAP in every patient indicates that there must be alternative explanations in these individuals.

The measles hypothesis of Crohn's disease is now discredited [48].

2.2
Defective Neutrophil Function Drives the Disease

Although Crohn's disease presents as a condition characterized by excessive inflammation, mounting evidence suggests that these patients in fact possess an impaired acute inflammatory response. In vivo, they exhibit markedly delayed recruitment of neutrophils to the sites of breaches in an epithelial layer, as demonstrated in the skin window model of acute inflammation [104]. This defect does not occur in inflammatory disease controls (such as patients with ulcerative colitis or RA), nor does it relate to Crohn's disease activity or use of medication. In assays of chemotaxis in vitro [85], Crohn's neutrophils migrate normally. This suggests an alteration in the inflammatory milieu rather than an intrinsic failure of leukocyte motility; the causative agents remain unidentified. Defects have also been reported in other areas of neutrophil biology, including reduced ability to generate superoxide through their respiratory burst in both active and quiescent disease [25] and attenuated bactericidal capacity [118]. Recently, a preliminary clinical trial hinted at efficacy of GM-CSF (granulocyte/macrophage colony stimulating factor) in the treatment of Crohn's disease [31].

Our hypothesis (DJBM and AWS) then is that impaired neutrophil migration or possibly function leads to persistence of antigenic or other organic material within the bowel wall (Fig. 1). The importance of gut luminal contents in the generation of Crohn's lesions has been unequivocally demonstrated by experiments examining the effects of diversion and reintroduction of the faecal stream to distal bowel [99]. In healthy individuals, bacteria and other intestinal contents that breach the mucosal barrier induce rapid neutrophil migration to the site of insult, leading to phagocytosis, digestion and eradication of the extraneous material. This may tie in with the recent discoveries of susceptibility polymorphisms in Crohn's patients in the genes for CARD15 [60, 88] and the endotoxin-sensing proteins CD14 [64] and TLR4 [44], as these provide some of the earliest recognition determinants for bacteria both in leukocytes and within the bowel. Failure of clearance could lead to accumulation of debris, which could then be surrounded and engulfed predominantly by macrophages, provoking the chronic inflammatory, granulomatous pic-

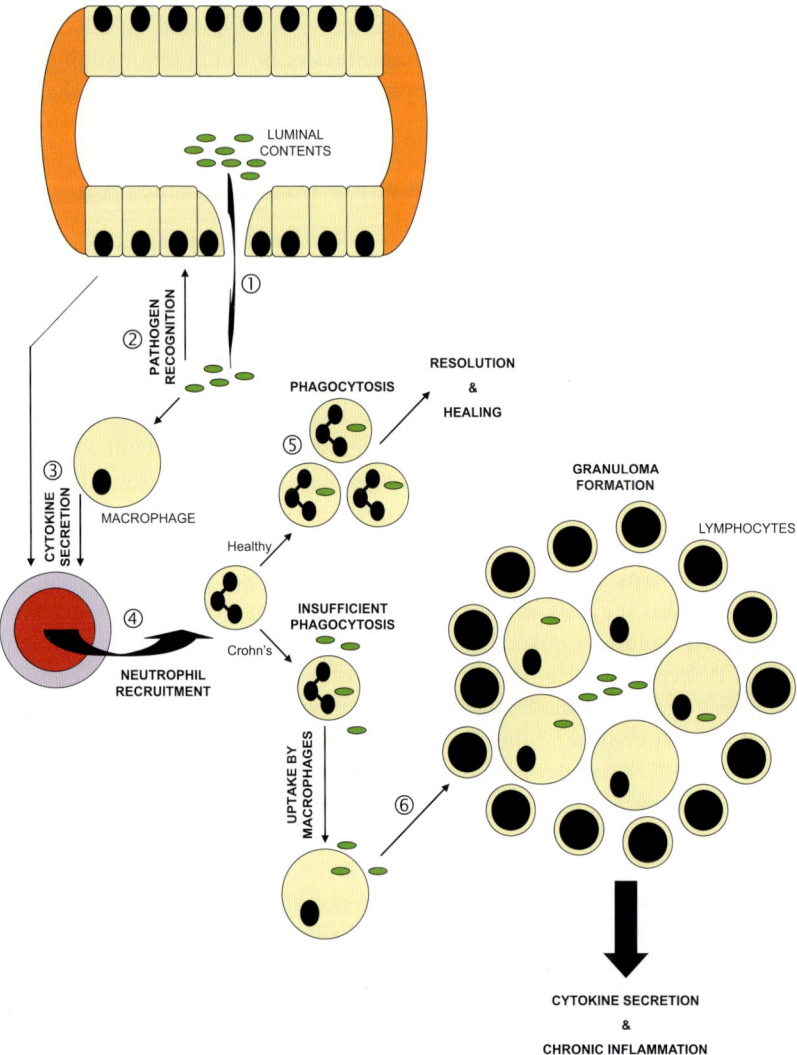

ture so characteristic of this disease. Indeed, bacterial DNA can be detected within the macrophages of Crohn's granulomata [100]. Parallels may be drawn with tuberculosis, in which failure to destroy the microbe leads to its persistence within macrophages. This persistence is followed by the formation of granulomata and a lymphocyte-driven chronic inflammation similar to that observed in Crohn's disease.

Fig. 1 Hypothesis: failure of neutrophil accumulation leads to persistence of debris and granuloma formation within the bowel wall. Bowel luminal contents ingress into the bowel wall through defects in the epithelial barrier (*1*). Detection of this extraneous material by receptors (including CARD15 and toll-like receptors) on macrophages and enterocytes (*2*) leads to cytokine secretion (*3*) and subsequent extravasation of neutrophils (*4*). In healthy individuals, sufficient numbers of neutrophils are recruited to phagocytose and degrade the debris (*5*). The acute inflammatory response resolves and healing follows. In Crohn's patients, impaired neutrophil migration leads to persistence of the offending stimulus. This becomes surrounded and engulfed by macrophages with resultant granuloma formation (*6*). The activated leukocytes within this structure, however, secrete pro-inflammatory cytokines driving a secondary chronic inflammation in active disease

The bowel disease observed in congenital disorders of neutrophil biology provides a compelling precedent for suspecting such a mechanism. Patients with chronic granulomatous disease, a primary immunodeficiency characterized by defective killing and digestion of microbes by neutrophils [95], can often develop a colitis macroscopically and microscopically indistinguishable from that seen in Crohn's disease [111]. Similar pathology also occurs in other neutrophil disorders, including glycogen storage disease-Ib [32], leukocyte adhesion deficiency [26], Chediak-Higashi syndrome [61], and various neutropaenias [40, 67, 108, 113]. A defective inflammatory response also appears consistent with epidemiological observations. The rapidly rising incidence of Crohn's disease in the Western world parallels an increase in the standards of food hygiene [35]. Endemic intestinal infestation and infection, as seen in the tropics where the disease remains exceedingly rare, might prime the bowel for an effective response to subsequent insult; this could also explain the benefits observed in patients treated with helminths [109]. We can also consider smoking, which is associated with a fourfold increase in the risk of developing Crohn's disease [16], and which dramatically reduces mucosal blood flow and consequent delivery of inflammatory cells [38].

A partial failure of acute inflammation could also account for much of the data cited in support of microbiological causes of Crohn's disease. The immune response could be of sufficient magnitude to prevent overwhelming infection but not total eradication of bacteria from the bowel wall. Indeed, the evidence for MAP can be interpreted to imply abnormal persistence rather than increased rates of acquisition. An important control experiment frequently omitted in such studies would be to determine the pathogen specificity of the findings. In fact, the failure to clear bacteria appears nonspecific, in that *Bacteroides vulgatus*, *Escherichia coli* [100], *Listeria monocytogenes* [73], and various *Yersinia* [68] and *Chlamydia* species have all been reported at increased frequencies in Crohn's patients. Whether or not any of these subsequently contribute to the pathogenesis remains unresolved, but their presence may merely represent a marker of the underlying immunodeficiency disease process that we hypothesize.

In our opinion, therefore, the evidence argues against a pathogenic role for any specific microbial species, but instead for an insufficiency in innate immunity that impairs clearance of foreign material in the bowel. Consequent accumulation of these bacteria and their products may then drive the chronic inflammation associated with active disease.

3
Ankylosing Spondylitis and the Other Spondyloarthritides

AS is of particular interest here because, on one side, a chronic immune response against self-antigens is assumed to be crucial for the immunopathology and, on the other, bacteria seem necessary to trigger the disease [107]. The chronic inflammation of AS primarily affects the spine and the sacroiliac joints, but extraspinal structures such as peripheral joints, the enthesis (insertion of tendons/ligaments at bone), the eye (uveitis) and the aorta can also be involved. Histology [9, 12] and magnetic resonance imaging [11] suggest that the primary site of inflammation is the cartilage/bone interphase. Mononuclear cell infiltrates occur mainly in cartilage and the subchondral bone. In early and active sacroiliitis, T cells and macrophages dominate these infiltrates, implicating a specific cellular immune response [9].

AS is strongly associated with the MHC class I antigen HLA-B27, found in 90%–95% of patients [15], and the prevalence of HLA-B27 in populations correlates with the prevalence of AS. Approximately 5% of HLA-B27-positve individuals develop ankylosing spondylitis during their lifetime [13], the majority before the age of 45 years. Animal models together with epidemiological and genetic studies in humans clearly indicate a direct role of HLA-B27 rather than an alternative linked gene. Among other possibilities, presentation of still unknown pathogenic peptides to $CD8^+$ T cells has been suggested to explain this association [66].

3.1
Absence of Persistent Microbial Antigen

As frequently occurs in suspected autoimmune diseases, there is no direct evidence of an autoimmune process. Cartilage has been proposed as the most likely target of any such response [76, 81]. It cannot be excluded that microbial antigens persist in the diverse structures involved, but this does not seem likely. Furthermore, biopsies from the sacroiliac joints have proved negative for candidate bacteria by PCR [14].

The cartilage-derived candidate autoantigens most investigated in animal models are collagen type II and proteoglycan, the major components of cartilage and other periarticular structures. While the collagen II-induced arthritis model resembles RA, animals immunized with proteoglycan show features typical of AS [5, 121]. The G1 globular domain of aggrecan, the major proteoglycan protein, has been identified as immunodominant in this model. The proteoglycan link protein has been suggested as another candidate. These proteins also occur in the eye and the aorta, and a T cell response against both has also been demonstrated in human arthritides, including AS, RA and juvenile chronic arthritis. We could also recently demonstrate a $CD4^+$ [122] and a $CD8^+$ [123] T cell response to aggrecan-derived peptides in the peripheral blood from AS patients, although this was not HLA-B27 restricted. We subsequently used computer prediction to screen all cartilage proteins for candidate peptides likely to stimulate HLA-B27-restricted $CD8^+$ T cells [3]. From this we isolated approximately 120 nonameric peptides, which were then tested for in vitro stimulation of $CD8^+$ T cells from patient synovial fluid. We identified one peptide from collagen type VI that was stimulatory in five out of seven patients. All these data are compatible with a cartilage-directed autoimmune response in the disease pathogenesis, but proof for this is still lacking and we shall investigate this question further.

3.2
The Triggering Infection

Among all the candidate autoimmune diseases, AS possesses the best evidence of bacterial infection as a crucial trigger. In 1%–4% of individuals with infection of the gastrointestinal tract with *Enterobacteriae* or the urogenital tract with *Chlamydia trachomatis*, a so-called reactive arthritis develops in the following 6 weeks. Between 30%–70% of these patients are positive for HLA-B27, and among these patients 20%–40% develop the full clinical picture of AS 10–20 years after the initial infection [70].

Similarly, 10%–20% of patients with inflammatory bowel disease (IBD) develop peripheral arthritis at some time during the course of their disease. AS has been reported in between 5%–10% of patients with IBD with those positive for HLA-B27 at especially high risk: in one study of 231 Crohn's patients, 54% of HLA-B27-positive patients developed AS compared to 2.6% of those who were negative [93]. Thus, at least half of the HLA-B27-positive IBD patients will develop ankylosing spondylitis that cannot be differentiated from the primary form of the disease. Stimulation of the immune system in IBD by translocated gut bacteria therefore might well trigger AS, and T cells primed in the gut could recognize related bacteria or cross-reacting self-antigens in the joints [79]. When the T cell repertoire from an inflamed joint was compared with gut biopsies from a patient who had both IBD and arthritis, the same antigen specificities were found in both compartments. Furthermore, the $CD8^+$ T cell receptor repertoire matched that of lymphocytes from patients with ReA [78], supporting the concept that there may be common dominant bacterial antigens in AS and related diseases. Finally, although fewer than 10% of AS patients complain of preceding infections or IBD, infections with ReA-associated bacteria and gut lesions in IBD patients are often subclinical [107].

3.3
Antibiotics Inhibit Triggering

The crucial question is whether an autoimmune disease runs an independent course after the initial bacterial trigger or whether it requires chronic interaction. Unfortunately, good studies have not been conducted on the effect of healing of gut lesions in Crohn's disease or in AS. One interesting study suggests that treatment with antibiotics can prevent development of AS or related conditions. Patients with an acute enteral ReA treated for 3 months with ciprofloxacin did not benefit during the first 12 months of follow-up [119]. However, 11 out of 27 (45%) patients from the placebo group had developed chronic rheumatic diseases when re-evaluated after 4–7 years, compared to only 2 out of 26 (7.7%) of the patients who originally received antibiotic treatment [120]. Furthermore, all rheumatic manifestations in the former but not the latter group manifested AS-type features and occurred in HLA-B27-positive individuals. At last we have data indicating that uncontrolled bacterial infection can cause AS manifestations and that an initial infection controlled by antibiotics cannot do so; nevertheless, this must occur in the context of HLA-B27.

This interpretation is supported by additional indirect evidence. In the 1940s and 1950s, arthritis associated with urogenital infections was associated with development of ankylosing spondylitis in Sweden in a higher percentage than 20–30 years later [89]. Long-term antibiotic treatment was the main difference between the management of these groups. Similarly, AS and related diseases were more severe in lower social classes with poorer hygiene (without a refrigerator) in North Africa [22]. AS starts at an earlier age and runs a more severe course in countries such as Mexico [69], China [58], and North Africa [54] as compared with Western Europe. Furthermore, the first generation of immigrants from North Africa to France suffered more severe

AS than does the second (B. Amor, unpublished observations). All these data indicate that persistent or repeated infection, mostly probably gut-derived, makes an important contribution to the pathogenesis and severity of AS. The mechanisms that lead from infection to autoimmunity in AS have not yet been defined.

4
Regulatory Mechanisms in Autoimmunity

Supposing that autoimmunity is not the root cause of a disease, does that end the matter? Even when the production of autoantibodies or autoreactive T cells clearly depends on the continued presence of the infecting organism or its residual antigen, it would be rash to conclude that self-antigens play no part. Their involvement might be secondary resulting from any of several known mechanisms, including epitope spreading [37, 91], polyclonal activation of T or B cells by parasite mitogen [23], and loss of downregulation [84]. Earlier discussions of downregulation have been superseded by the discovery of the new mechanisms listed in Table 2, all of which play a role in TCR-transgenic models of autoimmunity as shown. In humans, inactivation of the Treg marker FoxP3 gene causes the IPEX (immune dysregulation, polyendocrinopathy, enteropathy, X-linked syndrome) syndrome [6]. The role of the adaptor molecule Cbl-1 in modulating autoimmunity is particularly well mapped out. Additional but less well-documented molecules that could be added to this list include SOCS-1/2, GRAIL, Delta/Serrate/Notch, Neuropilin-1 and SATB1. Taken together, these mechanisms make it unlikely that the border in the immune system between self and non-self is as sharp as had once been supposed. True, deletion of self-reactive T cells (negative selection) in the thymus and in the periphery still carries the main responsibility for tolerance-of-self, but it no longer stands alone. Clearly disruption of any of these suppressive mechanisms might cause autoimmunity, and any of them might be disrupted by infection.

Table 2 Downregulatory mechanisms revealed in TCR-transgenic models of autoimmunity

Tregs (CD25 CD4 T cells) [18, 34]
CTLA4 ligation [34]
T cells secreting: TGF-beta [39]; IL-4, IL10 [10]; IL12 [83]
Cbl-1 activity [4, 20, 51]

4.1
Downregulation Occurs Within Dendritic Cell Clusters

Regulatory clusters of cells within the immune system probably play an important part in regulating autoimmunity, as is argued from the studies listed in Table 3. Each dendritic cell (DC) located within lymph node or spleen, together with the cluster of T cells that forms around it, comprises an autonomous regulatory unit. Within the cluster, signals pass between the DC and its surrounding T cells via the immunological synapse. Cytokines signal between all cell types in the cluster (paracrine activity), but at normal levels of activity each cluster forms an autonomous unit with little endocrine transmission of signals between clusters. T cells within a cluster signal to one another not only via cytokines but also via the DC itself (Tada's term "epicrine" activity applies). As shown in Fig. 2, each cluster operates as a democracy in which the outcome is determined by voting among its constituent cells according

Table 3 Regulatory mechanisms within dendritic cell clusters

DC, Th(autoimmune), Th(bystander)	Cell frequency effect in vivo [17, 102]
DC, Th(naïve), Th(anergic bystanders)	Human cells in vitro [74]
DC, Th(naïve), Th1, Th2	Gene gun immunization in vivo [24]
DC, Th(naïve), Th2	Chimera in vivo [2]
DC, Th, Treg	Mathematical model [72]
DC, Th, Treg	IL-2R blockade, mathematical model [101]

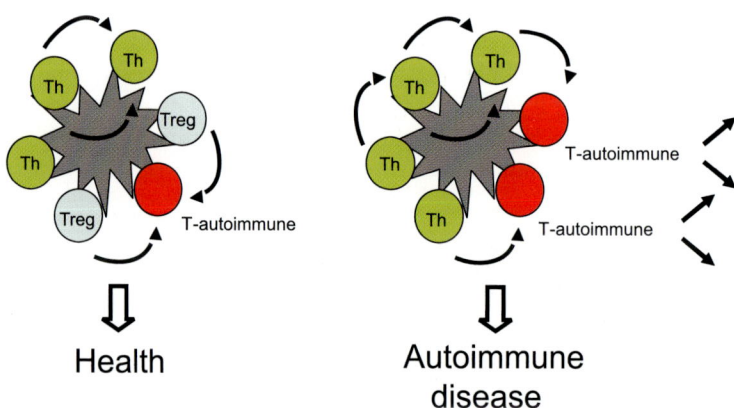

Fig. 2 Majority rule in the autonomous T cell cluster. The quantitative effect of excess activated T cells or lack of downregulatory T cells could cause autoimmunity

to their number and level of activation. In health, potentially autoreactive T cells are too minor a population to generate a response, and in addition may be outvoted by suppressive T cells in accordance with the models referred to in Table 3. Infection might increase the proportion of activated cells, thus allowing potentially autoreactive T cells to join in the response. When the infection dies down, autoimmune disease will ensue if activated autoreactive T cells remain in sufficient numbers. In addition, infection might reduce the proportion of functional suppressive T cells. We would be the first to admit that evidence for this hypothesis is sketchy (although growing). Mathematical modelling as an approach to systems biology is beginning to provide critical insight, and surely has much more to contribute. The key question is whether the democratic model provides sufficient stability to maintain autoimmunity within what are after all stringent limits.

4.2
Arenas Where Downregulation May Operate

Where can we hope to learn more about secondary mechanisms that might provide a window for infection-dependent autoimmunity? Table 4 lists conditions where these might be expected to operate, and indeed in several cases have been found to do so.

Finally, it is well established that one way or another infection influences susceptibility to autoimmune disease. Two comprehensive reviews discuss

Table 4 Systems known or likely to involve downregulation

Autoimmunity driven by monoclonal T or B cells	Collagen induced arthritis [65]
	Experimental allergic encephalomyelitis [39, 83]
	Optic neuritis [8]
	Neuritis [90, 116]
	Diabetes [33, 43]
	Gastritis [1, 18]
	Lupus [59]
	Epithelial [80]
Long-term transplant survival, particularly when incompatible only at minor antigens	Cardiac, mouse [106] human [77]
	Renal, human [56, 96]
Models of fluctuating autoimmunity	EAE in SJL mice [45]
	Arthritis post-cell transfer [57]
	Arthritis induced by type IX cartilage [75]
Immunological genes associated with autoimmune disease	T1D [29]

the range of mechanisms that may underlie this association [7, 97]. To this discussion, we would add only that attractive as the hygiene hypothesis is to explain the association, it should not be accepted uncritically [117].

4.3
Fear of Autoimmunity Can Hold Up Vaccine Development

On a more negative note, a mistaken belief in autoimmunity can hold up vaccine development, as Kierszenbaum cogently argues for Chagas' disease [63]. This is a disease where a vaccine is much needed: high disease prevalence in particular areas, lack of effective symptomatic treatment and lack of effective anti-parasite measures. Meningococcus B is another instance. Conjugate vaccine against Meningococcus C composed of capsular polysaccharide conjugated to a protein carrier is effective and now widely used. A similar vaccine against Men B has not been developed because of the danger presented by expression of a cross-reactive polysaccharide in neural tissue (Table 5). Instead, several serogroup B vaccines based on outer membrane vesicles have been shown to be immunogenic and reasonably effective in adults and older children, but the protection offered by them is chiefly strain-specific.

Table 5 Where threat of autoimmunity impedes vaccine development

Pathogen	Cross-reactivity ("mimicry")
Trypanosoma cruzii	Heart [63]
Meningococcus B	Neural [42]
Borrelia burgdorferi	Joints and elsewhere (Lyme disease) [41]

In summary, direct evidence for a primary role for infection in many of the suspected autoimmune disease remains lacking. Whilst microbial species and their antigens appear to influence the development of inflammation, these must occur within the context of a susceptible immune system. Although secondary self-reactive immunopathology may occur during an acute insult, no proof has been presented that infection can establish a long-lasting autonomous immune response in these conditions.

References

1. Alderuccio F, Cataldo V, van Driel IR et al. (2000) Tolerance and autoimmunity to a gastritogenic peptide in TCR transgenic mice. Int Immunol 12:343–352
2. Alpan O, Bachelder E, Isil E et al. (2004) 'Educated' dendritic cells act as messengers from memory to naive T helper cells. Nat Immunol 5:615–622

3. Atagunduz P, Appel H, Kuon W et al. (2005) HLA-B27 restricted CD8+ T cell response to cartilage-derived self peptides in ankylosing spondylitis. J Arthritis Rheum 52:892–901
4. Bachmaier K, Krawczyk C, Sasaki T et al. (2000) Negative regulation of lymphocyte activation and autoimmunity by the molecular adaptor Cbl-b. Nature 403:211–216
5. Bardos T, Szabo Z, Czipri M et al. (2005) A longitudinal study on an autoimmune murine model of ankylosing spondylitis. Ann Rheum Dis 64:981–987
6. Bennett CL, Christie J, Ramsdell F et al. (2001) The immune dysregulation, polyendocrinopathy, enteropathy, X-linked syndrome (IPEX) is caused by mutations of FOXP3. Nat Genet 27:20–21
7. Benoist C, Mathis D (2001) Autoimmunity provoked by infection: how good is the case for T cell epitope mimicry? Nat Immunol 2:797–801
8. Bettelli E, Pagany M, Weiner HL et al. (2003) Myelin oligodendrocyte glycoprotein-specific T cell receptor transgenic mice develop spontaneous autoimmune optic neuritis. J Exp Med 197:1073–1081
9. Bollow MFT, Fischer T, Reisshauer H et al. (2000) Quantitative analyses of sacroiliac biopsies in spondyloarthropathies: T cells and macrophages predominate in early and active sacroiliitis: cellularity correlates with the degree of enhancement detected by magnetic resonance imaging. Ann Rheum Dis 59:135–140
10. Brand DD, Myers LK, Whittington KB et al. (2002) Detection of early changes in autoimmune T cell phenotype and function following intravenous administration of type II collagen in a TCR-transgenic model. J Immunol 168:490–498
11. Braun J, Bollow M, Eggens U et al. (1994) Use of dynamic magnetic resonance imaging with fast imaging in the detection of early and advanced sacroiliitis in spondylarthropathy patients. Arthritis Rheum 37:1039–1045
12. Braun J, Bollow M, Neure L et al. (1995) Use of immunohistologic and in situ hybridization techniques in the examination of sacroiliac joint biopsy specimens from patients with ankylosing spondylitis. Arthritis Rheum 38:499–505
13. Braun J, Bollow M, Remlinger G et al. (1998) Prevalence of spondylarthropathies in HLA-B27 positive and negative blood donors. Arthritis Rheum 41:58–67
14. Braun J, Tuszewski M, Ehlers S et al. (1997) Nested polymerase chain reaction strategy simultaneously targeting DNA sequences of multiple bacterial species in inflammatory joint diseases. II. Examination of sacroiliac and knee joint biopsies of patients with spondyloarthropathies and other arthritides. J Rheumatol 24:1101–1105
15. Brewerton DA, Hart FD, Nichols A et al (1973) Ankylosing spondylitis and HL-A 27. Lancet 28:904–907
16. Bridger S, Lee JC, Bjarnasson I et al. (2002) In siblings with similar genetic susceptibility for inflammatory bowel disease, smokers tend to develop Crohn's disease and non-smokers develop ulcerative colitis. Gut 51:21–25
17. Brunner MC, Mitchison NA, Schneider SC et al. (1994) Immunoregulation mediated by T-cell clusters. Folia Biol (Praha) 40:359–369
18. Candon S, McHugh RS, Foucras G et al. (2004) Spontaneous organ-specific Th2-mediated autoimmunity in TCR transgenic mice. J Immunol 172:2917–2924
19. Chacon O, Bermudez LE, Barletta RG (2004) Johne's disease, inflammatory bowel disease, and Mycobacterium paratuberculosis. Annu Rev Microbiol 58:329–363

20. Chiang YJ, Kole HK, Brown K et al. (2000) Cbl-b regulates the CD28 dependence of T-cell activation. Nature 403:216–220
21. Chiodini RJ, Van Kruiningen HJ, Thayer WR et al. (1988) Spheroplastic phase of mycobacteria isolated from patients with Crohn's disease. J Clin Microbiol. 24:357–363
22. Claudepierre P, Gueguen A, Ladjouze A et al (1995) Predictive factors of severity of spondyloarthropathy in North Africa. Br J Rheumatol 34:1139–1145
23. Cooper PJ (1996) Autoimmunity and onchocerciasis. Lancet 347:404
24. Creusot RJ, Mitchison NA (2004) How DCs control cross-regulation between lymphocytes. Trends Immunol 25:126–131
25. Curran FT, Allan RN (1991) Superoxide production by Crohn's disease neutrophils. Gut 32:399–402
26. D'Agata ID, Paradis K, Chad Z et al. (1996) Leucocyte adhesion deficiency presenting as a chronic ileocolitis. Gut 39:605–608
27. Dalziel TK (1913) Chronic intestinal enteritis. BMJ ii:1068–1070
28. Daniel-Ribeiro CT, Zanini G (2000) Autoimmunity and malaria: what are they doing together? Acta Trop 76:205–221
29. Dean L, McEntyre JR (2004). The genetic landscape of diabetes [Internet]. National Library of Medicine (US), NCBI, Bethesda, MD
30. Deshpande SP, Lee S, Zheng M et al. (2001) Herpes simplex virus-induced keratitis: evaluation of the role of molecular mimicry in lesion pathogenesis. J Virol 75:3077–3088
31. Dieckgraefe BK, Korzenik J (2002) Treatment of active Crohn's disease with recombinant human granulocyte-macrophage colony-stimulating factor. Lancet 360:1478–1480
32. Dieckgraefe BK, Korzenik JR, Husain A et al (2002) Association of glycogen storage disease 1b and Crohn disease: results of a North American survey. Eur J Pediatr 161: S88–S92
33. DiPaolo RJ, Unanue ER (2001) The level of peptide-MHC complex determines the susceptibility to autoimmune diabetes: studies in HEL transgenic mice. Eur J Immunol 31:3453–3459
34. Eggena MP, Walker LS, Nagabhusanam V et al. (2004) Cooperative roles of CTLA-4 and regulatory T cells in tolerance to an islet cell antigen. J Exp Med 199:1725–1730
35. Ekbom A, Montgomery SM (2004) Environmental risk factors (excluding tobacco and microorganisms): critical analysis of old and new hypotheses. Best Pract Res Clin Gastroenterol. 18:497–508
36. El Zaatari, FA, Osato MS (2001) Etiology of Crohn's disease: the role of Mycobacterium avium paratuberculosis. Trends Mol Med 7:247–252
37. Ellmerich S, Takacs K, Mysko M et al. (2004) Disease-related epitope spread in a humanized T cell receptor transgenic model of multiple sclerosis. Eur J Immunol 34:1839–1848
38. Emmanuel AV, Kamm MA (1999) Laser Doppler measurement of rectal mucosal blood flow. Gut 45:64–69
39. Faria AM, Maron R, Ficker SM et al. (2003) Oral tolerance induced by continuous feeding: enhanced up-regulation of transforming growth factor-beta/interleukin-10 and suppression of experimental autoimmune encephalomyelitis. J Autoimmun 20:135–145

40. Fata F, Myers P AJ, Grinberg M et al. (1997) Cyclic neutropenia in Crohn's ileocolitis: efficacy of granulocyte colony-stimulating factor. J Clin Gastroenterol 24:253–256
41. Fikrig E, Barthold SW, Kantor FS et al. (1992) Long-term protection of mice from Lyme disease by vaccination with OspA. Infect Immun 60:773–777
42. Finne J, Bitter-Suermann D, Goridis C et al. (1987) An IgG monoclonal antibody to group B meningococci cross-reacts with developmentally regulated polysialic acid units of glycoproteins in neural and extraneural tissues. J Immunol 138:4402–4407
43. Forster I, Hirose R, Arbeit JM et al. (1995) Limited capacity for tolerization of $CD4^+$ T cells specific for a pancreatic beta cell neo-antigen. Immunity 2:573–285
44. Franchimont D, Vermeire S (2004) Deficient host-bacteria interactions in inflammatory bowel disease? The toll-like receptor (TLR)-4. Asp299gly polymorphism is associated with Crohn's disease and ulcerative colitis. Gut 53:987–992
45. Fritz RB, Chou CH, McFralin DE (1983) Relapsing murine experimental allergic encephalomyelitis induced by myelin basic protein. J Immunol 130:1024–1026
46. Gale EA, Atkinson M (2004) A piece of nucleic acid surrounded by controversy: coxsackievirus and the causes of Type 1 diabetes. Diabet Med 21:503–506
47. Gallin MY, Jacobi AB, Buttner DW et al. (1995) Human autoantibody to defensin: disease association with hyperreactive onchocerciasis (sowda). J Exp Med. 182:41–47
48. Ghosh S, Armitage E, Wilson D et al. (2001) Detection of persistent measles virus infection in Crohn's disease: current status of experimental work. Gut 48:748–752
49. Good MF (1995) What can a worm teach us about autoimmunity? Lancet 346:1311–1312
50. Green J, Casabonne D, Newton R (2004) Coxsackie B virus serology and Type 1 diabetes mellitus: a systematic review of published case-control studies. Diabet Med. 21:507–514
51. Gronski MA, Boulter JM, Moskophidis D et al. (2004) TCR affinity and negative regulation limit autoimmunity. Nat Med 10:1234–1239
52. Gui GP, Thomas PR, Tizard ML et al. (1997) Two-year-outcomes analysis of Crohn's disease treated with rifabutin and macrolide antibiotics. J Antimicrob Chemother 39:393–400
53. Guilherme L, Kalil J (2004) Rheumatic fever: from sore throat to autoimmune heart lesions. Int Arch Allergy Immunol 134:56–64
54. Hajjaj-Hassouni N, Maetzel A, Dougados M (1993) Comparison of patients evaluated for spondyloarthropathy in France and Morocco. Rev Rhum Ed Fr 60:420–425
55. Hermon-Taylor J, Barnes N, Clarke C et al. (1998) Mycobacterium paratuberculosis cervical lymphadenitis, followed five years later by terminal ileitis similar to Crohn's disease. BMJ 316:449–453
56. Hernandez-Fuentes MP, Lechler RI (2005) Chronic graft loss. Contrib Nephrol 146:54–64
57. Hesse M, Mitchison NA (2000) Relapsing arthritis induced by cell transfer from collagen-immunised mice. Autoimmunity 32:27–32
58. Huang F, Zhang J, Zju J et al. (2003) Juvenile spondyloarthropathies: the Chinese experience. Rheum Dis Clin North Am 29:531–547
59. Hueber W, Zeng D, Strober S et al. (2004) Interferon-alpha-inducible proteins are novel autoantigens in murine lupus. Arthritis Rheum 50:3239–3249

60. Hugot JP, Chamaillard M, Zouali H et al. (2001) Association of NOD2 leucine-rich repeat variants with susceptibility to Crohn's disease. Nature 411:599–603
61. Ishii E, Matui T, Iida M et al. (1987) Chediak-Higashi syndrome with intestinal complication. Report of a case. J Clin Gastroenterol 9:556–558
62. Kalil J, Cunha-Neto E (1996) Autoimmunity in Chagas disease cardiomyopathy: fulfilling the criteria at last? Parasitol Today 12:396–399
63. Kierszenbaum F (2003) Views on the autoimmunity hypothesis for Chagas disease pathogenesis. FEMS Immunol Med Microbiol 37:1–11
64. Klein W, Tromm A, Griga T et al. (2002) A polymorphism in the CD14 gene is associated with Crohn disease. Scand J Gastroenterol 37:189–191
65. Kouskoff V, Korganow AS, Duchatelle V et al. (1996) Organ-specific disease provoked by systemic autoimmunity. Cell 87:811–822
66. Kuon W, Sieper J (2003) Identification of HLA-B27-restricted peptides in reactive arthritis and other spondyloarthropathies: computer algorithms and fluorescent activated cell sorting analysis as tools for hunting of HLA-B27-restricted chlamydial and autologous crossreactive peptides involved in reactive arthritis and ankylosing spondylitis. Rheum Dis Clin North Am 29:595–611
67. Lamport RD, Katz S, Eskreis D (1992) Crohn's disease associated with cyclic neutropenia. Am J Gastroenterol. 87:1638–1642
68. Lamps LW, Madhusudhan KT, Havens JM et al. (2003) Pathogenic Yersinia DNA is detected in bowel and mesenteric lymph nodes from patients with Crohn's disease. Am J Surg Pathol 27:220–227
69. Lau CS, Burgos-Vargas R, Louthrenoo W et al. (1998) Features of spondyloarthritis around the world. Rheum Dis Clin North Am 24:753–770
70. Leirisalo-Repo M (1998) Prognosis, course of disease, and treatment of the spondyloarthropathies. Rheum Dis Clin North Am 24:737–751
71. Leon JS, Daniels MD, Toriello KM et al. (2004) A cardiac myosin-specific autoimmune response is induced by immunization with Trypanosoma cruzi proteins. Infect Immun 72:3410–3417
72. Leon K, Faro J, Lage A et al (2004) Inverse correlation between the incidences of autoimmune disease and infection predicted by a model of T cell mediated tolerance. J Autoimmun 22:31–42
73. Liu Y, Van Kruiningen HJ, West AB et al. (1995) Immunocytochemical evidence of Listeria, Escherichia coli, and Streptococcus antigens in Crohn's disease. Gastroenterology 108:1396–1404
74. Lombardi G, Sidhu S, Batchelor RJ et al. (1994) Anergic T cells as suppressor cells in vitro. Science 264:1587–1589
75. Lu S, Carlsen S, Hansson AS et al. (2002) Immunization of rats with homologous type XI collagen leads to chronic and relapsing arthritis with different genetics and joint pathology than arthritis induced with homologous type II collagen. J Autoimmun 18:199–211
76. Maksymowych WP (2000) Ankylosing spondylitis—at the interface of bone and cartilage. J Rheumatol 27:2295–2301
77. Manavalan JS, Kim-Schulze S, Scotto L et al. (2004) Alloantigen specific CD8+CD28– FOXP3+ T suppressor cells induce ILT3+ ILT4+ tolerogenic endothelial cells, inhibiting alloreactivity. Int Immunol 16:1055–1068

78. May E, Dulphy N, Fauendorf E et al. (2002) Conserved TCR beta chain usage in reactive arthritis: evidence for selection by a putative HLA-B27-associated autoantigen. Tissue Antigens 60:299–308
79. May E, Marker-Hermann E, Wittig BM et al. (2000) Identical T-cell expansions in the colon mucosa and the synovium of a patient with enterogenic spondyloarthropathy. Gastroenterology 119:1745–1755
80. McGargill MA, Mayerova D, Stefanski HE et al. (2002) A spontaneous CD8. T cell-dependent autoimmune disease to an antigen expressed under the human keratin 14 promoter. J Immunol 169:2141–7
81. McGonagle D, Emery P (1999) Classification of inflammatory arthritis. Lancet 353:671
82. Meilof JF, Van der Lelij A, Rokeach LA et al. (1993) Autoimmunity and filariasis. Autoantibodies against cytoplasmic cellular proteins in sera of patients with onchocerciasis. J Immunol 151:5800–9
83. Mendel I, Natarajan K, Ben-Nun A et al (2004) A novel protective model against experimental allergic encephalomyelitis in mice expressing a transgenic TCR-specific for myelin oligodendrocyte glycoprotein. J Neuroimmunol 10–21
84. Mitchison NA (1993) A walk round the edges of self tolerance. Ann Rheum Dis 52: S3–5
85. Morain CO, Segal AA, Walker D et al. (1981) Abnormalities of neutrophil function do not cause the migration defect in Crohn's disease. Gut 22:817–822
86. Nahar IK, Shojania K (2003) Infliximab treatment of rheumatoid arthritis and Crohn's disease. Ann Pharmacother 37:1256–1265
87. Naser SA, Ghobrial G, Romero C et al. (2004) Culture of Mycobacterium avium subspecies paratuberculosis from the blood of patients with Crohn's disease. Lancet 364:1039–1044
88. Ogura Y, Bonen DK, Inohara N et al. (2001) A frameshift mutation in NOD2 associated with susceptibility to Crohn's disease. Nature 411:603–606
89. Olhagen B (1983) Urogenital syndromes and spondarthritis. Br J Rheumatol 22:33–40
90. Oono T, Fukui Y, Masuko S et al. (2001) Organ-specific autoimmunity in mice whose T cell repertoire is shaped by a single antigenic peptide. J Clin Invest 108:1589–1596
91. Pette M, Fujita K, Wilkinson D et al. (1990) Myelin autoreactivity in multiple sclerosis: recognition of myelin basic protein in the context of HLA-DR2 products by T lymphocytes of multiple-sclerosis patients and healthy donors. Proc Natl Acad Sci U S A 87:7968–7972
92. Pontes-de-Carvalho L, Santana CC, Soares MB et al. (2002) Experimental chronic Chagas' disease myocarditis is an autoimmune disease preventable by induction of immunological tolerance to myocardial antigens. J Autoimmun 18:131–138
93. Purrmann J, Zeidler H, Bertrams J et al. (1988) HLA antigens in ankylosing spondylitis associated with Crohn's disease. Increased frequency of the HLA phenotype B27,B44. J Rheumatol 15:1658–1661
94. Quirke P (2001) Mycobacterium avium subspecies paratuberculosis is a cause of Crohn's disease. Gut 49:757–760
95. Reeves EP, Lu H, Jacobs HL et al. (2002) Killing activity of neutrophils is mediated through activation of proteases by K+ flux. Nature 416:291–297

96. Rodriguez DS, Jankowska-Gan E, Haynes LD et al. (2004) Immune regulation and graft survival in kidney transplant recipients are both enhanced by human leukocyte antigen matching. Am J Transplant 4:537–543
97. Rose NR (1998) The role of infection in the pathogenesis of autoimmune disease. Semin Immunol 10:5–13
98. Rose NR, Hill SL (1996) The pathogenesis of postinfectious myocarditis. Clin Immunol Immunopathol. 80: S92–S99
99. Rutgeerts P, Goboes K, Peeters M et al. (1991) Effect of faecal stream diversion on recurrence of Crohn's disease in the neoterminal ileum. Lancet 338:771–774
100. Ryan P, Kelly RG, Lee G et al. (2004) Bacterial DNA within granulomas of patients with Crohn's disease—detection by laser capture microdissection and PCR. Am J Gastroenterol 99:1539–1543
101. Scheffold A, Hühn J, Hoffer T (2005) Regulation of CD4+CD25+Treg activity: it takes (IL-) two to tango. Europ J Immunol 35:1336–1341
102. Schneider SC, Mitchison NA (1995) Self-reactive T cell hybridomas and tolerance. Same range of antigen dose dependence but higher numbers of self-reactive T cell hybridomas from mice in which self-tolerance has been broken by antiserum treatment. J Immunol 154:3796–3805
103. Schwimmbeck PL, Badorff C, Rohn G et al. (1996) The role of sensitized T-cells in myocarditis and dilated cardiomyopathy. Int J Cardiol 54:117–125
104. Segal AW, Loewi G (1976) Neutrophil dysfunction in Crohn's disease. Lancet 2:219–221
105. Shafran I, Kugler L, El-Zaateri LA et al. (2002) Open clinical trial of rifabutin and clarithromycin therapy in Crohn's disease. Dig Liver Dis 34:22–28
106. Sho M, Yamada A, Najafian M et al. (2002) Physiological mechanisms of regulating alloimmunity: cytokines, CTLA-4, CD25+ cells, and the alloreactive T cell clone size. J Immunol 169:3744–3751
107. Sieper J, Braun J (1995) Pathogenesis of spondylarthropathies. Persistent bacterial antigen, autoimmunity, or both? Arthritis Rheum 38:1547–1554
108. Stevens C, Peppercorn MA, Grand RJ (1991) Crohn's disease associated with autoimmune neutropenia. J Clin Gastroenterol 13:328–330
109. Summers RW, Elliott DE, Urban JF Jr et al (2005) Trichuris suis therapy in Crohn's disease. Gut 54:87–90
110. Tarleton RL, Zhang L, Downs MO (1997) "Autoimmune rejection" of neonatal heart transplants in experimental Chagas disease is a parasite-specific response to infected host tissue. Proc Natl Acad Sci U S A 94:3932–3937
111. Thrasher AJ, Keep NH, Wientjes F et al. (1994) Chronic granulomatous disease. Biochim Biophys Acta 1227:1–24
112. Van Kruiningen HJ (1999) Lack of support for a common etiology in Johne's disease of animals and Crohn's disease in humans. Inflamm Bowel Dis 5:183–191
113. Vannier JP, Arnaud-Battandier F, Ricour C et al. (1982) Chronic neutropenia and Crohn's disease in childhood. Report of 2 cases. Arch Fr Pediatr 39:367–370
114. Varela-Calvino R, Ellis R, Sgarbi G et al. (2002) Characterization of the T-cell response to coxsackievirus B4: evidence that effector memory cells predominate in patients with type 1 diabetes. Diabetes 51:1745–1753

115. Verjans GM, Remeijer L, Mooy CM et al. (2000) Herpes simplex virus-specific T cells infiltrate the cornea of patients with herpetic stromal keratitis: no evidence for autoreactive T cells. Invest Ophthalmol Vis Sci 41:2607–2612
116. Waldner H, Whitters MJ, Sobel RA et al. (2000) Fulminant spontaneous autoimmunity of the central nervous system in mice transgenic for the myelin proteolipid protein-specific T cell receptor. Proc Natl Acad Sci U S A 97:3412–3417
117. Wieringa MH, Vermeire PA, Brunekreef B et al. (2001) Increased occurrence of asthma and allergy: critical appraisal of studies using allergic sensitization, bronchial hyper-responsiveness and lung function measurements. Clin Exp Allergy 31:1553–1563
118. Worsaae N, Staehr JK (1982) Impaired in vitro function of neutrophils in Crohn's disease. Scand J Gastroenterol 17:91–96
119. Yli-Kerttula T, Luukkainen R, Yli-Kerttula U et al. (2000) Effect of a three-month course of ciprofloxacin on the outcome of reactive arthritis. Ann Rheum Dis 59:565–570
120. Yli-Kerttula T, Luukkainen R, Yli-Kerttula U et al. (2003) Effect of a three-month course of ciprofloxacin on the late prognosis of reactive arthritis. Ann Rheum 62:880–884
121. Zhang Y (2003) Animal models of inflammatory spinal and sacroiliac joint diseases. Rheum Dis Clin North Am 29:631–645
122. Zhao ZS, Granucci F, Yeh L (1998) Molecular mimicry by herpes simplex virus-type 1: autoimmune disease after viral infection. Science 279:1344–1347
123. Zou J, Appel H, Rudwaleit M et al. (2004) Analysis of the CD8+ T cell response to the G1 domain of aggrecan in ankylosing spondylitis. Ann Rheum Dis 64:722–729
124. Zou J, Zhang Y, Rudwaleit M et al. (2003) Predominant cellular immune response to the cartilage autoantigenic G1 aggrecan in ankylosing spondylitis and rheumatoid arthritis. Rheumatology (Oxford) 42:846–855

The Systemic Autoinflammatory Diseases: Inborn Errors of the Innate Immune System

S. Brydges (✉) · D. L. Kastner

Genetics and Genomics Branch, National Institute of Arthritis and Musculoskeletal and Skin Diseases, National Institutes of Health, Bethesda, MD 20892-1820, USA
brydgess@mail.nih.gov

1	Introduction	128
2	Familial Mediterranean Fever	130
3	Syndrome of Pyogenic Arthritis, Pyoderma Gangrenosum, and Acne	133
4	The Cryopyrinopathies: Familial Cold Autoinflammatory Syndrome, Muckle-Wells Syndrome, and Neonatal-Onset Multisystem Inflammatory Disease	135
5	Blau Syndrome	139
6	TNF Receptor-Associated Periodic Syndrome	141
7	Hyperimmunoglobulinemia D with Periodic Fever Syndrome	145
8	Concluding Remarks	148
References		149

Abstract The autoinflammatory syndromes are a newly recognized group of immune disorders that lack the high titers of self-reactive antibodies and T cells characteristic of classic autoimmune disease. Nevertheless, patients with these illnesses experience unprovoked inflammatory disease in the absence of underlying infection. Here we discuss recent advances in eight Mendelian autoinflammatory diseases. The causative genes and the proteins they encode play a critical role in the regulation of innate immunity. Both pyrin and cryopyrin, the proteins mutated in familial Mediterranean fever and the cryopyrinopathies, respectively, are involved in regulation of the pro-inflammatory cytokine, IL-1β, and may influence the activity of the transcription factor, NFκB. NOD2, the Blau syndrome protein, shares certain domains with cryopyrin and appears to be a sensor of intracellular bacteria. PSTPIP1, mutated in the syndrome of pyogenic arthritis with pyoderma gangrenosum and acne, interacts both with pyrin and a protein tyrosine phosphatase to regulate innate and adaptive immune responses. Somewhat unexpectedly, mutations in the p55 TNF receptor lead not to immunodeficiency but to dramatic inflammatory disease, the mechanisms of which are still under investigation. Finally, the discovery of the genetic basis of the hyperimmunoglobulinemia D with periodic fever syndrome has provided a fascinating but incompletely understood link between cholesterol biosynthesis and autoinflammation. In this manuscript, we summarize the current state of the art with regard to the diagnosis, pathogenesis, and treatment of these inborn errors of the innate immune system.

1
Introduction

Systemic autoinflammatory diseases are a relatively newly recognized category of illnesses, characterized by seemingly unprovoked inflammation in the absence of an infectious etiology. As these disorders lack the high titers of autoantibodies and self-reactive T lymphocytes characteristic of the more conventional autoimmune diseases, autoinflammation is considered a defect in the regulation of innate immunity (McDermott et al. 1999; Galon et al. 2000; Hull et al. 2003; Stojanov and Kastner 2005). Among the conditions first recognized as autoinflammatory were the hereditary periodic fever syndromes, which present with recurrent or in some cases fluctuating fevers and localized inflammation, often involving the skin, joints, or serosal membranes. Between flares, patients may experience few overt symptoms, although biochemical evidence of inflammation may continue at a subclinical level. Several other classes of autoinflammatory disease have subsequently been proposed, including pyogenic disorders such as the syndrome of pyogenic arthritis with pyoderma gangrenosum and acne (PAPA), and granulomatous disorders such as Blau syndrome and Crohn's disease.

The present review will focus on the six known hereditary periodic fevers, as well as PAPA and Blau syndromes, all of which are inherited as single-gene Mendelian illnesses (Table 1). Within the last several years, the six genes underlying these eight disorders have all been cloned (French FMF Consortium 1997; International FMF Consortium 1997; Drenth et al. 1999; Houten et al. 1999a; McDermott et al. 1999; Hoffman et al. 2001a; Miceli-Richard et al. 2001; Aganna et al. 2002; Aksentijevich et al. 2002; Dode et al. 2002; Feldmann et al. 2002; X. Wang et al. 2002; Wise et al. 2002). Identification of these genes has not only shed light on newly recognized pathways regulating innate immunity, but has uncovered heretofore unrecognized pathophysiologic connections among these disparate clinical conditions.

Table 1 Autoinflammatory disease genes and their protein products

	Disease						
	FMF	PAPA	FCAS MWS NOMID	Blau	TRAPS	HIDS
Locus	MEFV	PSTPIP1/*CD2BP1*	CIAS1	NOD2/CARD15	TNFRSF1A	MVK
Chromosomal location	16p13.3	15q24	1q44	16q12	12p13.2	12q24
Gene structure	10 exons	15 exons	9 exons	12 exons	10 exons	11 exons
Protein size	781 a.a.	416 a.a.	920–1034 a.a. (depending on number of LRRs)	1040 a.a.	455 a.a.	396 a.a.
Protein name	Pyrin/ marenostrin	PSTPIP1, CD2BP1,	Cryopyrin, NALP3, PYPAF1, CATERPILLER1.1	NOD2, CARD15,	TNFRSF1A, P55, CD120a, TNFR1	MK
Domains	PYD, Coiled-coil, B-box, B30.2/rfp/SPRY	Fer-CIP4, Coiled-coil, SH3, PEST	PYD, NACHT, LRR (7–11)	CARD (2), NACHT, LRR (10)	CRD (4), DD	ATP-binding
Putative function(s)	Regulation of pro-inflammatory cytokine release, NF-κB activation, apoptosis	Regulation of protein phosphorylation, upstream regulator of pyrin, immune synapse construction	Regulation of proinflammatory cytokine release, NF-κB activation, apoptosis	Intracellular sensor of bacterial products, signal transduction	Binds TNF, NF-κB activation, regulation of leukocyte apoptosis	Phosphorylates mevalonic acid, cholesterol synthesis, isoprenoid synthesis

An updated list of mutations for each of these genes is available online at http://fmf.igh.cnrs.fr/infevers/

2
Familial Mediterranean Fever

Familial Mediterranean fever (FMF) is a recessively inherited periodic fever syndrome with carrier rates as high as 1:3 to 1:5 among individuals of Armenian, Jewish, Arab, or Turkish descent (Aksentijevich et al. 1999; Stoffman et al. 2000; Gershoni-Baruch et al. 2001; Kogan et al. 2001; Touitou 2001; Yilmaz et al. 2001; Al-Alami et al. 2003), thus raising the possibility of heterozygote selection. FMF is characterized by 1- to3-day febrile episodes with abdominal pain, pleurisy, arthritis, or a characteristic erysipeloid rash. Between attacks, patients feel comparatively well, despite evidence of subclinical inflammation (Tunca et al. 1999; Korkmaz et al. 2002; Duzova et al. 2003). Although sometimes debilitating during flares, the arthritis is usually nondeforming and none of the febrile symptoms are life-threatening. However, continuous elevation of inflammatory markers during and between attacks may lead to the tissue deposition of a misfolded fragment of the acute phase protein, serum amyloid A. This type of systemic amyloidosis frequently resulted in renal failure and early death before the era of colchicine prophylaxis.

Both the acute attacks and the amyloidosis of FMF can usually be prevented with colchicine (Dinarello et al. 1974; Zemer et al. 1974, 1986, 1991). Although colchicine is known to destabilize microtubules at high doses in vitro, the mechanism by which it prevents FMF attacks is incompletely understood. Colchicine is concentrated in granulocytes (Ben-Chetrit and Levy 1998), the major effector cells in acute FMF attacks, and its therapeutic benefit in FMF may be related to its effects on cell-surface adhesion molecules (Cronstein et al. 1995), leukocyte migration (Dinarello et al. 1976), or even the fact that the protein mutated in FMF can bind microtubules (Mansfield et al. 2001).

FMF is caused by over 50 mutations in the *MEFV* (<u>ME</u>diterranean <u>Fe</u>ver) gene, which are available online at http://fmf.igh.cnrs.fr/infevers/ (Touitou et al. 2004). Although most mutations show recessive inheritance patterns, a sizable percentage of patients with single identifiable mutations evince symptoms of FMF. In rare cases, dominant inheritance within families has been documented (Booth et al. 2000), and it is possible that modifier genes may sometimes allow the expression of the FMF phenotype in other patients harboring a single mutation.

The coding sequence of *MEFV* subsumes ten exons, oriented $5' \rightarrow 3'$, centromere $\rightarrow$ telomere, covering approximately 15 kb on chromosome 16p13.3 (International FMF Consortium 1997). The approximately 3.7-kb transcript encodes a 781-amino acid protein called pyrin (International FMF Consortium 1997) or marenostrin (French FMF Consortium 1997). Pyrin is mainly expressed in granulocytes, cytokine-activated monocytes, dendritic cells, and in fibroblasts derived from skin, peritoneum, and synovium (Centola et al. 2000; Matzner et al. 2000; Diaz et al. 2004), consistent with the predominant role of granulocytes in (FMF)!FMF inflammation and the anatomic distribution of attacks. Endogenous pyrin is cytoplasmic in monocytes but predominantly nuclear in granulocytes, dendritic cells, and synovial fibroblasts (Diaz et al. 2004). Recent in vitro data suggest that the interaction of pyrin with the 14.3.3 protein may play a role in controlling subcellular localization of pyrin (Jeru et al. 2005).

The pyrin protein consists of a 92-amino acid N-terminal PYRIN domain (Bertin and DiStefano 2000), also denoted PYD (Martinon et al. 2001), PAAD (Pawlowski et al. 2001), or DAPIN (Staub et al. 2001), a B-box zinc finger, a coiled-coil region, and a C-terminal B30.2/rfp/SPRY domain (Vernet et al. 1993; Henry et al. 1998; Seto et al. 1999). PYD is a member of the death domain fold superfamily (Fairbrother et al. 2001; Richards et al. 2001), which also includes death domains (DDs), death effector domains (DEDs), and caspase recruitment domains (CARDs). DD fold superfamily motifs have three-dimensional structures consisting of a specific orientation of six alpha helices, enabling homotypic protein interactions via electrostatic effects (Eliezer 2003; Hiller et al. 2003; Liepinsh et al. 2003; Liu et al. 2003). The B-box and coiled-coil regions also mediate protein–protein interactions (Centola et al. 1998; Shoham et al. 2003).

Consistent with the probable functions of its subunits, pyrin is capable of interacting with several other proteins. Through cognate N-terminal PYD interactions, pyrin binds the bipartite adaptor protein ASC (apoptosis-associated speck-like protein with a CARD) (Masumoto et al. 1999; Richards et al. 2001). ASC also contains a CARD domain and is able to bind caspase-1 (IL-1β-converting enzyme [ICE]) via CARD–CARD homotypic interactions (Martinon et al. 2002; Srinivasula et al. 2002; L. Wang et al. 2002). In vitro, contact with ASC enables multimerization and autocatalysis of caspase-1 zymogen into its p20 and p10 enzymatic subunits. Caspase-1 then cleaves the inactive, 31-kDa IL-1β precursor to its active, secreted 17-kDa form. Secreted IL-1β is a potent proinflammatory mediator.

Studies of $ASC^{-/-}$ mice indicate that ASC is essential for activation of caspase-1 and IL-1β secretion following stimulation with bacterial lipopolysaccharide or the intracellular bacterium *Salmonella typhimurium* (Mariathasan et al. 2004). In vivo, ASC participates in macromolecular complexes denoted inflammasomes to activate caspase-1 (Martinon and Tschopp 2004). The first inflammasome described contains ASC, a PYD and CARD-containing protein called NALP1, and caspases-1 and -5 (Martinon et al. 2002). A second inflammasome, to be discussed at greater length below, includes cryopyrin (also called NALP3), ASC, two molecules of caspase-1, and another protein denoted Cardinal (Agostini et al. 2004).

The effects of pyrin's interaction with ASC are complex and incompletely understood. In mice expressing a truncated form of pyrin, caspase-1 and IL-1β activation were shown to be increased, whereas ectopic expression of pyrin in mouse monocytic RAW cells led to suppression of IL-1β production, thus suggesting an inhibitory role for pyrin in caspase-1 activation, possibly by sequestering ASC (Fig. 1) (Chae et al. 2003). In contrast, in a more recent study of transfected human embryonic kidney cells, pyrin was found to potentiate ASC-dependent IL-1β production (Yu et al. 2005). In transfection systems in which ASC is not present, pyrin appears to suppress IL-1β production (Stehlik et al. 2003).

Pyrin has variously been found to have an inhibitory effect (Dowds et al. 2003; Masumoto et al. 2003), a context-dependent effect that could either be stimulatory or inhibitory (Stehlik et al. 2002), or no effect (Yu et al. 2005)

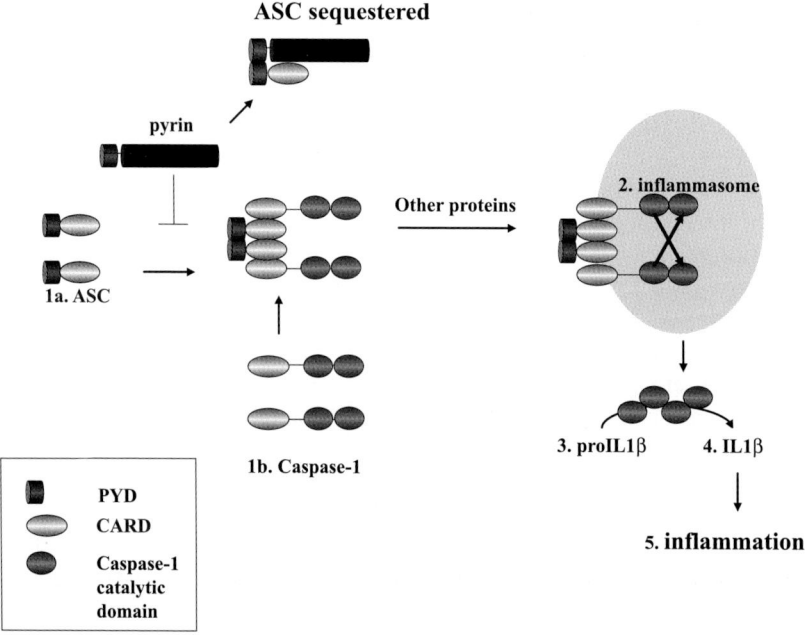

Fig. 1 The sequestration hypothesis of pyrin function. Pyrin inhibits inflammatory signals by binding and sequestering ASC, which forms a multimolecular inflammasome complex by associating with caspase-1 and other proteins. The inflammasome allows activation of caspase-1 and subsequent cleavage of proIL-1β to its active, secreted form

on NF-κB activation in cell lines, depending on the precise experimental conditions. Through its PYD, ASC has been shown to interact with the IκB kinase complex (IKK), an upstream regulator of NF-κB activation, and high levels of ASC suppress NF-κB activation (Stehlik et al. 2002). Possibly, the relative amounts of pyrin and ASC may affect their interactions with one another as well as with IKK, thereby tipping the balance either toward or against NF-κB activation.

Defective apoptosis may also play a role in the pathogenesis of FMF. Peritoneal macrophages from mice expressing the aforementioned truncated pyrin are deficient in apoptosis, possibly prolonging the inflammatory response by allowing activated cells to survive (Chae et al. 2003). Nevertheless, in some in vitro systems pyrin appears to exert an ASC-dependent anti-apoptotic effect (Richards et al. 2001; Dowds et al. 2003; Masumoto et al. 2003).

Although it appears that the impact of pyrin on various inflammatory pathways may depend on experimental if not physiologic conditions, it is clear that the interaction between pyrin and ASC is crucial for several of these effects. Perhaps reflecting the importance of PYD cognate interactions for pyrin's function, FMF-associated mutations in this N-terminal domain are very rare. In contrast, mutations in the C-terminal B30.2/rfp/SPRY domain are extremely common, and, given the high carrier frequency for FMF among certain human populations, appear to have been selected, perhaps by a pathogen or group of pathogens. Moreover, there is evidence that the wild-type sequence of the human B30.2/rfp/SPRY domain has been selected over primate evolution (Schaner et al. 2001). These observations have fueled speculation that the B30.2/rfp/SPRY domain of pyrin might bind certain intracellular pathogen-associated molecular patterns (PAMPs) (Schaner et al. 2001; Yu et al. 2005), although there is currently no direct experimental evidence to support this hypothesis. It is intriguing to note that the B30.2/rfp/SPRY domain of another protein, TRIM5α, blocks infection of certain retroviruses, and has undergone positive selection in primate evolution similar to pyrin (Perron et al. 2004; Song et al. 2005).

3
Syndrome of Pyogenic Arthritis, Pyoderma Gangrenosum, and Acne

As noted above, the B-box and coiled-coil motifs of pyrin are also protein interaction domains, mediating binding to proline-serine-threonine phosphatase interacting protein 1 (PSTPIP1) (Shoham et al. 2003), also known as CD2-binding protein 1 (CD2BP1) (Li et al. 1998). PSTPIP1 is a 416-amino acid protein encoded on chromosome 15q24 (Wise et al. 2002). PSTPIP1 consists of an N-terminal Fer-CIP4 domain (Aspenstrom 1997), followed by a coiled-coil region, and finally an SH3 domain at the C-terminus (Fig. 2). Both the coiled-coil and the SH3 motif are necessary for interaction with pyrin (Shoham et al. 2003).

Patients with certain mutations in the coiled-coil domain of PSTPIP1 have a condition called the syndrome of pyogenic arthritis, pyoderma gangrenosum, and acne (PAPA), an autosomal dominant disease associated with deforming, sterile arthropathy, severe cutaneous ulcers with pathergic reactions at sites of minor trauma (pyoderma gangrenosum), and cystic acne (Wise et al. 2002). PAPA mutations in PSTPIP1 attenuate its association with protein tyrosine phosphatase with a PEST (proline, glutamate, serine, threonine) domain (PTP-PEST) (Spencer et al. 1997; Wise et al. 2002; Badour et al. 2004), resulting in hyperphosphorylation of PSTPIP1 (Cote et al. 2002). Hyperphosphorylation in turn increases the strength of the interaction between pyrin and PSTPIP1 (Shoham et al. 2003), perhaps preventing pyrin from exerting negative regulatory effects on the innate immune response.

Consistent with a major role for the pyrin–PSTPIP1 interaction in the pathogenesis of PAPA syndrome, both proteins are expressed at high levels in neutrophils (Shoham et al. 2003), and neutrophils are the major effector cell in this disorder (Lindor et al. 1997), as is the case for FMF. Moreover, cell lines co-transfected with pyrin and PAPA-associated PSTPIP1 mutants secreted significantly more IL-1β than cells co-transfected with pyrin and wild-type PSTPIP1 (Shoham et al. 2003), and peripheral blood leukocytes from a patient with clinically active PAPA syndrome were found to secrete high levels of IL-1β when cultured in vitro. These results are consistent with

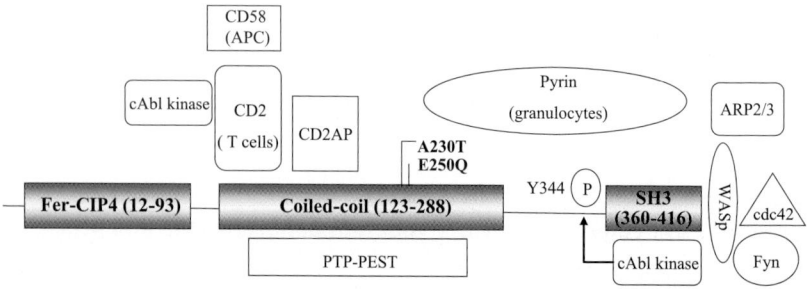

Fig. 2 Protein schematic of PSTPIP1, showing the domains and binding partners. PSTPIP1 interacts with a variety of proteins involved in immune regulation, including PTP-PEST, pyrin, CD2, and WASp. Also shown are the main kinases responsible for phosphorylation events (Fyn, cAbl), as well as proteins involved in actin polymerization (cdc42, Arp2/3)

the hypothesis that PAPA-associated PSTPIP1 mutants exert their effects in neutrophils by inducing the sequestration of pyrin, with consequent excessive IL-1β production.

PSTPIP1 may also play a role in the regulation of the adaptive immune response. In T lymphocytes, PSTPIP1 interacts with several key molecules implicated in the formation of the "immunologic synapse" in antigen recognition (Badour et al. 2003a, b, 2004). Recent studies have clearly demonstrated a necessary role for PSTPIP1 in coupling the CD2 T cell membrane receptor with the Wiskott-Aldrich syndrome protein (WASp), thereby linking CD2 engagement with WASp-induced actin polymerization and synapse formation. This process is, in part, regulated by the phosphorylation status of both CD2 (Li et al. 1998) and WASp (Cote et al. 2002), with PTP-PEST playing a negative regulatory role (Badour et al. 2004). Although PAPA-associated mutations in PSTPIP1 do not affect its interaction with either CD2 or WASp (Wise et al. 2002), they may nevertheless accentuate immunologic synapse formation in T cells by limiting the participation of PTP-PEST in the macromolecular complex. The ramifications of these potential perturbations in the adaptive immune response for the granulocyte-mediated pathology of PAPA syndrome remain to be determined. The predicted lesion in dephosphorylation of the CD2-PSTPIP1-WASp complex might also lead to as yet undocumented increased resistance to viral or intracellular bacterial pathogens in PAPA patients, or to increased susceptibility to contact-induced delayed-type hypersensitivity reactions.

4
The Cryopyrinopathies: Familial Cold Autoinflammatory Syndrome, Muckle-Wells Syndrome, and Neonatal-Onset Multisystem Inflammatory Disease

Similar to pyrin and PSTPIP1, many other proteins involved in the regulation of innate immunity consist of multiple protein interaction domains. A second disease-associated molecule containing an N-terminal PYD is denoted cryopyrin (Hoffman et al. 2001b), so named for its N-terminal PYD and to reflect its association with cold-induced urticaria. This protein is also known as NALP3 (Aganna et al. 2002; Tschopp et al. 2003), PYPAF1 (Manji et al. 2002), or caterpiller 1.1 (Harton et al. 2002; O'Connor et al. 2003; Ting and Davis 2004). Mutations in this protein cause three separate disease entities that vary in severity. Familial cold autoinflammatory syndrome (FCAS, also known as familial cold urticaria, familial polymorphous cold eruption, and cold hypersensitivity) is a relatively mild febrile syndrome characterized by episodic fever, rash, and arthralgia, precipitated by exposure to cold temperature. The rash resembles urticaria, but biopsies show a neutrophilic infiltrate and the absence of mast cells (Hoffman et al. 2001b). Muckle-Wells syndrome (MWS) is a more severe illness with more prominent joint involvement, bilateral progressive hearing loss, and increased risk of systemic amyloidosis. Febrile episodes are often longer than those with FCAS, and there is usually no association with cold temperature. Finally, neonatal onset multisystem inflammatory disease (NOMID; also called chronic infantile neurological, cutaneous, and articular syndrome, CINCA [Prieur et al. 1987]) is potentially the most serious cryopyrinopathy, with continuous symptoms fluctuating in intensity. Many patients with NOMID/CINCA develop a bilateral deforming arthropathy due to overgrowth of the epiphyses of the long bones (Prieur and Griscelli 1981; Hassink and Goldsmith 1983; Hashkes and Lovell 1997; Prieur 2001). Besides daily rash and fever, patients may have hepatosplenomegaly, aseptic meningitis, bilateral hearing loss, vision loss, and mental retardation. Growth retardation and reduced reproductive potential are common. Mortality has been estimated at 20% by age 20 (Prieur et al. 1987; Hashkes and Lovell 1997).

Although the cryopyrinopathies have been separated into three distinct conditions, there is a continuous spectrum of pathology from mild (FCAS) to severe (NOMID/CINCA), with some mutations associated with more than one syndrome and wide variation in manifestations among individuals with the same diagnosis. NOMID/CINCA patients in particular fall into various disease subgroups, with some experiencing severe joint disease and central nervous system involvement, and others with milder arthropathy and few or no mental disabilities. All three syndromes are inherited in an autosomal dominant fashion (Hoffman et al. 2001a; Aganna et al. 2002; Aksentijevich et al. 2002; Dode et al. 2002), although de novo mutations have been documented, especially in NOMID/CINCA, and it appears likely that additional modifier genes influence the observed phenotype, as is the case with FMF.

The cryopyrin protein, encoded on chromosome 1q44, consists of an N-terminal PYD, followed by a NACHT (neuronal apoptosis inhibitor protein, CIITA, HET-E, and TP1, also called NBS: nucleotide-binding site [Koonin and Aravind 2000]) domain, and 7–11 C-terminal leucine-rich repeats (LRR), depending on the splice isoform. Mutations associated with disease are missense substitutions mainly found in the NACHT domain (Neven et al. 2004). The NACHT contains various conserved motifs, including an ATP/GTPase-specific P loop and a Mg^{++} binding site (the Walker A and B domains, respectively) (Walker et al. 1982). The NACHT domain is homologous to a domain in APAF-1 (Zou et al. 1997), a protein that activates the pro-apoptotic enzyme, caspase-9, by oligomerization and ATP binding (Acehan et al. 2002).

To date four NOMID/CINCA-associated mutations cluster around the NACHT metal ion-binding site, and many others line the nucleotide-binding cleft (Albrecht et al. 2003; Neven et al. 2004), suggesting that this motif regulates the function of cryopyrin in inflammatory cells. Cryopyrin is expressed in polymorphonuclear cells, consistent with the principal role of neutrophils in the urticaria-like lesions, as well as in cultured chondrocytes, which may explain the arthropathy observed in NOMID/CINCA (Feldmann et al. 2002).

Similar to pyrin, cryopyrin has been shown to associate with ASC via PYD–PYD homotypic interactions (Manji et al. 2002), thus potentially implicating cryopyrin in the regulation of cytokine production (L. Wang et al. 2002), NF-κB activation (Manji et al. 2002; Stehlik et al. 2002; Dowds et al. 2003), and apoptosis (Dowds et al. 2003). Cryopyrin (NALP3) forms a proinflammatory molecular platform called the NALP3 inflammasome (Fig. 3) by complexing with ASC and another protein called Cardinal, thereby bringing two molecules of caspase-1 into close proximity to induce autocatalysis and consequent IL-1β and IL-18 activation (Agostini et al. 2004). Disease-associated mutations in *CIAS1* cause spontaneous IL1β production by patients' peripheral blood monocytes (Agostini et al. 2004) and transfected cell lines (Dowds et al. 2004). As noted above, under some conditions pyrin may compete with cryopyrin for ASC, thereby limiting IL-1β production.

As is the case for pyrin, cryopyrin's effect on NFκB activation is controversial. In the presence of ASC, cryopyrin may activate NF-κB (Manji et al. 2002; Dowds et al. 2003), inhibit TNF-induced NF-κB induction (O'Connor et al. 2003), exert a context-dependent effect on NF-κB activation (Stehlik et al. 2002), or have no effect on NF-κB (Yu et al. 2005). The possible ASC-dependent effect of cryopyrin on NF-κB may be mediated by the indirect interaction of ASC with the IKK complex through RICK/Rip2/CARDIAK (Inohara et al. 1998; McCarthy et al. 1998; Thome et al. 1998), or through a direct interaction of ASC with IKK (Stehlik et al. 2002). Transfected cryopyrin mutants have increased NF-κB stimulatory activity, but only if ASC is present (Dowds et al. 2004). Without ASC, cryopyrin and its mutants suppress NF-κB activity. The currently available data suggest a complex picture in which the stoichiometric relationships of multiple interacting proteins may determine the effect of cryopyrin on NF-κB activation under varying conditions.

The molecular mechanism by which NACHT-domain mutations in cryopyrin lead to autoinflammatory disease is still under investigation. One attractive hypothesis is based on the possible intramolecular interaction of the NACHT domain and LRRs (Fig. 3). Deletion of the C-terminal LRRs is necessary to detect optimal association of cryopyrin with Cardinal, suggesting the possibility of an autoinhibitory effect of the LRRs on NACHT-mediated inflammasome assembly (Agostini et al. 2004). By this hypothesis, disease-associated mu-

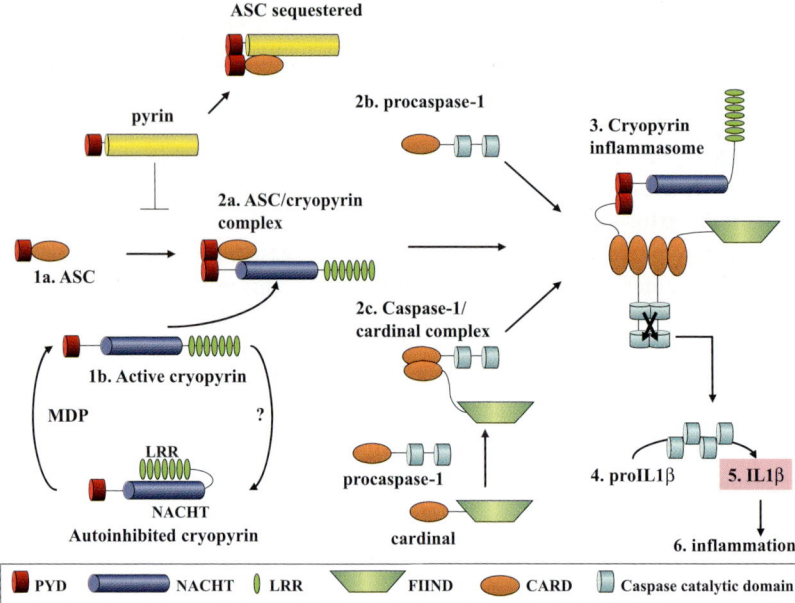

Fig. 3 Formation of the cryopyrin inflammasome. When not sequestered by pyrin, ASC can complex with cryopyrin once cryopyrin is freed from autoinhibition. Caspase-1 and Cardinal also bind the ASC–cryopyrin complex, leading to caspase-1 activation by induced proximity and cleavage and secretion of IL-1β

tations in cryopyrin's NACHT domain might somehow attenuate the autoinhibitory interaction, leading to constitutive activation or a lowered threshold for assembly of an active inflammasome.

Recent studies have focused on the possible role of bacterial PAMPs in the activation of the NALP3 inflammasome. Based on the known ability of PAMPs to activate toll-like receptors (TLRs) through their extracellular LRRs (Medzhitov and Janeway 1998; Takeda et al. 2003), it is attractive to speculate that intracellular proteins such as cryopyrin, with a NACHT and LRR domain (now denoted NLR proteins [Martinon and Tschopp 2005]), might also be activated by LRR interactions with PAMPs. Martinon and colleagues (2004) have recently shown that muramyl dipeptide (MDP), a peptidoglycan motif found in the cell wall of Gram-positive and Gram-negative bacteria, may activate the NALP3 inflammasome, likely by releasing LRR-mediated autoinhibition. Moreover, macrophages from a patient with MWS were found to show increased IL-1β secretion in the presence of MDP. Adding an element of complexity to the picture, disease-associated cryopyrin mutations also increase the affinity of the PYD for ASC (Dowds et al. 2004).

Studies on cryopyrin-null mice also suggest a role for cryopyrin in sensing pro-inflammatory signals. One study showed activation of the inflammasome and subsequent caspase-1 cleavage and IL-1β secretion in response to bacterial RNA, a response abrogated in cryopyrin-null mice (Kanneganti et al. 2006). A second study found that the monosodium urate crystals responsible for gout-associated inflammation were also able to trigger caspase-1 activation and secretion of IL-1β from a cultured monocytic cell line. Pretreating cells with colchicine, commonly used to treat gout attacks, blocked IL-1β maturation. Cryopyrin-null mice were unable to upregulate IL-1β secretion (Martinon et al. 2006). Finally, a third study using cryopyrin-null mice showed that substances perturbing intracellular potassium concentrations, such as ATP and certain bacterial toxins, were also able to activate caspase-1 via the cryopyrin inflammosome (Mariathasan et al. 2006).

Although cryopyrin may potentially regulate innate immunity through a number of pathways, including cytokine production, NF-κB activation, and apoptosis, therapeutic trials targeting IL-1β suggest a primary role for this cytokine in the pathogenesis of FCAS, MWS, and NOMID/CINCA. Relatively short-term studies of the IL-1β receptor antagonist anakinra show great promise in all three conditions (Dailey et al. 2004; Frenkel et al. 2004; Hawkins et al. 2004a, b; Hoffman et al. 2004). These clinical trials demonstrated a significant impact of anakinra on fever, rash, and acute-phase proteins in all three disorders, and on the central nervous system manifestations in NOMID/CINCA (Dailey et al. 2004).

5
Blau Syndrome

Combinations of PYD, CARD, NACHT, and/or LRR domains are found in over 20 other proteins encoded in the human genome (Tschopp et al. 2003; Ting and Davis 2004; Martinon and Tschopp 2005), many of which are expressed in immune tissues. One such molecule is the NOD2/CARD15 protein, which contains two N-terminal CARD domains, followed by a NACHT domain and ten LRR motifs (Fig. 4). Mutations in the LRR of NOD2/CARD15 were first associated with Crohn's disease, one of two common forms of inflammatory bowel disease (Hugot et al. 2001; Ogura et al. 2001). Crohn's disease is a multifactorial disorder characterized by fever, diarrhea, abdominal pain, granulomatous lesions in the gastrointestinal tract, and, at times, extraintestinal manifestations in the skin, joints, and eyes. Subsequently, LRR variants of NOD2/CARD15 were associated with psoriatic arthritis (Rahman et al. 2003), another genetically complex inflammatory disorder.

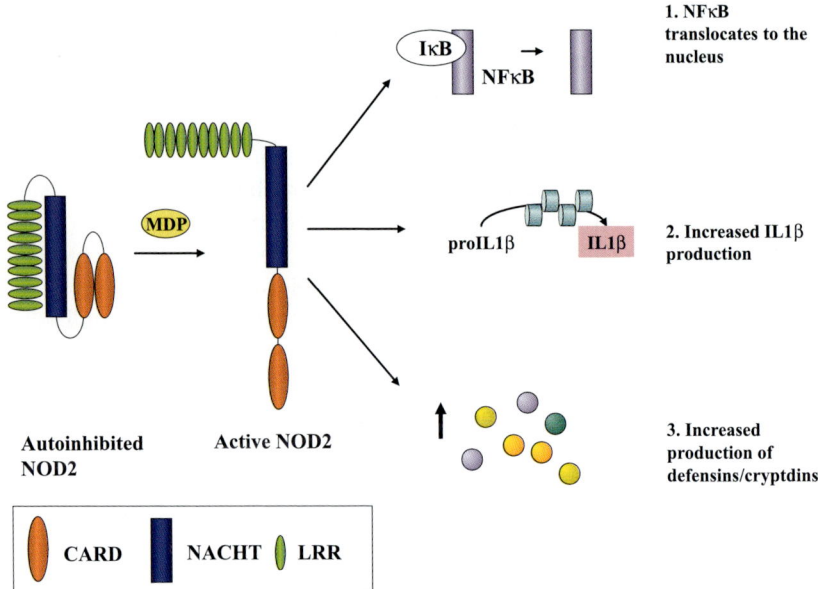

Fig. 4 Physiologic role of NOD2/CARD15. NOD2 is normally in an autoinhibited conformation. Upon binding MDP, NOD2 is released from autoinhibition and may impact inflammation in several ways, including activation of NFκB, IL1β production, and/or increased production of defensins/cryptdins

In contrast, mutations in the NACHT domain of NOD2/CARD15 have been shown to cause Blau syndrome (BS) (Miceli-Richard et al. 2001), a rare autosomal dominant disorder characterized by early-onset granulomatous arthritis, rash, and uveitis with camptodactyly (permanent contractures of the digits) (Blau 1985; Jabs et al. 1985; Miller 1986; Raphael et al. 1993). More recently, mutations in the NACHT domain of NOD2/CARD15 have been found to cause a clinically similar disorder, early-onset sarcoidosis (EOS) (Kanazawa et al. 2005).

Even though they share a common underlying gene, BS/EOS and CD exhibit important clinical differences. BS/EOS patients present with granulomatous lesions in sterile sites such as the eye and the joints, and, as such, BS/EOS is clearly autoinflammatory. In contrast, although CD patients sometimes develop arthritis, uveitis, or even pyoderma gangrenosum, the primary lesion of CD is in the intestine, and the clinical phenotype may well be influenced by intestinal flora.

NOD2/CARD15 is expressed primarily in myeloid cells, as well as Paneth cells in the small intestine, and activated intestinal epithelial cells (Eckmann and Karin 2005). As is the case for cryopyrin, MDP stimulates NOD2/CARD15-mediated NF-κB activation (Girardin et al. 2003; Inohara et al. 2003), and a common CD-associated mutation of the LRR abrogates this effect, suggesting that NOD2/CARD15 also senses intracellular bacteria through this domain. NOD2/CARD15-mediated NF-κB activation occurs through several pathways (Eckmann and Karin 2005), including the induction of CARD–CARD cognate interactions with RICK/Rip2/CARDIAK, leading to IKK activation (Abbott et al. 2004).

The physiologic role of NOD2/CARD15 and the consequent effects of CD-associated mutations, remain unclear. Recent studies of Nod2/Card15-deficient mice demonstrated increased susceptibility to orally administered bacterial pathogens and a deficiency in cryptdins, a subgroup of intestinal anti-microbial peptides (Kobayashi et al. 2005). Moreover, mice harboring a CD-associated Nod2/Card15 mutant exhibited increased NF-κB activation in response to MDP and accentuated secretion of IL-1β (Maeda et al. 2005). These data suggest a proinflammatory role for NOD2/CARD15, with CD mutations representing activating, "gain-of-function" variants. Nevertheless, yet another study of Nod2-deficient mice suggested an anti-inflammatory role for normal NOD2/CARD15, inhibiting TLR-2-stimulated NF-κB activation, with CD-associated mutations representing a loss of this negative regulatory function (Watanabe et al. 2004). Although both models predict increased inflammatory activation in peripheral blood monocytes from CD patients, in fact the opposite has been observed (Li et al. 2004).

Consistent with the autosomal dominant pattern of inheritance for BS, and with the presence of BS lesions in aseptic sites, BS-associated NOD2/CARD15 mutations are gain-of-function variants that result in MDP-independent constitutive activation of NF-κB (Chamaillard et al. 2003a, b; Tanabe et al. 2004). It is interesting to note that the NOD2/CARD15 codon at which two different BS mutations have been identified is in a position in the NACHT domain homologous to the location of the MWS/FCAS-associated R260W mutation in cryopyrin (Chamaillard et al. 2003a). Similarly, EOS-associated NOD2/CARD15 mutations are also associated with increased basal NF-κB activity (Kanazawa et al. 2005).

6
TNF Receptor-Associated Periodic Syndrome

The tumor necrosis factor (TNF) receptor-associated periodic syndrome (TRAPS) is a dominantly inherited periodic fever syndrome caused by mutations in the 55-kDa TNF receptor gene (*TNFRSF1A*), encoded on chromosome

12p13 (McDermott et al. 1999; Hull et al. 2002). The receptor protein is variously denoted TNFRSF1A, TNFRI, p55, or CD120a. Prior to the discovery of the causative mutations from which this disorder takes its name, this condition was clinically described in a large Irish/Scottish kindred (Williamson et al. 1982; McDermott et al. 1997), prompting the name familial Hibernian fever. With the benefit of molecular genetics, it is now clear that this clinical syndrome, with associated *TNFRSF1A* mutations, is found worldwide, and hence the ethnically neutral, mechanistically unifying TRAPS nomenclature was proposed (McDermott et al. 1999). TRAPS is now the second most common hereditary periodic fever syndrome, with over 45 mutations having been described (http://fmf.igh.cnrs.fr/infevers/).

TRAPS patients suffer febrile episodes of variable duration but at times lasting more than 1 week (Hull et al. 2002), longer than the attacks of FMF, HIDS, FCAS, or MWS. As is the case for FMF, fever may be accompanied by serosal inflammation, most commonly sterile peritonitis or pleurisy. In addition, many patients have cutaneous symptoms consisting of migratory areas of macular erythema on the torso or limb(s). Frequently, patients complain of myalgia underlying areas of rash. Ocular inflammation, most commonly conjunctivitis and/or periorbital edema, may also be part of the febrile attacks. Laboratory findings include leukocytosis, thrombocytosis, elevations in the C-reactive protein and serum amyloid A, and an accelerated erythrocyte sedimentation rate. Up to 10% of patients may eventually develop systemic amyloidosis (Aksentijevich et al. 2001).

The TNF receptor p55 protein is expressed nearly ubiquitously, thus differentiating it from the TNF p75 receptor, which is expressed mainly on leukocytes and endothelial cells. Trimers of TNF bind the p55 receptor (Banner et al. 1993), which then oligomerizes and transduces signals into the cell (Engelmann et al. 1990). These signals can be proinflammatory, upregulating expression of adhesion molecules and proinflammatory cytokines and promoting lymphocyte activation, or pro-apoptotic, activating caspases (Chen and Goeddel 2002). Emphasizing the importance of the p55 receptor in signal transduction, mice with disruptions in *TNFRSF1* have a severely reduced ability to mount inflammatory responses (Pfeffer et al. 1993; Peschon et al. 1998).

Key aspects of signal transduction through the p55 receptor, beginning with receptor aggregation by TNF trimers, are illustrated in Fig. 5 (Chen and Goeddel 2002). The cytoplasmic tails of the p55 trimer contain DD motifs (MacEwan 2002), which allow interaction with TNFR-associated DD proteins (TRADDs). TRADDs subsequently recruit TNFR-associated factor 2 (TRAF2) proteins, receptor-interacting protein (RIP), and cellular inhibitor of apoptosis proteins (cIAP) into the complex. Fas-associated DD protein (FADD) binds

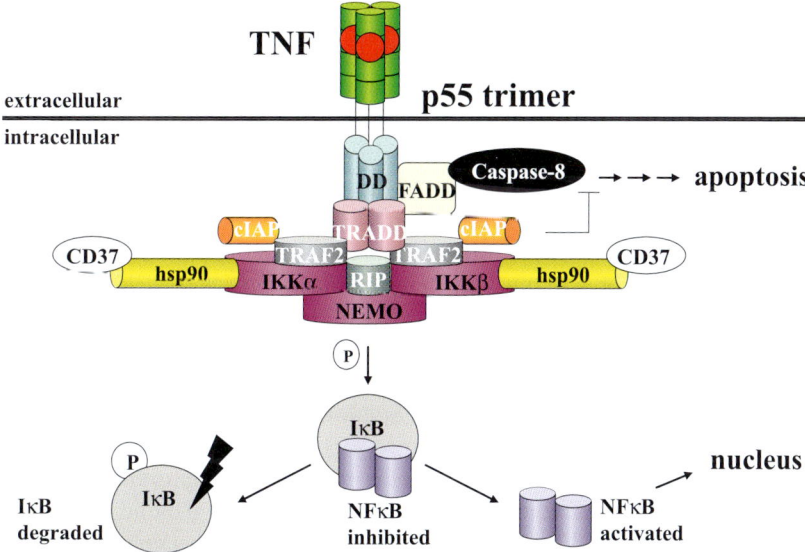

Fig. 5 Signaling through the p55 TNF receptor. Trimers of TNF bind trimerized receptor via moieties in the second and third receptor CARD domains. Binding transduces signals into the cell via the TNF receptor death domains (*DDs*). The DDs recruit various intracellular proteins involved in NFκB activation and cell death

TRADD and recruits caspase-8, promoting apoptosis, whereas TRAF2 binds cIAP and the IKK complex (IKKα, IKKβ, and IKKγ [NEMO]), promoting NFκB activation and cell survival. Two additional proteins, hsp90 and CD37, are also recruited to facilitate shuttling of NFκB into the nucleus.

The extracellular portion of p55 consists of four cysteine-rich domains (CRDs), each containing six conserved cysteine residues, allowing formation of three intramolecular disulfide bonds per domain (Banner et al. 1993). CRDs 2 and 3 make up the ligand-binding region of p55, while a region in CRD1 appears to mediate ligand-independent oligomerization. This region has been termed the preligand binding assembly domain (PLAD) and is essential for proper TNF binding and signal transduction (Chan et al. 2000). Following signal transduction, metalloproteases cleave the receptor in its extracellular portion, close to the membrane (Schall et al. 1990; Wallach et al. 1991; Brakebusch et al. 1994; Mullberg et al. 1995). Normally, receptor cleavage seems to accomplish two things: first, removal of the ligand-binding domain prevents continued signaling into the cell and helps limit the immune response, and second, cleavage creates a soluble pool of receptors that compete with membrane-bound receptors for ligand binding, further attenuating the immune response.

TRAPS-associated mutations are located exclusively in the extracellular region, nearly all in CRDs 1 and 2. About half of the known mutations causing TRAPS are missense substitutions at cysteine residues, thus disrupting disulfide bonds. Unpaired cysteine residues may allow improper folding of the receptor and interchain disulfide bonds between two receptors to occur, possibly interfering with receptor clearance, ligand binding, and/or signal transduction. Emphasizing the importance of the cysteine residues, mutations at cysteines tend to predispose patients to more severe disease, with an increased risk of systemic amyloidosis (Aksentijevich et al. 2001). At the time of this writing, no patients have been identified with null mutations, mutations in the transmembrane or intracellular domains of TNFRSF1A, or mutations in the p75 TNF receptor.

With the initial description of TRAPS, studies of a family with the C52F *TNFRSF1A* mutation demonstrated impaired activation-induced in vitro shedding of mutant p55 receptors, but not of the normal p75 receptors (McDermott et al. 1999). Binding of radiolabeled TNF to C52F peripheral blood leukocytes was not significantly different from normals, and there was no evidence for constitutive IL-6 production in vitro. Moreover, in a panel of 27 individuals harboring four different *TNFRSF1A* mutations, serum levels of soluble p55 receptors between attacks were roughly half of those observed in unaffected relatives, and during attacks were much less than those observed in patients with active rheumatoid arthritis or systemic lupus erythematosus. Taken together, these data gave rise to the "shedding hypothesis," which proposed that the autoinflammatory phenotype of TRAPS is due to defective cleavage of p55 ectodomains from the cell surface.

Subsequently, shedding defects were documented for a number of other TRAPS mutations, including H22Y, C30S, C33G, P46L, T50M, T50K, F112I, and I170N, which is very close to the actual cleavage site (Aksentijevich et al. 2001; Nevala et al. 2002; Aganna et al. 2003; Kriegel et al. 2003). Nevertheless, as the spectrum of TRAPS mutations expanded, it became clear that impaired receptor cleavage could not be documented for a number of disease-associated variants, including T37I, ΔD42, C52R, a splice mutation, N65I, and R92Q (Aksentijevich et al. 2001; Aganna et al. 2003), and that in some cases receptor shedding defects are cell type-dependent (Huggins et al. 2004).

Recent studies indicate a number of other functional abnormalities in mutant p55 TNF receptors. These include impaired intracellular trafficking, with consequent trapping of mutant receptor in the endoplasmic reticulum (Todd et al. 2004), reduced affinity for TNF (Todd et al. 2004), decreased TNF-induced leukocyte apoptosis (Siebert et al. 2005), and constitutive activation of NF-κB (Yousaf et al. 2005). It is quite possible that certain pathogenic mechanisms may be more relevant to some mutations than to others, and that more than one mechanism may be operative for some, if not all, mutations. This broader concept of pathogenesis may explain why TNF inhibition with the TNFR:Fc fusion protein etanercept is effective in reducing, although usually not totally eliminating, clinical and laboratory evidence of inflammation in TRAPS (Hull et al. 2002, 2003; Drewe et al. 2003).

7
Hyperimmunoglobulinemia D with Periodic Fever Syndrome

Hyperimmunoglobulinemia D with periodic fever syndrome (HIDS), also called Dutch type periodic fever, is an autosomal recessive disorder caused by mutations in *MVK*, which encodes mevalonate kinase (MK) (Drenth et al. 1999; Houten et al. 1999a; Valle 1999). HIDS patients have episodes of fever, lymphadenopathy, abdominal pain, arthralgia, and/or rash that last about 4–8 days, approximately every 4–8 weeks, though these time periods vary (Drenth et al. 1994). The rash has no predilection for the lower legs, unlike that of FMF, nor is it usually migratory, like that seen in TRAPS. Patients may also suffer from diarrhea, nausea, headache, and malaise during attacks. Generally the disease presents in infancy. Biochemical markers found in some but not all HIDS patients include elevated serum IgD levels (Drenth et al. 1994) and increased mevalonate concentration in the urine during febrile attacks (Drenth et al. 1999; Houten et al. 1999a; Frenkel et al. 2001; Kelley and Takada 2002). Attacks can be triggered by physical exertion, emotional stress, or vaccinations. Amyloidosis is a rare complication in HIDS (Ostuni et al. 1996; Obici et al. 2004).

HIDS was first described in 1984 (van der Meer et al. 1984), and 15 years later two independent groups, using complementary positional and functional approaches, identified *MVK* as the HIDS susceptibility locus (Drenth et al. 1999; Houten et al. 1999a). The MK enzyme is involved in the biosynthesis of cholesterol and nonsterol isoprenoids (Fig. 6). Mutations in *MVK* are also responsible for a second inherited disease, mevalonic aciduria (MA) (Hoffmann et al. 1986; Kelley 2000). Besides inflammatory symptoms similar to those of HIDS, MA patients exhibit mental retardation, ataxia, failure to thrive, myopathy, and cataracts (Hoffmann et al. 1993). Thus HIDS may be considered a mild presentation of MA.

MVK phosphorylates mevalonic acid in a pathway that leads to production of cholesterol, isoprenylated proteins, dolichol, isopentenyl tRNAs, heme A, ubiquinone, and sterols (Goldstein and Brown 1990; Brown and Goldstein 1997; Valle 1999) (Fig. 6). HIDS patients have some residual MVK activity (1%–7% of normal controls (Houten et al. 1999a, 2001)), whereas

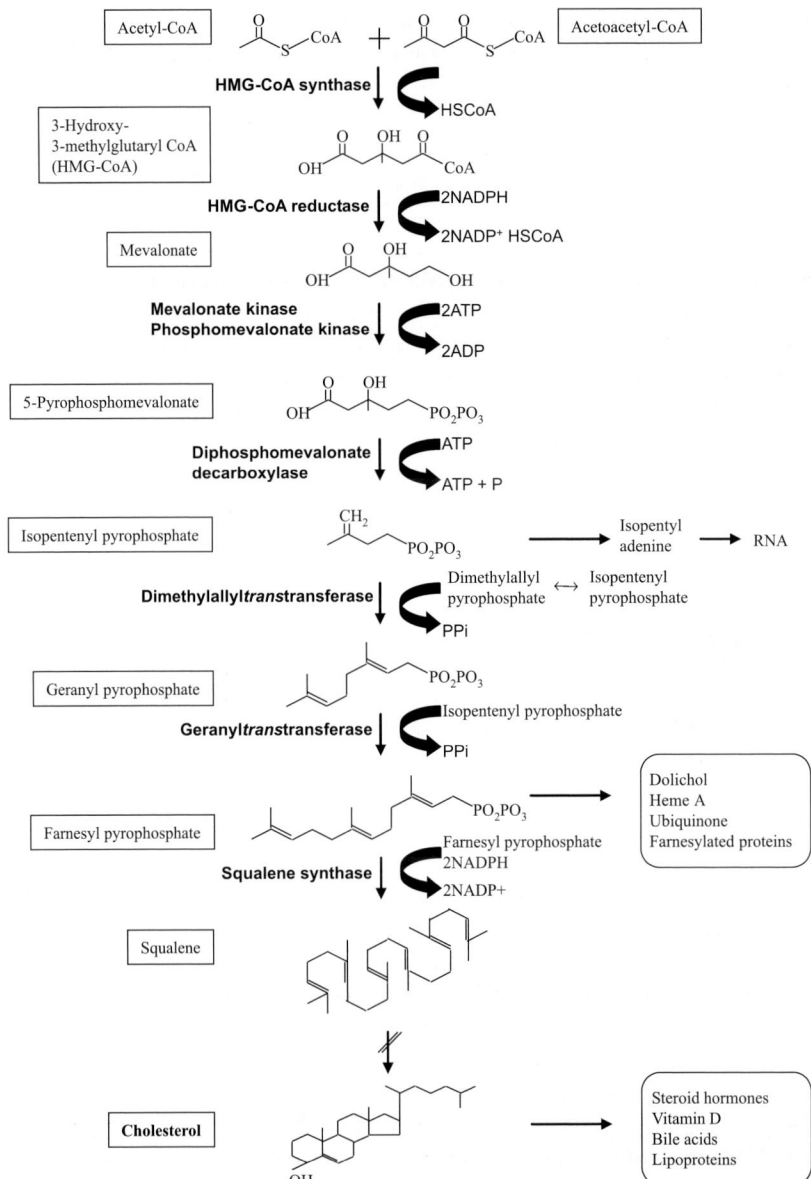

Fig. 6 The mevalonate pathway. This biochemical pathway leads to production of cholesterol, vitamin D and steroid hormones, as well as dolichol, heme, farnesylated proteins, and ubiquinone. Mevalonate kinase, mutated in HIDS and mevalonic aciduria, catalyzes the transfer of a phosphate group to mevalonic acid

activity is unmeasurable in MA patients (Hoffmann et al. 1993; Houten et al. 1999b), consistent with the more severe phenotype characteristic of MA.

Mutations associated with HIDS are scattered nearly throughout the *MVK* coding sequence, with over 35 different substitutions tabulated online (http://fmf.igh.cnrs.fr/infevers/). The vast majority of HIDS patients have at least one copy of the V377I substitution (Cuisset et al. 2001; Houten et al. 2001), and most are compound heterozygotes for V377I and a second mutation. Although some HIDS patients are homozygous for V377I, they tend to have milder disease presentations, suggesting that V377I is a low penetrance allele (Simon et al. 2003).

Just how loss of activity of the MK enzyme leads to an autoinflammatory phenotype is unclear. Elevated mevalonate levels do not appear to cause fever, as MA patients have much higher levels than HIDS patients, yet MA inflammatory episodes occur at about the same frequency and intensity as those of HIDS. Further, two patients with MA treated with lovastatin, an inhibitor of HMGR, developed flares despite reduced levels of mevalonate (Hoffmann et al. 1993). HIDS symptoms are also unlikely to be triggered by low cholesterol, as patients' cholesterol levels are usually in the low normal range (Simon and Drenth 1999).

Studies examining the function of MK carrying HIDS-associated mutations indicate the enzyme's activity is temperature sensitive (Houten et al. 2002). The V377I mutation decreases the protein's stability at high temperatures. When produced in *Escherichia coli,* the V377I MK variant showed approximately 20% of control activity at 30°C, 5% at 37°C, and almost no activity at 40°C. Likely the protein is misfolded under normal, in vivo conditions, and degraded during episodes of fever.

Surprisingly, protein isoprenylation in HIDS patients is normal (Houten et al. 2003), indicating that compensatory mechanisms exist to circumvent low enzymatic activity. MK-deficient cells appear to continue flux through the pathway by maintaining very high intracellular levels of mevalonate, possibly through the induction of 3-hydroxy-3-methylglutaryl-CoA reductase (HMGR), the enzyme just upstream of MK. One hypothesis for the pathogenesis of HIDS suggests that fever resulting from minor stimuli such as vaccinations or upper respiratory infections might reduce the activity of mutant MK, leading to a transient drop in isoprenylated compounds, stimulating an upregulation of HMGR activity, which increases intracellular mevalonate concentration to maintain movement through the pathway (Houten et al. 2003). Due to the very high levels of mevalonate maintained within cells, there is substantial leakage, accounting for the elevated urine mevalonate seen during attacks.

Possibly, a transient decrease in isoprenoids may trigger HIDS symptoms. In one study, IL1β secretion was accentuated in HIDS cells, an effect potentiated by lovastatin and relieved by addition of mevalonate, farnesol, and geranyl-geranyl (Frenkel et al. 2002). Small GTP-binding proteins in the Rho, Ras, and Rab families are important intermediates in signal transduction and require prenylation for function (Sinensky 2000). These intermediates may form a link between the mevalonate pathway and the inflammatory symptoms of HIDS.

The elevation in IgD common in HIDS patients may be an epiphenomenon, though one study indicated that IgD can cause proinflammatory responses in monocytes in vitro (Drenth et al. 1996). HIDS patients with normal IgD levels have been documented (Saulsbury 2003). In addition, elevated IgD levels may not precede inflammatory attacks and attack severity is not correlated with IgD concentration (Drenth et al. 1994). Further, other diseases involving chronic inflammation, including sarcoidosis and tuberculosis (Drenth et al. 1994), also cause elevations in IgD. Nevertheless, patients with HIDS may exhibit IgD levels much higher than those seen in other conditions, although the connection with the mevalonate pathway remains enigmatic.

8
Concluding Remarks

As noted by Sir William Harvey, a detailed understanding of rare disorders often informs our understanding of normal physiology. Molecular analysis of the autoinflammatory syndromes described in this manuscript has provided important new insights into the regulation of innate immunity. In the case of FMF and the cryopyrinopathies, positional cloning led to the discovery of novel genes and proteins that define new pathways for the regulation of cytokine production, NF-κB activation, and apoptosis. For PAPA syndrome and HIDS, the underlying genes were already in the databases at the time the causal relationship was discovered, but the connection with autoinflammatory disease was quite unexpected. Even for BS/EOS and TRAPS, for which the underlying genes were already known to be important regulators of inflammation, there have been important mechanistic lessons. Recognition of the molecular basis of these autoinflammatory disorders has provided the conceptual underpinnings for marked improvements in the treatment of the cryopyrinopathies and TRAPS. Continued study of these and other related conditions is likely to lead to further advances in diagnosis, pathogenesis, and treatment that are likely to extend far beyond the patients with these uncommon but fascinating illnesses.

References

Abbott DW, Wilkins A, Asara JM, Cantley LC (2004) The Crohn's disease protein NOD2, requires RIP2 in order to induce ubiquitinylation of a novel site on NEMO Curr Biol 14:2217–2227

Acehan D, Jiang X, Morgan DG, Heuser JE, Wang X, Akey CW (2002) Three-dimensional structure of the apoptosome: implications for assembly, procaspase-9 binding, and activation. Mol Cell 9:423–432

Aganna E, Martinon F, Hawkins PN, Ross JB, Swan DC, Booth DR, Lachmann HJ, Bybee A, Gaudet R, Woo P et al (2002) Association of mutations in the NALP3/CIAS1/PYPAF1 gene with a broad phenotype including recurrent fever, cold sensitivity, sensorineural deafness, and AA amyloidosis. Arthritis Rheum 46:2445–2452

Aganna E, Hammond L, Hawkins PN, Aldea A, McKee SA, van Amstel HK, Mischung C, Kusuhara K, Saulsbury FT, Lachmann HJ et al (2003) Heterogeneity among patients with tumor necrosis factor receptor-associated periodic syndrome phenotypes. Arthritis Rheum 48:2632–2644

Agostini L, Martinon F, Burns K, McDermott MF, Hawkins PN, Tschopp J (2004) NALP3 forms an IL-1beta-processing inflammasome with increased activity in Muckle-Wells autoinflammatory disorder. Immunity 20:319–325

Aksentijevich I, Torosyan Y, Samuels J, Centola M, Pras E, Chae JJ, Oddoux C, Wood G, Azzaro MP, Palumbo G et al (1999) Mutation and haplotype studies of familial Mediterranean fever reveal new ancestral relationships and evidence for a high carrier frequency with reduced penetrance in the Ashkenazi Jewish population. Am J Hum Genet 64:949–962

Aksentijevich I, Galon J, Soares M, Mansfield E, Hull K, Oh HH, Goldbach-Mansky R, Dean J, Athreya B, Reginato AJ et al (2001) The tumor-necrosis-factor receptor-associated periodic syndrome: new mutations in TNFRSF1A, ancestral origins, genotype-phenotype studies, and evidence for further genetic heterogeneity of periodic fevers. Am J Hum Genet 69:301–314

Aksentijevich I, Nowak M, Mallah M, Chae JJ, Watford WT, Hofmann SR, Stein L, Russo R, Goldsmith D, Dent P et al (2002) De novo CIAS1 mutations, cytokine activation, and evidence for genetic heterogeneity in patients with neonatal-onset multisystem inflammatory disease (NOMID): a new member of the expanding family of pyrin-associated autoinflammatory diseases. Arthritis Rheum 46:3340–3348

Al-Alami JR, Tayeh MK, Najib DA, Abu-Rubaiha ZA, Majeed HA, Al-Khateeb MS, El-Shanti HI (2003) Familial Mediterranean fever mutation frequencies and carrier rates among a mixed Arabic population. Saudi Med J 24:1055–1059

Albrecht M, Domingues FS, Schreiber S, Lengauer T (2003) Structural localization of disease-associated sequence variations in the NACHT and LRR domains of PYPAF1 and NOD2. FEBS Lett 554:520–528

Aspenstrom P (1997) A Cdc42 target protein with homology to the non-kinase domain of FER has a potential role in regulating the actin cytoskeleton. Curr Biol 7:479–487

Badour K, Zhang J, Shi F, McGavin MK, Rampersad V, Hardy LA, Field D, Siminovitch KA (2003a) The Wiskott-Aldrich syndrome protein acts downstream of CD2 and the CD2AP and PSTPIP1 adaptors to promote formation of the immunological synapse. Immunity 18:141–154

Badour K, Zhang J, Siminovitch KA (2003b) The Wiskott-Aldrich syndrome protein: forging the link between actin and cell activation. Immunol Rev 192:98–112

Badour K, Zhang J, Shi F, Leng Y, Collins M, Siminovitch KA (2004) Fyn and PTP-PEST-mediated regulation of Wiskott-Aldrich syndrome protein (WASp) tyrosine phosphorylation is required for coupling T cell antigen receptor engagement to WASp effector function and T cell activation. J Exp Med 199:99–112

Banner DW, D'Arcy A, Janes W, Gentz R, Schoenfeld HJ, Broger C, Loetscher H, Lesslauer W (1993) Crystal structure of the soluble human 55 kd TNF receptor-human TNF beta complex: implications for TNF receptor activation. Cell 73:431–445

Ben-Chetrit E, Levy M (1998) Does the lack of the P-glycoprotein efflux pump in neutrophils explain the efficacy of colchicine in familial Mediterranean fever and other inflammatory diseases? Med Hypotheses 51:377–380

Bertin J, DiStefano PS (2000) The PYRIN domain: a novel motif found in apoptosis and inflammation proteins. Cell Death Differ 7:1273–1274

Blau EB (1985) Familial granulomatous arthritis, iritis, and rash. J Pediatr 107:689–693

Booth DR, Gillmore JD, Lachmann HJ, Booth SE, Bybee A, Soyturk M, Akar S, Pepys MB, Tunca M, Hawkins PN (2000) The genetic basis of autosomal dominant familial Mediterranean fever. Q J Med 93:217–221

Brakebusch C, Varfolomeev EE, Batkin M, Wallach D (1994) Structural requirements for inducible shedding of the p55 tumor necrosis factor receptor. J Biol Chem 269:32488–32496

Brown MS, Goldstein JL (1997) The SREBP pathway: regulation of cholesterol metabolism by proteolysis of a membrane-bound transcription factor. Cell 89:331–340

Centola M, Aksentijevich I, Kastner DL (1998) The hereditary periodic fever syndromes: molecular analysis of a new family of inflammatory diseases. Hum Mol Genet 7:1581–1588

Centola M, Wood G, Frucht DM, Galon J, Aringer M, Farrell C, Kingma DW, Horwitz ME, Mansfield E, Holland SM et al (2000) The gene for familial Mediterranean fever MEFV, is expressed in early leukocyte development and is regulated in response to inflammatory mediators. Blood 95:3223–3231

Chae JJ, Komarow HD, Cheng J, Wood G, Raben N, Liu PP, Kastner DL (2003) Targeted disruption of pyrin, the FMF protein, causes heightened sensitivity to endotoxin and a defect in macrophage apoptosis. Mol Cell 11:591–604

Chamaillard M, Girardin SE, Viala J, Philpott DJ (2003a) Nods Nalps and Naip: intracellular regulators of bacterial-induced inflammation. Cell Microbiol 5:581–592

Chamaillard M, Philpott D, Girardin SE, Zouali H, Lesage S, Chareyre F, Bui TH, Giovannini M, Zaehringer U, Penard-Lacronique V et al (2003b) Gene-environment interaction modulated by allelic heterogeneity in inflammatory diseases. Proc Natl Acad Sci U S A 100:3455–3460

Chan FK, Chun HJ, Zheng L, Siegel RM, Bui KL, Lenardo MJ (2000) A domain in TNF receptors that mediates ligand-independent receptor assembly and signaling. Science 288:2351–2354

Chen G, Goeddel DV (2002) TNF-R1 signaling: a beautiful pathway. Science 296:1634–1635

Cote JF, Chung PL, Theberge JF, Halle M, Spencer S, Lasky LA, Tremblay ML (2002) PSTPIP is a substrate of PTP-PEST and serves as a scaffold guiding PTP-PEST toward a specific dephosphorylation of WASP J Biol Chem 277:2973–2986

Cronstein BN, Molad Y, Reibman J, Balakhane E, Levin RI, Weissmann G (1995) Colchicine alters the quantitative and qualitative display of selectins on endothelial cells and neutrophils. J Clin Invest 96:994–1002

Cuisset L, Drenth JP, Simon A, Vincent MF, van der Velde Visser S, van der Meer JW, Grateau G, Delpech M (2001) Molecular analysis of MVK mutations and enzymatic activity in hyper-IgD and periodic fever syndrome. Eur J Hum. Genet 9:260–266

Dailey NJ, Aksentijevich I, Chae JJ, Wesley R, Snyder C, Magalnick M, Watford WT, Gelabert A, Jones J, Pham T-H et al (2004) Interleukin-1 receptor antagonist anakinra in the treatment of neonatal onset multisystem inflammatory disease. Arthritis Rheum 50:S440

Diaz A, Hu C, Kastner DL, Schaner P, Reginato AM, Richards N, Gumucio DL (2004) Lipopolysaccharide-induced expression of multiple alternatively spliced MEFV transcripts in human synovial fibroblasts: a prominent splice isoform lacks the C-terminal domain that is highly mutated in familial Mediterranean fever. Arthritis Rheum 50:3679–3689

Dinarello CA, Wolff SM, Goldfinger SE, Dale DC, Alling DW (1974) Colchicine therapy for familial Mediterranean fever. A double-blind trial. N Engl J Med 291:934–937

Dinarello CA, Chusid MJ, Fauci AS, Gallin JI, Dale DC, Wolff SM (1976) Effect of prophylactic colchicine therapy on leukocyte function in patients with familial Mediterranean fever. Arthritis Rheum 19:618–622

Dode C, Le Du N, Cuisset L, Letourneur F, Berthelot JM, Vaudour G, Meyrier A, Watts RA, Scott DG, Nicholls A et al (2002) New mutations of CIAS1 that are responsible for Muckle-Wells syndrome and familial cold urticaria: a novel mutation underlies both syndromes. Am J Hum Genet 70:1498–1506

Dowds TA, Masumoto J, Chen FF, Ogura Y, Inohara N, Nunez G (2003) Regulation of cryopyrin/Pypaf1 signaling by pyrin, the familial Mediterranean fever gene product. Biochem Biophys Res Commun 302:575–580

Dowds TA, Masumoto J, Zhu L, Inohara N, Nunez G (2004) Cryopyrin-induced interleukin 1beta secretion in monocytic cells: enhanced activity of disease-associated mutants and requirement for ASC. J Biol Chem 279:21924–21928

Drenth JP, Haagsma CJ, van der Meer JW (1994) Hyperimmunoglobulinemia D and periodic fever syndrome. The clinical spectrum in a series of 50 patients. International Hyper-IgD Study Group. Medicine (Baltimore) 73:133–144

Drenth JP, Goertz J, Daha MR, van der Meer JW (1996) Immunoglobulin D enhances the release of tumor necrosis factor-alpha, and interleukin-1 beta as well as interleukin-1 receptor antagonist from human mononuclear cells. Immunology 88:355–362

Drenth JP, Cuisset L, Grateau G, Vasseur C, van de Velde-Visser SD, de Jong JG, Beckmann JS, van der Meer JW, Delpech M (1999) Mutations in the gene encoding mevalonate kinase cause hyper-IgD and periodic fever syndrome. International Hyper-IgD Study Group. Nat Genet 22:178–181

Drewe E, McDermott EM, Powell PT, Isaacs JD, Powell RJ (2003) Prospective study of anti-tumour necrosis factor receptor superfamily 1B fusion protein, and case study of anti-tumour necrosis factor receptor superfamily 1A fusion protein, in tumour necrosis factor receptor associated periodic syndrome (TRAPS): clinical and laboratory findings in a series of seven patients. Rheumatology (Oxford) 42:235–239

Duzova A, Bakkaloglu A, Besbas N, Topaloglu R, Ozen S, Ozaltin F, Bassoy Y, Yilmaz E (2003) Role of A-SAA in monitoring subclinical inflammation and in colchicine dosage in familial Mediterranean fever. Clin Exp Rheumatol 21:509–514

Eckmann L, Karin M (2005) NOD2 and Crohn's disease: loss or gain of function? Immunity 22:661–667

Eliezer D (2003) Folding pyrin into the family. Structure (Camb) 11:1190–1191

Engelmann H, Holtmann H, Brakebusch C, Avni YS, Sarov I, Nophar Y, Hadas E, Leitner O, Wallach D (1990) Antibodies to a soluble form of a tumor necrosis factor (TNF) receptor have TNF-like activity. J Biol Chem 265:14497–14504

Fairbrother WJ, Gordon NC, Humke EW, O'Rourke KM, Starovasnik MA, Yin JP, Dixit VM (2001) The PYRIN domain: a member of the death domain-fold superfamily. Protein Sci 10:1911–1918

Feldmann J, Prieur AM, Quartier P, Berquin P, Certain S, Cortis E, Teillac-Hamel D, Fischer A, de Saint Basile G (2002) Chronic infantile neurological cutaneous and articular syndrome is caused by mutations in CIAS1, a gene highly expressed in polymorphonuclear cells and chondrocytes. Am J Hum Genet 71:198–203

French FMF Consortium (1997) A candidate gene for familial Mediterranean fever. Nat Genet 17:25–31

Frenkel J, Houten SM, Waterham HR, Wanders RJ, Rijkers GT, Duran M, Kuijpers TW, van Luijk W, Poll-The BT, Kuis W (2001) Clinical and molecular variability in childhood periodic fever with hyperimmunoglobulinaemia D. Rheumatology (Oxford) 40:579–584

Frenkel J, Rijkers GT, Mandey SH, Buurman SW, Houten SM, Wanders RJ, Waterham HR, Kuis W (2002) Lack of isoprenoid products raises ex vivo interleukin-1beta secretion in hyperimmunoglobulinemia D and periodic fever syndrome. Arthritis Rheum 46:2794–2803

Frenkel J, Wulffraat NM, Kuis W (2004) Anakinra in mutation-negative NOMID/CINCA syndrome: comment on the articles by Hawkins et al and Hoffman and Patel. Arthritis Rheum 50:3738–3739; author reply 3739–3740

Galon J, Aksentijevich I, McDermott MF, O'Shea JJ, Kastner DL (2000) TNFRSF1A mutations and autoinflammatory syndromes. Curr Opin Immunol 12:479–486

Gershoni-Baruch R, Shinawi M, Leah K, Badarnah K, Brik R (2001) Familial Mediterranean fever: prevalence, penetrance and genetic drift. Eur J Hum Genet 9:634–637

Girardin SE, Boneca IG, Viala J, Chamaillard M, Labigne A, Thomas G, Philpott DJ, Sansonetti PJ (2003) Nod2 is a general sensor of peptidoglycan through muramyl dipeptide (MDP) detection. J Biol Chem 278:8869–8872

Goldstein JL, Brown MS (1990) Regulation of the mevalonate pathway. Nature 343:425–430

Harton JA, Linhoff MW, Zhang J, Ting JP (2002) Cutting edge: CATERPILLER: a large family of mammalian genes containing CARD, pyrin, nucleotide-binding, and leucine-rich repeat domains. J Immunol 169:4088–4093

Hashkes PJ, Lovell DJ (1997) Recognition of infantile-onset multisystem inflammatory disease as a unique entity. J Pediatr 130:513–515

Hassink SG, Goldsmith DP (1983) Neonatal onset multisystem inflammatory disease. Arthritis Rheum 26:668–673

Hawkins PN, Bybee A, Aganna E, McDermott MF (2004a) Response to anakinra in a de novo case of neonatal-onset multisystem inflammatory disease. Arthritis Rheum 50:2708–2709

Hawkins PN, Lachmann HJ, Aganna E, McDermott MF (2004b) Spectrum of clinical features in Muckle-Wells syndrome and response to anakinra. Arthritis Rheum 50:607–612

Henry J, Mather IH, McDermott MF, Pontarotti P (1998) B30.2-like domain proteins: update and new insights into a rapidly expanding family of proteins. Mol Biol Evol 15:1696–1705

Hiller S, Kohl A, Fiorito F, Herrmann T, Wider G, Tschopp J, Grutter MG, Wuthrich K (2003) NMR structure of the apoptosis- and inflammation-related NALP1 pyrin domain. Structure (Camb) 11:1199–1205

Hoffman HM, Mueller JL, Broide DH, Wanderer AA, Kolodner RD (2001a) Mutation of a new gene encoding a putative pyrin-like protein causes familial cold autoinflammatory syndrome and Muckle-Wells syndrome. Nat Genet 29:301–305

Hoffman HM, Wanderer AA, Broide DH (2001b) Familial cold autoinflammatory syndrome: phenotype and genotype of an autosomal dominant periodic fever. J Allergy Clin Immunol 108:615–620

Hoffman HM, Rosengren S, Boyle DL, Cho JY, Nayar J, Mueller JL, Anderson JP, Wanderer AA, Firestein GS (2004) Prevention of cold-associated acute inflammation in familial cold autoinflammatory syndrome by interleukin-1 receptor antagonist. Lancet 364:1779–1785

Hoffmann G, Gibson KM, Brandt IK, Bader PI, Wappner RS, Sweetman L (1986) Mevalonic aciduria–an inborn error of cholesterol and nonsterol isoprene biosynthesis. N Engl J Med 314:1610–1614

Hoffmann GF, Charpentier C, Mayatepek E, Mancini J, Leichsenring M, Gibson KM, Divry P, Hrebicek M, Lehnert W, Sartor K et al (1993) Clinical and biochemical phenotype in 11 patients with mevalonic aciduria. Pediatrics 91:915–921

Houten SM, Kuis W, Duran M, de Koning TJ, van Royen-Kerkhof A, Romeijn GJ, Frenkel J, Dorland L, de Barse MM, Huijbers WA et al (1999a) Mutations in MVK, encoding mevalonate kinase, cause hyperimmunoglobulinaemia D and periodic fever syndrome. Nat Genet 22:175–177

Houten SM, Romeijn GJ, Koster J, Gray RG, Darbyshire P, Smit GP, de Klerk JB, Duran M, Gibson KM, Wanders RJ et al (1999b) Identification and characterization of three novel missense mutations in mevalonate kinase cDNA causing mevalonic aciduria, a disorder of isoprene biosynthesis. Hum Mol Genet 8:1523–1528

Houten SM, Koster J, Romeijn GJ, Frenkel J, Di Rocco M, Caruso U, Landrieu P, Kelley RI, Kuis W, Poll-The BT et al (2001) Organization of the mevalonate kinase (MVK) gene and identification of novel mutations causing mevalonic aciduria and hyperimmunoglobulinaemia D and periodic fever syndrome. Eur J Hum Genet 9:253–259

Houten SM, Frenkel J, Rijkers GT, Wanders RJ, Kuis W, Waterham HR (2002) Temperature dependence of mutant mevalonate kinase activity as a pathogenic factor in hyper-IgD and periodic fever syndrome. Hum Mol Genet 11:3115–3124

Houten SM, Schneiders MS, Wanders RJ, Waterham HR (2003) Regulation of isoprenoid/cholesterol biosynthesis in cells from mevalonate kinase-deficient patients. J Biol Chem 278:5736–5743

Huggins ML, Radford PM, McIntosh RS, Bainbridge SE, Dickinson P, Draper-Morgan KA, Tighe PJ, Powell RJ, Todd I (2004) Shedding of mutant tumor necrosis factor receptor superfamily 1A associated with tumor necrosis factor receptor-associated periodic syndrome: differences between cell types. Arthritis Rheum 50:2651–2659

Hugot JP, Chamaillard M, Zouali H, Lesage S, Cezard JP, Belaiche J, Almer S, Tysk C, O'Morain CA, Gassull M et al (2001) Association of NOD2 leucine-rich repeat variants with susceptibility to Crohn's disease. Nature 411:599–603

Hull KM, Drewe E, Aksentijevich I, Singh HK, Wong K, McDermott EM, Dean J, Powell RJ, Kastner DL (2002) The TNF receptor-associated periodic syndrome (TRAPS): emerging concepts of an autoinflammatory disorder. Medicine (Baltimore) 81:349–368

Hull KM, Shoham N, Chae JJ, Aksentijevich I, Kastner DL (2003) The expanding spectrum of systemic autoinflammatory disorders and their rheumatic manifestations. Curr Opin Rheumatol 15:61–69

Inohara N, del Peso L, Koseki T, Chen S, Nunez G (1998) RICK, a novel protein kinase containing a caspase recruitment domain, interacts with CLARP and regulates CD95-mediated apoptosis. J Biol Chem 273:12296–12300

Inohara N, Ogura Y, Fontalba A, Gutierrez O, Pons F, Crespo J, Fukase K, Inamura S, Kusumoto S, Hashimoto M et al (2003) Host recognition of bacterial muramyl dipeptide mediated through NOD2. Implications for Crohn's disease. J Biol Chem 278:5509–5512

International FMF Consortium (1997) Ancient missense mutations in a new member of the RoRet gene family are likely to cause familial Mediterranean fever. Cell 90:797–807

Jabs DA, Houk JL, Bias WB, Arnett FC (1985) Familial granulomatous synovitis, uveitis, and cranial neuropathies. Am J Med 78:801–804

Jeru I, Papin S, L'Hoste S, Duquesnoy P, Cazeneuve C, Camonis J, Amselem S (2005) Interaction of pyrin with 14.3.3 in an isoform-specific and phosphorylation-dependent manner regulates its translocation to the nucleus. Arthritis Rheum 52:1848–1857

Kanazawa N, Okafuji I, Kambe N, Nishikomori R, Nakata-Hizume M, Nagai S, Fuji A, Yuasa T, Manki A, Sakurai Y et al (2005) Early-onset sarcoidosis and CARD15 mutations with constitutive nuclear factor-kappaB activation: common genetic etiology with Blau syndrome. Blood 105:1195–1197

Kanneganti T-D, Özören N, Body-Malapel M, Amer A, Park J-H, Franchi L, Whitfield J, Barchet W, Colonna M, Vandenabeele P, Bertin J, Coyle A, Grant EP, Akira S, Núñez G (2006) Bacterial RNA and small antiviral compounds activate caspase-1 through cryopyrin/Nalp3. Nature (in press)

Kelley RI (2000) Inborn errors of cholesterol biosynthesis. Adv Pediatr 47:1–53

Kelley RI, Takada I (2002) Hereditary periodic fever. N Engl J Med 346:1415–1416; author reply 1415–1416

Kobayashi KS, Chamaillard M, Ogura Y, Henegariu O, Inohara N, Nunez G, Flavell RA (2005) Nod2-dependent regulation of innate and adaptive immunity in the intestinal tract. Science 307:731–734

Kogan A, Shinar Y, Lidar M, Revivo A, Langevitz P, Padeh S, Pras M, Livneh A (2001) Common MEFV mutations among Jewish ethnic groups in Israel: high frequency of carrier and phenotype III states and absence of a perceptible biological advantage for the carrier state. Am J Med Genet 102:272–276

Koonin EV, Aravind L (2000) The NACHT family—a new group of predicted NTPases implicated in apoptosis and MHC transcription activation. Trends Biochem Sci 25:223–224

Korkmaz C, Ozdogan H, Kasapcopur O, Yazici H (2002) Acute phase response in familial Mediterranean fever. Ann Rheum Dis 61:79–81

Kriegel MA, Huffmeier U, Scherb E, Scheidig C, Geiler T, Kalden JR, Reis A, Lorenz HM (2003) Tumor necrosis factor receptor-associated periodic syndrome characterized by a mutation affecting the cleavage site of the receptor: implications for pathogenesis. Arthritis Rheum 48:2386–2388

Li J, Nishizawa K, An W, Hussey RE, Lialios FE, Salgia R, Sunder-Plassmann R, Reinherz EL (1998) A cdc15-like adaptor protein (CD2BP1) interacts with the CD2 cytoplasmic domain and regulates CD2-triggered adhesion. EMBO J 17:7320–7336

Li J, Moran T, Swanson E, Julian C, Harris J, Bonen DK, Hedl M, Nicolae DL, Abraham C, Cho JH (2004) Regulation of IL-8 and IL-1beta expression in Crohn's disease associated NOD2/CARD15 mutations. Hum Mol Genet 13:1715–1725

Liepinsh E, Barbals R, Dahl E, Sharipo A, Staub E, Otting G (2003) The death-domain fold of the ASC PYRIN domain, presenting a basis for PYRIN/PYRIN recognition. J Mol Biol 332:1155–1163

Lindor NM, Arsenault TM, Solomon H, Seidman CE, McEvoy MT (1997) A new autosomal dominant disorder of pyogenic sterile arthritis, pyoderma gangrenosum, and acne: PAPA syndrome. Mayo Clin Proc 72:611–615

Liu T, Rojas A, Ye Y, Godzik A (2003) Homology modeling provides insights into the binding mode of the PAAD/DAPIN/pyrin domain, a fourth member of the CARD/DD/DED domain family. Protein Sci 12:1872–1881

MacEwan DJ (2002) TNF receptor subtype signalling: differences and cellular consequences. Cell Signal 14:477–492

Maeda S, Hsu LC, Liu H, Bankston LA, Iimura M, Kagnoff MF, Eckmann L, Karin M (2005) Nod2 mutation in Crohn's disease potentiates NF-kappaB activity and IL-1beta processing. Science 307:734–738

Manji GA, Wang L, Geddes BJ, Brown M, Merriam S, Al-Garawi A, Mak S, Lora JM, Briskin M, Jurman M et al (2002) PYPAF1, a PYRIN-containing Apaf1-like protein that assembles with ASC and regulates activation of NF-kappa B J Biol Chem 277:11570–11575

Mansfield E, Chae JJ, Komarow HD, Brotz TM, Frucht DM, Aksentijevich I, Kastner DL (2001) The familial Mediterranean fever protein, pyrin, associates with microtubules and colocalizes with actin filaments. Blood 98:851–859

Mariathasan S, Newton K, Monack DM, Vucic D, French DM, Lee WP, Roose-Girma M, Erickson S, Dixit VM (2004) Differential activation of the inflammasome by caspase-1 adaptors ASC and Ipaf. Nature 430:213–218

Mariathasan S, Weiss DS, Newton K, McBride J, O'Rourke K, Roose-Girma M, Lee P, Weinrauch Y, Monack DM, Dixit VM (2006) Cryopyrin activates the inflammasome in response to toxins and ATP. Nature (in press)

Martinon F, Tschopp J (2004) Inflammatory caspases: linking an intracellular innate immune system to autoinflammatory diseases. Cell 117:561–574

Martinon F, Tschopp J (2005) NLRs join TLRs as innate sensors of pathogens. Trends Immunol 26:447–454

Martinon F, Hofmann K, Tschopp J (2001) The pyrin domain: a possible member of the death domain-fold family implicated in apoptosis and inflammation. Curr Biol 11:R118–120

Martinon F, Burns K, Tschopp J (2002) The inflammasome: a molecular platform triggering activation of inflammatory caspases and processing of proIL-beta. Mol Cell 10:417–426

Martinon F, Agostini L, Meylan E, Tschopp J (2004) Identification of bacterial muramyl dipeptide as activator of the NALP3/cryopyrin inflammasome. Curr Biol 14:1929–1934

Martinon F, Pétrilli V, Mayor A, Tardivel A, Tschopp J (2006) Gout-associated uric acid crystals activate the NALP3 inflammasome. Nature (in press)

Masumoto J, Taniguchi S, Ayukawa K, Sarvotham H, Kishino T, Niikawa N, Hidaka E, Katsuyama T, Higuchi T, Sagara J (1999) ASC, a novel 22-kDa protein, aggregates during apoptosis of human promyelocytic leukemia HL-60 cells. J Biol Chem 274:33835–33838

Masumoto J, Dowds TA, Schaner P, Chen FF, Ogura Y, Li M, Zhu L, Katsuyama T, Sagara J, Taniguchi S et al (2003) ASC is an activating adaptor for NF-kappa B and caspase-8-dependent apoptosis. Biochem Biophys Res Commun 303:69–73

Matzner Y, Abedat S, Shapiro E, Eisenberg S, Bar-Gil-Shitrit A, Stepensky P, Calco S, Azar Y, Urieli-Shoval S (2000) Expression of the familial Mediterranean fever gene and activity of the C5a inhibitor in human primary fibroblast cultures. Blood 96:727–731

McCarthy JV, Ni J, Dixit VM (1998) RIP2 is a novel NF-kappaB-activating and cell death-inducing kinase. J Biol Chem 273:16968–16975

McDermott EM, Smillie DM, Powell RJ (1997) Clinical spectrum of familial Hibernian fever: a 14-year follow-up study of the index case and extended family. Mayo Clin Proc 72:806–817

McDermott MF, Aksentijevich I, Galon J, McDermott EM, Ogunkolade BW, Centola M, Mansfield E, Gadina M, Karenko L, Pettersson T et al (1999) Germline mutations in the extracellular domains of the 55 kDa TNF receptor TNFR1, define a family of dominantly inherited autoinflammatory syndromes. Cell 97:133–144

Medzhitov R, Janeway CA Jr (1998) An ancient system of host defense. Curr Opin Immunol 10:12–15

Miceli-Richard C, Lesage S, Rybojad M, Prieur AM, Manouvrier-Hanu S, Hafner R, Chamaillard M, Zouali H, Thomas G, Hugot JP (2001) CARD15 mutations in Blau syndrome. Nat Genet 29:19–20

Miller JJ 3rd (1986) Early-onset "sarcoidosis" and "familial granulomatous arthritis (arteritis)": the same disease. J Pediatr 109:387–388

Mullberg J, Durie FH, Otten-Evans C, Alderson MR, Rose-John S, Cosman D, Black RA, Mohler KM (1995) A metalloprotease inhibitor blocks shedding of the IL-6 receptor and the p60 TNF receptor. J Immunol 155:5198–5205

Nevala H, Karenko L, Stjernberg S, Raatikainen M, Suomalainen H, Lagerstedt A, Rauta J, McDermott MF, Peterson P, Pettersson T et al (2002) A novel mutation in the third extracellular domain of the tumor necrosis factor receptor 1 in a Finnish family with autosomal-dominant recurrent fever. Arthritis Rheum 46:1061–1066

Neven B, Callebaut I, Prieur AM, Feldmann J, Bodemer C, Lepore L, Derfalvi B, Benjaponpitak S, Vesely R, Sauvain MJ et al (2004) Molecular basis of the spectral expression of CIAS1 mutations associated with phagocytic cell-mediated autoinflammatory disorders CINCA/NOMID, MWS, and FCU. Blood 103:2809–2815

O'Connor W Jr, Harton JA, Zhu X, Linhoff MW, Ting JP (2003) CIAS1/cryopyrin/PYPAF1/NALP3/CATERPILLER 1.1 is an inducible inflammatory mediator with NF-kappa B suppressive properties. J Immunol 171:6329–6333

Obici L, Manno C, Muda AO, Picco P, D'Osualdo A, Palladini G, Avanzini MA, Torres D, Marciano S, Merlini G (2004) First report of systemic reactive (AA) amyloidosis in a patient with the hyperimmunoglobulinemia D with periodic fever syndrome. Arthritis Rheum 50:2966–2969

Ogura Y, Inohara N, Benito A, Chen FF, Yamaoka S, Nunez G (2001) Nod2, a Nod1/Apaf-1 family member that is restricted to monocytes and activates NF-kappaB J Biol Chem 276:4812–4818

Ostuni P, Vertolli U, Marson P (1996) Atypical hypergammaglobulinaemia D syndrome with amyloidosis: an overlap with familial Mediterranean fever? Clin Rheumatol 15:610–612

Pawlowski K, Pio F, Chu Z, Reed JC, Godzik A (2001) PAAD—a new protein domain associated with apoptosis, cancer and autoimmune diseases. Trends Biochem Sci 26:85–87

Perron MJ, Stremlau M, Song B, Ulm W, Mulligan RC, Sodroski J (2004) TRIM5alpha mediates the postentry block to N-tropic murine leukemia viruses in human cells. Proc Natl Acad Sci U S A 101:11827–11832

Peschon JJ, Torrance DS, Stocking KL, Glaccum MB, Otten C, Willis CR, Charrier K, Morrissey PJ, Ware CB, Mohler KM (1998) TNF receptor-deficient mice reveal divergent roles for p55 and p75 in several models of inflammation. J Immunol 160:943–952

Pfeffer K, Matsuyama T, Kundig TM, Wakeham A, Kishihara K, Shahinian A, Wiegmann K, Ohashi PS, Kronke M, Mak TW (1993) Mice deficient for the 55 kd tumor necrosis factor receptor are resistant to endotoxic shock, yet succumb to L monocytogenes infection. Cell 73:457–467

Prieur AM, Griscelli C (1981) Arthropathy with rash, chronic meningitis, eye lesions, and mental retardation. J Pediatr 99:79–83

Prieur AM, Griscelli C, Lampert F, Truckenbrodt H, Guggenheim MA, Lovell DJ, Pelkonnen P, Chevrant-Breton J, Ansell BM (1987) A chronic, infantile, neurological, cutaneous and articular (CINCA) syndrome. A specific entity analysed in 30 patients. Scand J Rheumatol Suppl 66:57–68

Prieur AM (2001) A recently recognised chronic inflammatory disease of early onset characterised by the triad of rash, central nervous system involvement and arthropathy. Clin Exp Rheumatol 19:103-106

Rahman P, Bartlett S, Siannis F, Pellett FJ, Farewell VT, Peddle L, Schentag CT, Alderdice CA, Hamilton S, Khraishi M et al (2003) CARD15: a pleiotropic autoimmune gene that confers susceptibility to psoriatic arthritis. Am J Hum Genet 73:677-681

Raphael SA, Blau EB, Zhang WH, Hsu SH (1993) Analysis of a large kindred with Blau syndrome for HLA, autoimmunity, and sarcoidosis. Am J Dis Child 147:842-848

Richards N, Schaner P, Diaz A, Stuckey J, Shelden E, Wadhwa A, Gumucio DL (2001) Interaction between pyrin and the apoptotic speck protein (ASC) modulates ASC-induced apoptosis. J Biol Chem 276:39320-39329

Saulsbury FT (2003) Hyperimmunoglobulinemia D and periodic fever syndrome (HIDS) in a child with normal serum IgD, but increased serum IgA concentration. J Pediatr 143:127-129

Schall TJ, Lewis M, Koller KJ, Lee A, Rice GC, Wong GH, Gatanaga T, Granger GA, Lentz R, Raab H et al (1990) Molecular cloning and expression of a receptor for human tumor necrosis factor. Cell 61:361-370

Schaner P, Richards N, Wadhwa A, Aksentijevich I, Kastner D, Tucker P, Gumucio D (2001) Episodic evolution of pyrin in primates: human mutations recapitulate ancestral amino acid states. Nat Genet 27:318-321

Seto MH, Liu HL, Zajchowski DA, Whitlow M (1999) Protein fold analysis of the B30.2-like domain. Proteins 35:235-249

Shoham NG, Centola M, Mansfield E, Hull KM, Wood G, Wise CA, Kastner DL (2003) Pyrin binds the PSTPIP1/CD2BP1 protein, defining familial Mediterranean fever and PAPA syndrome as disorders in the same pathway. Proc Natl Acad Sci U S A 100:13501-13506

Siebert S, Amos N, Fielding CA, Wang EC, Aksentijevich I, Williams BD, Brennan P (2005) Reduced tumor necrosis factor signaling in primary human fibroblasts containing a tumor necrosis factor receptor superfamily 1A mutant. Arthritis Rheum 52:1287-1292

Simon A, Drenth JP (1999) Genes associated with periodic fevers highlighted at Dutch workshop. Lancet 354:2141

Simon A, Mariman EC, van der Meer JW, Drenth JP (2003) A founder effect in the hyperimmunoglobulinemia D and periodic fever syndrome. Am J Med 114:148-152

Sinensky M (2000) Recent advances in the study of prenylated proteins. Biochim Biophys Acta 1484:93-106

Song B, Javanbakht H, Perron M, Park do H, Stremlau M, Sodroski J (2005) Retrovirus restriction by TRIM5alpha variants from Old World and New World primates. J Virol 79:3930-3937

Spencer S, Dowbenko D, Cheng J, Li W, Brush J, Utzig S, Simanis V, Lasky LA (1997) PSTPIP: a tyrosine phosphorylated cleavage furrow-associated protein that is a substrate for a PEST tyrosine phosphatase. J Cell Biol 138:845-860

Srinivasula SM, Poyet JL, Razmara M, Datta P, Zhang Z, Alnemri ES (2002) The PYRIN-CARD protein ASC is an activating adaptor for caspase-1. J Biol Chem 277:21119-21122

Staub E, Dahl E, Rosenthal A (2001) The DAPIN family: a novel domain links apoptotic and interferon response proteins. Trends Biochem Sci 26:83–85

Stehlik C, Fiorentino L, Dorfleutner A, Bruey JM, Ariza EM, Sagara J, Reed JC (2002) The PAAD/PYRIN-family protein ASC is a dual regulator of a conserved step in nuclear factor kappaB activation pathways. J Exp Med 196:1605–1615

Stehlik C, Lee SH, Dorfleutner A, Stassinopoulos A, Sagara J, Reed JC (2003) Apoptosis-associated speck-like protein containing a caspase recruitment domain is a regulator of procaspase-1 activation. J Immunol 171:6154–6163

Stoffman N, Magal N, Shohat T, Lotan R, Koman S, Oron A, Danon Y, Halpern GJ, Lifshitz Y, Shohat M (2000) Higher than expected carrier rates for familial Mediterranean fever in various Jewish ethnic groups. Eur J Hum Genet 8:307–310

Stojanov S, Kastner DL (2005) Familial autoinflammatory diseases: genetics, pathogenesis and treatment. Curr Opin Rheumatol 17:586–599

Takeda K, Kaisho T, Akira S (2003) Toll-like receptors. Annu Rev Immunol 21:335–376

Tanabe T, Chamaillard M, Ogura Y, Zhu L, Qiu S, Masumoto J, Ghosh P, Moran A, Predergast MM, Tromp G et al (2004) Regulatory regions and critical residues of NOD2 involved in muramyl dipeptide recognition. EMBO J 23:1587–1597

Thome M, Hofmann K, Burns K, Martinon F, Bodmer JL, Mattmann C, Tschopp J (1998) Identification of CARDIAK, a RIP-like kinase that associates with caspase-1. Curr Biol 8:885–888

Ting JP, Davis BK (2004) CATERPILLER: a novel gene family important in immunity, cell death, and diseases. Annu Rev Immunol 23:387–414

Todd I, Radford PM, Draper-Morgan KA, McIntosh R, Bainbridge S, Dickinson P, Jamhawi L, Sansaridis M, Huggins ML, Tighe PJ et al (2004) Mutant forms of tumour necrosis factor receptor I that occur in TNF-receptor-associated periodic syndrome retain signalling functions but show abnormal behaviour. Immunology 113:65–79

Touitou I (2001) The spectrum of familial Mediterranean fever (FMF) mutations. Eur J Hum. Genet 9:473–483

Touitou I, Lesage S, McDermott M, Cuisset L, Hoffman H, Dode C, Shoham N, Aganna E, Hugot JP, Wise C et al (2004) Infevers: an evolving mutation database for autoinflammatory syndromes. Hum Mutat 24:194–198

Tschopp J, Martinon F, Burns K (2003) NALPs: a novel protein family involved in inflammation. Nat Rev Mol Cell Biol 4:95–104

Tunca M, Kirkali G, Soyturk M, Akar S, Pepys MB, Hawkins PN (1999) Acute phase response and evolution of familial Mediterranean fever. Lancet 353:1415

Valle D (1999) You give me fever. Nat Genet 22:121–122

Van der Meer JW, Vossen JM, Radl J, van Nieuwkoop JA, Meyer CJ, Lobatto S, van Furth R (1984) Hyperimmunoglobulinaemia D and periodic fever: a new syndrome. Lancet 1:1087–1090

Vernet C, Boretto J, Mattei MG, Takahashi M, Jack LJ, Mather IH, Rouquier S, Pontarotti P (1993) Evolutionary study of multigenic families mapping close to the human MHC class I region. J Mol Evol 37:600–612

Walker JE, Saraste M, Runswick MJ, Gay NJ (1982) Distantly related sequences in the alpha- and beta-subunits of ATP synthase, myosin, kinases and other ATP-requiring enzymes and a common nucleotide binding fold. EMBO J 1:945–951

Wallach D, Engelmann H, Nophar Y, Aderka D, Kemper O, Hornik V, Holtmann H, Brakebusch C (1991) Soluble and cell surface receptors for tumor necrosis factor. Agents Actions Suppl 35:51–57

Wang L, Manji GA, Grenier JM, Al-Garawi A, Merriam S, Lora JM, Geddes BJ, Briskin M, DiStefano PS, Bertin J (2002) PYPAF7, a novel PYRIN-containing Apaf1-like protein that regulates activation of NF-kappa B and caspase-1-dependent cytokine processing. J Biol Chem 277:29874–29880

Wang X, Kuivaniemi H, Bonavita G, Williams CJ, Tromp G (2002) High-resolution physical map for chromosome 16q12.1-q13, the Blau syndrome locus. BMC Genomics 3:24

Watanabe T, Kitani A, Murray PJ, Strober W (2004) NOD2 is a negative regulator of Toll-like receptor 2-mediated T helper type 1 responses. Nat Immunol 5:800–808

Williamson LM, Hull D, Mehta R, Reeves WG, Robinson BH, Toghill PJ (1982) Familial Hibernian fever. Q J Med 51:469–480

Wise CA, Gillum JD, Seidman CE, Lindor NM, Veile R, Bashiardes S, Lovett M (2002) Mutations in CD2BP1 disrupt binding to PTP PEST and are responsible for PAPA syndrome, an autoinflammatory disorder. Hum Mol Genet 11:961–969

Yilmaz E, Ozen S, Balci B, Duzova A, Topaloglu R, Besbas N, Saatci U, Bakkaloglu A, Ozguc M (2001) Mutation frequency of familial Mediterranean fever and evidence for a high carrier rate in the Turkish population. Eur J Hum Genet 9:553–555

Yousaf N, Gould DJ, Aganna E, Hammond L, Mirakian RM, Turner MD, Hitman GA, McDermott MF, Chernajovsky Y (2005) Tumor necrosis factor receptor I from patients with tumor necrosis factor receptor-associated periodic syndrome interacts with wild-type tumor necrosis factor receptor I and induces ligand-independent NF-kappaB activation. Arthritis Rheum 52:2906–2916

Yu JW, Wu J, Zhang Z, Datta P, Ibrahimi I, Taniguchi S, Sagara J, Fernandes-Alnemri T, Alnemri ES (2005) Cryopyrin and pyrin activate caspase-1, but not NF-kappaB, via ASC oligomerization. Cell Death Differ [Epub ahead of print]

Zemer D, Revach M, Pras M, Modan B, Schor S, Sohar E, Gafni J (1974) A controlled trial of colchicine in preventing attacks of familial Mediterranean fever. N Engl J Med 291:932–934

Zemer D, Pras M, Sohar E, Modan M, Cabili S, Gafni J (1986) Colchicine in the prevention and treatment of the amyloidosis of familial Mediterranean fever. N Engl J Med 314:1001–1005

Zemer D, Livneh A, Danon YL, Pras M, Sohar E (1991) Long-term colchicine treatment in children with familial Mediterranean fever. Arthritis Rheum 34:973–977

Zou H, Henzel WJ, Liu X, Lutschg A, Wang X (1997) Apaf-1, a human protein homologous to C elegans CED-4, participates in cytochrome c-dependent activation of caspase-3. Cell 90:405–413

Inefficient Clearance of Dying Cells and Autoreactivity

U. S. Gaipl[1] · A. Sheriff[1] · S. Franz[1] · L. E. Munoz[1] · R. E. Voll[2] · J. R. Kalden[1] · M. Herrmann[1] (✉)

[1] Institute for Clinical Immunology, Friedrich-Alexander-University of Erlangen-Nuremberg, Glückstrasse 4a, 91054 Erlangen, Germany
martin.herrmann@med3.imed.uni-erlangen.de

[2] IZKF Research Group N2, Nikolaus-Fiebiger Center of Molecular Medicine, Glückstr. 6, 91054 Erlangen, Germany

1	The Comeback of Dying Cells 162
2	Various Molecules Are Involved in the Clearance of Dying Cells 163
3	C-Reactive Protein and Dying Cells 164
4	Complement and DNase I Act as Back-up Molecules in the Clearance Process 165
5	Phosphatidylserine Exposure as One Early Membrane Change of Apoptotic Cells 165
6	Changes in the Glycoprotein Composition of Membranes of Apoptotic Cells 166
7	Impaired Clearance Functions and Autoimmunity 168
8	Heterogeneous and Intrinsic Clearance Defects in Some SLE Patients . . . 170
9	Conclusion 171
References 171

Abstract Dying cells were basically unnoticed by scientists for a long time and only came back into the spotlight roughly 10 years ago. The process of recognition and uptake of apoptotic and necrotic cells is complex and failures in this process can contribute to the pathogenesis of autoimmune diseases such as systemic lupus erythematosus (SLE). Here, we discuss the recognition and uptake molecules which are involved in an efficient clearance of dying cells in early and late phases of cell death. The exposure of phosphatidylserine (PS) is an early surface change of apoptosing cells recognized by several receptors and adaptor molecules. We demonstrated that dying cells have cell membranes with high lateral mobility of PS, which contribute to their efficient clearance. Changes of the glycoprotein composition of apoptotic cells occur later than the exposure of PS. We further observed that complement binding is an early event in necrosis and a rather late event in apoptosis. Complement, C-reactive protein (CRP), and serum DNase I act as back-up molecules in the clearance process. Finally, we discuss how the accumulation of secondary necrotic cells and cellular debris in the germinal centers of secondary lymph organs can lead to autoimmunity. It is reasonable to argue that clearance defects are major players in the development of autoimmune diseases such as SLE.

1
The Comeback of Dying Cells

About a decade ago scientists became aware that the disappearance of dead and dying cells is not just simple trash removal, and even more, that failure of removal has severe consequences and can lead to autoimmunity. The process of recognition and uptake of those cells is very complex and highly regulated. Cells can die in two main ways: apoptosis and necrosis. Apoptotic cells, which maintain their membrane integrity for a certain time, have to be cleared quickly and efficiently to prevent the release of tissue-damaging intracellular constituents, which consecutively initiates inflammation. Apoptosis is viewed as programmed cell death or cellular suicide and is characterized by specific morphological changes of the dying cells, including loss of membrane asymmetry, nuclear condensation, and DNA fragmentation. Apoptotic cells are rarely to found in vivo because of their rapid and efficient clearance by professional or even amateur phagocytes.

Necrotic cells need to be removed efficiently to limit organ damage and enable timely tissue repair. Apoptotic cells are normally cleared via an antiinflammatory pathway [19, 68]. In contrast to apoptotic cells, the uptake and removal of necrotic or lysed cells normally involves inflammation and an immune response. The morphological and biochemical characteristics of cells dying by necrosis differ markedly from those of cells dying by apoptosis [69]. Necrosis is characterized by swelling of cells and their organelles leading to the disruption of the cell membrane. The chromatin of a primary necrotic cell does not get fragmented, whereas it does in apoptotic cells [36]. The major difference between apoptotic and necrotic cells is the loss of membrane integrity in the latter. Cells dying by programmed cell death also get leaky, but only when they enter late stages of apoptosis. They are then called secondary necrotic cells. It has been shown that the high-mobility group B1 (HMGB1) protein that is "frozen" on the chromatin of apoptotic cells remains immobilized even under conditions of secondary necrosis, while in the case of primary necrotic cells it is released and acts as an inflammatory cytokine [60].

Therefore, even primary and secondary necrotic cells display different inflammatory signals. Another important regulator of inflammatory and immune responses is extracellular ATP. It can affect the functions of many cells via activation of P2 purinoceptors [15]. As one example, the semimaturation state of dendritic cells (DCs), characterized by the upregulation of co-stimulatory molecules and the inhibition of pro-inflammatory cytokines, can be caused by ATP released from necrotic cells [41]. ATP can be released by regulated exocytosis, traumatic cell lysis, or passive leakage from damaged cells.

2
Various Molecules Are Involved in the Clearance of Dying Cells

One major "eat me" signal for phagocytes on both apoptotic and necrotic cells is the exposure of phosphatidylserine (PS) [28]. Many receptors and adaptor molecules have been shown to contribute to the recognition and uptake of apoptotic cells by phagocytes (reviewed in [59]): collectin receptors, calreticulin/CD91, Fcγ-receptors, c-Mer, the β2-glycoprotein-1-receptor, integrins, lectins, CD14, the putative PS-receptor, ABC transporters, and scavenger receptors including CD36. Most of these receptors do not directly bind to apoptotic cells, rather the dying cells are engaged via bridging molecules (reviewed in [25]). Normally, apoptotic cells are efficiently taken up by phagocytes in the early phase of apoptosis. Defects in important recognition molecules for apoptotic cells can lead to autoimmunity [25]. Impaired clearance of apoptotic cell material or increased apoptosis has been implicated in the pathogenesis of systemic lupus erythematosus (SLE) [27, 38, 43]. Several gene-targeted mice that show defects in apoptosis and in the disposal of effete cells have been described to develop autoimmunity. In C1q-deficient mice, significantly greater numbers of glomerular apoptotic bodies were found and spontaneous development of autoantibodies was observed [9, 10]. DNase-I-deficient mice also display classical symptoms of SLE [46]. Mice with targeted deletion of the serum amyloid P component (SAP) gene have enhanced anti-DNA responses to immunization with extrinsic chromatin and spontaneously develop antinuclear autoimmunity [6]. SAP and DNase I are molecules that mask and digest autoantigens. Besides masking chromatin, SAP seems to function as an opsonin, enhancing phagocytosis of bound material [5]. Many other molecules like C1q or IgM [18] promote the clearance of dying cells [70]. Just recently, an impaired uptake of apoptotic B cells in the germinal centers in milk fat globule epidermal growth factor (EGF) factor 8 (MFG-E8)-deficient mice was observed [24]. MFG-E8 is a protein that binds to apoptotic cells by recognizing PS and that enhances the engulfment of apoptotic cells by macrophages. The above-mentioned molecules involved in the clearance of dying cells in mice also play important roles in human beings.

3
C-Reactive Protein and Dying Cells

C-reactive protein (CRP) is capable of binding to cells provided that they contain a substantial amount of lysophosphatidylcholine (lyso-PC) in the outer leaflet of their membranes, as in the case of dying cells. Once bound, CRP induces complement activation via the classical pathway, which in turn triggers the influx of neutrophils, decorates the surface of the ligand with opsonizing complement fragments and enhances phagocytosis of the cells that have bound CRP and complement. CRP also interacts with Fc receptors on phagocytic cells and acts as an opsonin. Because the occurrence of lyso-PC is dependent on the exposure of PS, CRP, in this chronological view, efficiently decorates late apoptotic cells [67]. In addition to binding to the membrane of intact injured cells, CRP also binds to membranes and nuclear constituents of necrotic cells. Several nuclear constituents, including histones, small nuclear ribonucleoproteins, and ribonucleoprotein particles have been shown to bind CRP in a calcium-dependent fashion. Deposition of CRP to nuclei of necrotic cells at sites of inflammation has been observed, whereas CRP does not cross the plasma membrane of apoptotic cells. This might be considered another reasonable mechanism of fine tuning the differentiation between apoptosis and necrosis.

Characteristically, in human SLE, there is relative failure of the acute phase CRP response during active disease despite evident tissue inflammation [48]. Plasma and whole-body turnover studies of human CRP demonstrated that there was no evidence for accelerated clearance or catabolism of CRP [66]. The synthesis rate of CRP might thus be the only significant determinant of its plasma level.

Recently, a polymorphism at the C-reactive protein locus (CRP 4) has been detected in all 586 SLE families analyzed. It is located in the 3'-untranslated region (UTR). The significance of this polymorphism is not known. Since the stability of mRNA species depends on sequences within the 3'-UTR, it is of interest that CRP has a disproportionately long 3'-UTR. The mechanism which influences basal CRP expression remains to be established, but it may operate at the transcriptional or post-transcriptional stage, perhaps by specifying low levels of the protein [56]. A low CRP level could also be explained by IgG antibodies to CRP which are found in 78% of SLE patients [3] and may be able to deplete CRP.

4
Complement and DNase I Act as Back-up Molecules in the Clearance Process

An impaired uptake of apoptotic cells by human macrophages was observed in human serum depleted of specific complement components (C1q, C3) [42, 64]. We observed that complement binding is an early event in necrosis and a rather late event in the case of apoptosis. Complement components, mainly C1q, C3, and C4 act as back-up mechanism to clear apoptotic cells before they enter the dangerous stage of secondary necrosis [21, 22]. Disturbed clearance of nuclear DNA-protein complexes, remnants of dying cells, may initiate and propagate SLE [4, 54]. This is further substantiated by decreased levels of DNase I activity, as had been observed in the sera of SLE patients [14] and patients with other autoimmune diseases such as rheumatoid arthritis (RA) (U.S. Gaipl et al., unpublished data). DNase I, being the major serum nuclease, may be responsible for the degradation of chromatin accidentally released by inappropriately cleared dead cells [39]. Furthermore, DNase I acts together with C1q to efficiently degrade necrotic cell-derived chromatin [23]. A cooperation of DNase I with the plasminogen system was also suggested to contribute to a fast and effective breakdown of chromatin during necrosis [47]. The complement component C1q was found to be necessary for an effective uptake of degraded chromatin by monocyte-derived phagocytes [23] and acts together with soluble IgM in the clearance of dying cells [50]. We tested sera of autoimmune patients with regard to their ability to degrade necrotic cell-derived chromatin. A significant activity reduction of DNase I in sera of SLE and RA patients in comparison to normal healthy donors (NHDs) was observed. Most interestingly, SLE sera showed a strongly reduced degradation capacity of necrotic cell-derived chromatin in comparison to RA sera and NHD sera (U.S. Gaipl et al., unpublished data). This might be due to reduced complement activity detected mainly in the sera of SLE patients. We conclude that an additional protection from chromatin implicated in the development of autoimmune disorders such as SLE can be achieved by the C1q and DNase-I-dependent clearance of degraded chromatin.

5
Phosphatidylserine Exposure as One Early Membrane Change of Apoptotic Cells

Besides adaptor molecules such as complement, membrane changes in the very early phase of apoptosis serve as a recognition signal for phagocytes.

Those rapid surface changes include modifications of carbohydrates and exposure of anionic phospholipids, especially PS. The redistribution of PS both on phagocyte and prey is involved [40]. The protein annexin-V (AxV) preferentially binds PS with high affinity and inhibits apoptotic cell uptake by macrophages, most likely through interference with the availability of PS for recognition [11, 32]. Scientists started to look for the PS receptor. PS, being a phospholipid, could not be cloned and therefore Fadok's group started to produce monoclonal antibodies (Ab) against stimulated macrophages. The antigenic target of the monoclonal Ab 217 had hallmarks of a PSR, namely it recognized PS and blocked the engulfment of apoptotic cells [20]. Two other groups have reported phenotypes of PSR-deficient mice consistent with a role of the PSR in the removal of apoptotic cells [34, 35]. However, the essential role of the protein termed PSR in mediating the phagocytosis of dead cells has been questioned by a very recent study carefully investigating the phenotype of a third line of PSR-deficient mice [8]. Nevertheless, there is no doubt of PS itself and its putative receptor systems playing an important role in the uptake process of apoptotic and necrotic cells and in the modulation of immune responses in general. We showed that the availability of AxV at the site of dying tumor cell clearance disrupts their PS-dependent recognition and therefore abrogates immunosuppressive clearance. Indeed, addition of AxV strikingly heightened the immune response that apoptotic tumor cells elicit in vivo, including rejection of growing tumors [7]. An enigma exists with respect to the recognition and phagocytosis of PS exposing cells: viable PS exposing cells (e.g., activated B cells [16, 17], neutrophils in Barth syndrome [33], or monocytes [1]) are swallowed neither by amateur nor professional phagocytes. In contrast, apoptotic and necrotic PS exposing cells are efficiently taken up. We demonstrated that AxV binds to viable monocytes in a stochastic manner, whereas AxV binding to dying (apoptotic and necrotic) monocytes proceeds in a cooperative manner with a Hill coefficient as high as 10 [1]. We concluded that dying cells have cell membranes with high lateral mobility of PS and that AxV needs a critical density or clustering of PS molecules. It might also be that AxV needs a not yet defined co-factor that is only present on dying cells.

6
Changes in the Glycoprotein Composition of Membranes of Apoptotic Cells

Taken together, the exposure of PS is an early surface change of apoptosing cells recognized by several receptors and adaptor molecules [25, 58]. However, there are several reports showing that there are further membrane alterations during the later phases of apoptotic cell death leading to the recognition by additional adaptor molecules of apoptotic cells: the complement component C1q [10], surfactant protein A (SAP) and D (SPD) [61, 65], the long pentraxin PTX3 [55], and CRP. Furthermore, carbohydrate-binding proteins, the lectins, are also players of the innate immune system. Galactose- and mannose-specific receptors are discussed as having an important role for the recognition of dying cells [13]. We found that lectins recognizing the sugars mannose, frucose and N-actelyglucosamine bind to apoptotic cells during later phases of apoptosis. Compared to AxV, the binding of the lectins is delayed. A further difference is that viable cells also show a substantial binding of these lectins, which is increased markedly on apoptotic cells. The binding of AxV to apoptotic and necrotic cells is rather similar. This is in striking contrast to the lectin-binding capabilities, which is substantially higher in necrotic cells, when compared to apoptotic ones. The alteration in the exposure of carbohydrates is a feature of the late phases of apoptotic cell death and we conclude that it is a major membrane alteration preceding secondary necrosis. Examples of molecules and processes involved in the efficient clearance of dying cells and in the resolution of inflammation are summarized in Fig. 1.

Effective Clearance…

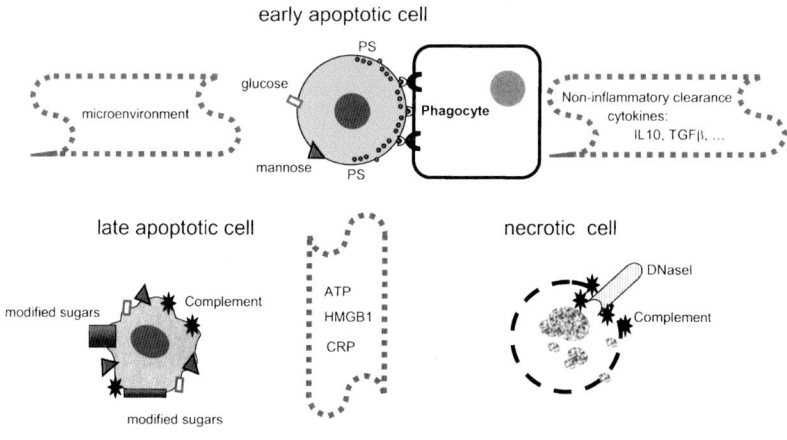

… No Autoimmunity!

Fig. 1 Pathways and examples of molecules involved in the clearance of apoptotic and necrotic cells. The figure illustrates surface changes and molecules involved in the recognition and uptake of dying cells and in the resolution of inflammation. *ATP* adenosine triphosphate, *CRP* C-reactive protein, *HMGB1* high mobility group B1 protein, *IL* interleukin; *PS* phosphatidylserine, *TGF* transforming growth factor

7
Impaired Clearance Functions and Autoimmunity

During necrotic as well as apoptotic cell death, autoantigens are cleaved or otherwise modified [12, 53]. These modifications may render cryptic epitopes immune-dominant [44, 45]. Dendritic cells may then acquire modified autoantigens such as apoptotic nuclei and chromatin and consequently autoreactive T cells can be activated (Fig. 2). Impaired clearance functions for dying cells may explain accumulation of apoptotic cells, and subsequently of secondary necrotic cells in various tissues of SLE patients [27, 49]. Increased levels of DNA and nucleosomes that have been observed in some SLE patients [51, 62] are most likely due to secondary necrotic cells, which are not able to retain this material. To investigate whether a defect in engulfment of apoptotic cell material can also be observed in germinal centers (GCs), we analyzed lymph node biopsies from SLE patients. A characteristic feature of the GC is the presence of specialized phagocytes, which under normal conditions remove apoptotic cells very efficiently in the early phases of apoptosis. These specialized macrophages are referred to as tingible body macrophages

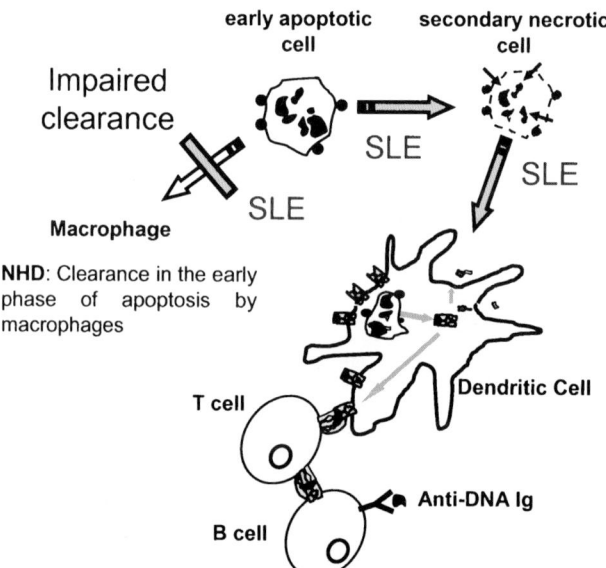

Fig. 2 Proposed mechanism for the etiopathogenesis of SLE (I). Defective scavenging of early apoptotic cells by macrophages enables access of late apoptotic cell-derived autoantigens (*arrows*) to dendritic cells and B cells. Antigen presentation occurs to potentially autoreactive T cells, which then become activated

(TBMs). Our data show that in a subgroup of patients with SLE, apoptotic cells accumulated in the GCs of the lymph nodes. The numbers of TBMs usually containing engulfed apoptotic nuclei were significantly reduced in these patients. In contrast to all controls, apoptotic material was observed associated with the surfaces of follicular dendritic cells (FDCs) [2]. There are three major locations where high rates of lymphocyte apoptosis can be observed: the thymus, the bone marrow, and the GCs of lymph nodes and spleen. In the case of GCs, it is of major importance to remove potential autoantigens, which could otherwise serve as antigen for affinity maturation of B cells [29]. In case of improperly ingested complement-binding apoptotic material, FDCs may serve as autoantigen repositories. This observation is in accordance with the extremely low phagocytic activity of FDCs [26]. The nuclear material on the surfaces of FDCs appears to be accessible for B cells. Therefore, we propose the following hypothesis for the induction of autoantibodies, at least in a subgroup of SLE patients: in the GC the apoptotic centrocytes are not adequately cleared in the early phase of the apoptotic cell death. This may be due to impaired phagocytic activity, or caused by

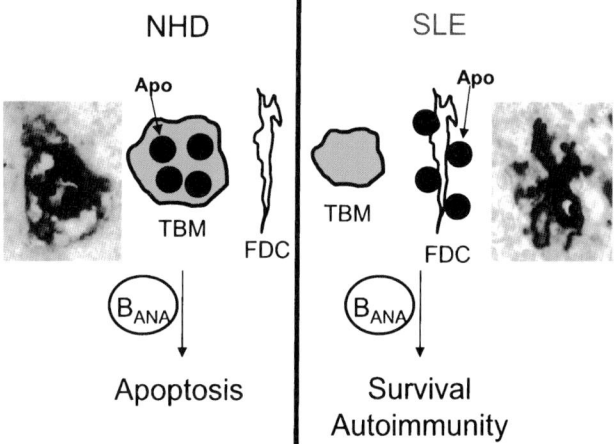

Fig. 3 Proposed mechanism for the etiopathogenesis of SLE (II). In the case of normal healthy donors (*NHD*) tingible body macrophages (*TBM*) efficiently take up apoptotic material (*left*). In the case of SLE (*right*), defective scavenging of apoptotic cells by TBM, which are absent or reduced in size, fails to sequester nuclear autoantigens (*Apo*). The small inserts show a typical TBM with engulfed apoptotic nuclei in the germinal centers of NHD and the accumulation of nuclear debris in the germinal centers of a patient with SLE. Follicular dendritic cell (FDC) -bound autoantigens (*Apo*) provide survival signals for B cells that had acquired nuclear reactivity during affinity maturation (B_{ANA}). These events challenge an important step to B cell tolerance

the absence of TBMs. Apoptosis can progress and the cells enter late stages of apoptotic cell death, including secondary necrosis. In this state, activation of the classical complement cascade may result in deposition of C3b on cell surfaces [21, 31, 42, 50]. Via C3b and its fragments, the apoptotic cells and nuclear debris can bind to CR2/CD21 on FDCs. Disintegrated apoptotic cells with lost membrane integrity give access to potential intracellular autoantigens. The latter can now provide a short-term survival signal for those B cells that have accidentally gained a B cell receptor reactive with nuclear antigens during the random process of somatic mutation. Under these conditions, B cell tolerance relies mainly on the presence of a functional T cell tolerance to nuclear autoantigens. Histone-specific T cells, able to provide in vitro help for dsDNA-specific B cells, have been detected in patients with SLE [4]. The presence of these cells in the mantle zone of the lymph node may be responsible for the activation of the autoreactive B cells and for the generation of plasma cells producing those nuclear antibodies that represent the humoral hallmark of SLE. Taken together, nuclear autoantigens bound to FDCs may provide a survival signal for autoreactive B cells, thereby overriding an important initial control mechanism of B cell tolerance (Fig. 3).

8
Heterogeneous and Intrinsic Clearance Defects in Some SLE Patients

Are clearance defects in SLE patients heterogeneous? We examined the uptake of various beads and dying cells by macrophages and granulocytes of SLE patients and NHD in vitro. We found that macrophages and/or granulocytes of some SLE patients showed a strongly reduced uptake of albumin beads, polyglobuline beads, apoptotic and necrotic cells, as well as degraded chromatin. Very interestingly, phagocytes from different SLE patients showed in part different phagocytic defects. The next step was and is to investigate whether the impaired clearance observed in certain SLE patients is an intrinsic defect. We isolated CD34 positive hematopoietic stem cells derived from the peripheral blood from SLE patients and NHD, respectively. SLE and NHD-derived stem cells showed similar proliferation in vitro. However, the differentiation into macrophages was reduced in SLE stem cell cultures. Many fewer macrophages differentiated from the CD34-positive stem cells and most of the SLE stem cell-derived macrophages showed reduced phagocytic capacity, were smaller, and died early. Factors responsible for the impaired differentiation rate are currently under investigation.

9
Conclusion

Autoimmune diseases affect large numbers of people worldwide. Genetic and environmental factors are thought to be involved in the etiopathogenesis of systemic autoimmune diseases such as SLE. Mechanisms that contribute to the development of SLE are T cell-dependent stimulation of B cells for the production of antinuclear antibodies [71], B cell overactivity (reviewed in [52]), anti-dsDNA as well as immune-complex-mediated organ damage [63], and increased amounts and abnormal presentation of potential autoantigens including nuclear antigens [27, 37]. The latter are accessible due to the impaired clearance of dying cells. Fc-receptor- and complement-mediated clearance defects have long been observed in patients with SLE [30, 57]. The concentration of CRP, a molecule also involved in the clearance of dying cells, is reduced in all SLE patients, especially during inflammatory phases [48]. Many molecule and receptor defects involved in the disposal of effete cells that contribute to the development of autoimmunity have been described. Therefore, it is reasonable to argue that clearance defects are major players in the development of autoimmune diseases such as SLE. The identification of the origin and causes of clearance defects is of major interest and the subject of ongoing investigation. The detection of defects in the clearance system may become important for the diagnosis of SLE and the molecules involved may become important biomarkers and therapeutic targets for autoimmune diseases.

Acknowledgements This work was supported by the Interdisciplinary Center for Clinical Research (IZKF) (project numbers A4 and N2) at the University Hospital of the University of Erlangen-Nuremberg, by Deutsche Forschungsgemeinschaft SFB 643 (project B5), by the research training grant GRK 592 from the German Research Society (DFG) to SF, by the Programme Alban, the European Union Programme of High Level Scholarships for Latin America, scholarship no. E04D047956VE to LM, by the European Commissions [E.U. (QLK3-CT-2002–02017_APOCLEAR)], and by the Lupus Erythemathodes Selbsthilfegemeinschaft e.V.

References

1. Appelt U, Sheriff A, Gaipl US, Kalden JR, Voll RE, Herrmann M (2005) Viable, apoptotic and necrotic monocytes expose phosphatidylserine: cooperative binding of the ligand annexin V to dying but not viable cells and implications for PS-dependent clearance. Cell Death Differ 12:194–196

2. Baumann I, Kolowos W, Voll RE, Manger B, Gaipl U, Neuhuber WL, Kirchner T, Kalden JR, Herrmann M (2002) Impaired uptake of apoptotic cells into tingible body macrophages in germinal centers of patients with systemic lupus erythematosus. Arthritis Rheum 46:191–201
3. Bell SA, Faust H, Schmid A, Meurer M (1998) Autoantibodies to C-reactive protein (CRP) and other acute-phase proteins in systemic autoimmune diseases. Clin Exp Immunol 113:327–332
4. Berden JH, Licht R, van Bruggen MC, Tax WJ (1999) Role of nucleosomes for induction and glomerular binding of autoantibodies in lupus nephritis. Curr Opin Nephrol Hypertens 8:299–306
5. Bharadwaj D, Mold C, Markham E, Du Clos TW (2001) Serum amyloid P component binds to Fc gamma receptors and opsonizes particles for phagocytosis. J Immunol 166:6735–6741
6. Bickerstaff MC, Botto M, Hutchinson WL, Herbert J, Tennent GA, Bybee A, Mitchell DA, Cook HT, Butler PJ, Walport MJ, Pepys MB (1999) Serum amyloid P component controls chromatin degradation and prevents antinuclear autoimmunity. Nat Med 5:694–697
7. Bondanza A, Zimmermann VS, Rovere-Querini P, Turnay J, Dumitriu IE, Stach CM, Voll RE, Gaipl US, Bertling W, Poschl E, Kalden JR, Manfredi AA, Herrmann M (2004) Inhibition of phosphatidylserine recognition heightens the immunogenicity of irradiated lymphoma cells in vivo. J Exp Med 200:1157–1165
8. Bose J, Gruber AD, Helming L, Schiebe S, Wegener I, Hafner M, Beales M, Kontgen F, Lengeling A (2004) The phosphatidylserine receptor has essential functions during embryogenesis but not in apoptotic cell removal. J Biol 3:15
9. Botto M, Dell'Agnola C, Bygrave AE, Thompson EM, Cook HT, Petry F, Loos M, Pandolfi PP, Walport MJ (1998) Homozygous C1q deficiency causes glomerulonephritis associated with multiple apoptotic bodies. Nat Genet 19:56–59
10. Botto M (2001) Links between complement deficiency and apoptosis. Arthritis Res 3:207–210
11. Callahan MK, Williamson P, Schlegel RA (2000) Surface expression of phosphatidylserine on macrophages is required for phagocytosis of apoptotic thymocytes. Cell Death Differ 7:645–653
12. Casciola-Rosen L, Andrade F, Ulanet D, Wong WB, Rosen A (1999) Cleavage by granzyme B is strongly predictive of autoantigen status: implications for initiation of autoimmunity. J Exp Med 190:815–826
13. Chionna A, Panzarini E, Pagliara P, De Luca A, Caforio S, Abbro L, Dini L (2003) Hepatic clearance of apoptotic lymphocytes: simply removal of waste cells? Eur J Histochem 47:97–104
14. Chitrabamrung S, Rubin RL, Tan EM (1981) Serum deoxyribonuclease I and clinical activity in systemic lupus erythematosus. Rheumatol Int 1:55–60
15. Di Virgilio F, Borea PA, Illes P (2001) P2 receptors meet the immune system. Trends Pharmacol Sci 22:5–7
16. Dillon SR, Mancini M, Rosen A, Schlissel MS (2000) Annexin V binds to viable B cells and colocalizes with a marker of lipid rafts upon B cell receptor activation. J Immunol 164:1322–1332
17. Dillon SR, Constantinescu A, Schlissel MS (2001) Annexin V binds to positively selected B cells [In Process Citation]. J Immunol 166:58–71

18. Ehrenstein MR, Cook HT, Neuberger MS (2000) Deficiency in serum immunoglobulin (Ig)M predisposes to development of IgG autoantibodies. J Exp Med 191:1253–1258
19. Fadok VA, Bratton DL, Frasch SC, Warner ML, Henson PM (1998) The role of phosphatidylserine in recognition of apoptotic cells by phagocytes. Cell Death Differ 5:551–562
20. Fadok VA, Bratton DL, Rose DM, Pearson A, Ezekewitz RA, Henson PM (2000) A receptor for phosphatidylserine-specific clearance of apoptotic cells. Nature 405:85–90
21. Gaipl US, Kuenkele S, Voll RE, Beyer TD, Kolowos W, Heyder P, Kalden JR, Herrmann M (2001) Complement binding is an early feature of necrotic and a rather late event during apoptotic cell death. Cell Death Differ 8:327–334
22. Gaipl US, Brunner J, Beyer TD, Voll RE, Kalden JR, Herrmann M (2003) Disposal of dying cells: a balancing act between infection and autoimmunity. Arthritis Rheum 48:6–11
23. Gaipl US, Beyer TD, Heyder P, Kuenkele S, Bottcher A, Voll RE, Kalden JR, Herrmann M (2004) Cooperation between C1q and DNase I in the clearance of necrotic cell-derived chromatin. Arthritis Rheum 50:640–649
24. Hanayama R, Tanaka M, Miyasaka K, Aozasa K, Koike M, Uchiyama Y, Nagata S (2004) Autoimmune disease and impaired uptake of apoptotic cells in MFG-E8-deficient mice. Science 304:1147–1150
25. Hart SP, Smith JR, Dransfield I (2004) Phagocytosis of opsonized apoptotic cells: roles for 'old-fashioned' receptors for antibody and complement. Clin Exp Immunol 135:181–185
26. Heinen E, Radoux D, Kinet-Denoel C, Moeremans M, De Mey J, Simar LJ (1985) Isolation of follicular dendritic cells from human tonsils and adenoids. III. Analysis of their Fc receptors. Immunology 54:777–784
27. Herrmann M, Voll RE, Zoller OM, Hagenhofer M, Ponner BB, Kalden JR (1998) Impaired phagocytosis of apoptotic cell material by monocyte-derived macrophages from patients with systemic lupus erythematosus. Arthritis Rheum 41:1241–1250
28. Hirt UA, Leist M (2003) Rapid, noninflammatory and PS-dependent phagocytic clearance of necrotic cells. Cell Death Differ 10:1156–1164
29. Janeway CA (1999) Immunobiology the immune system in health and disease. Current Biology Publications, New York, pp 339–358, 433–434
30. Kimberly RP, Meryhew NL, Runquist OA (1986) Mononuclear phagocyte function in SLE. I. Bipartite Fc- and complement-dependent dysfunction. J Immunol 137:91–96
31. Korb LC, Ahearn JM (1997) C1q binds directly and specifically to surface blebs of apoptotic human keratinocytes: complement deficiency and systemic lupus erythematosus revisited. J Immunol 158:4525–4528
32. Krahling S, Callahan MK, Williamson P, Schlegel RA (1999) Exposure of phosphatidylserine is a general feature in the phagocytosis of apoptotic lymphocytes by macrophages. Cell Death Differ 6:183–189
33. Kuijpers TW, Maianski NA, Tool AT, Becker K, Plecko B, Valianpour F, Wanders RJ, Pereira R, Van Hove J, Verhoeven AJ, Roos D, Baas F, Barth PG (2004) Neutrophils in Barth syndrome (BTHS) avidly bind annexin-V in the absence of apoptosis. Blood 5:5

34. Kunisaki Y, Masuko S, Noda M, Inayoshi A, Sanui T, Harada M, Sasazuki T, Fukui Y (2004) Defective fetal liver erythropoiesis and T lymphopoiesis in mice lacking the phosphatidylserine receptor. Blood 103:3362–3364
35. Li MO, Sarkisian MR, Mehal WZ, Rakic P, Flavell RA (2003) Phosphatidylserine receptor is required for clearance of apoptotic cells. Science 302:1560–1563
36. Lieberthal W, Levine JS (1996) Mechanisms of apoptosis and its potential role in renal tubular epithelial cell injury. Am J Physiol 271:F477–F488
37. Lorenz HM, Grunke M, Hieronymus T, Herrmann M, Kuhnel A, Manger B, Kalden JR (1997) In vitro apoptosis and expression of apoptosis-related molecules in lymphocytes from patients with systemic lupus erythematosus and other autoimmune diseases. Arthritis Rheum 40:306–317
38. Lorenz HM, Herrmann M, Winkler T, Gaipl U, Kalden JR (2000) Role of apoptosis in autoimmunity. Apoptosis 5:443–449
39. Macanovic M, Lachmann PJ (1997) Measurement of deoxyribonuclease I (DNase) in the serum and urine of systemic lupus erythematosus (SLE)-prone NZB/NZW mice by a new radial enzyme diffusion assay. Clin Exp Immunol 108:220–226
40. Marguet D (1999) Engulfment of apoptotic cells involves the redistribution of membrane phosphatidylserine on phagocyte and prey. [Record supplied by publisher]. Nat Cell Biol 1:454–456
41. Marteau F, Communi D, Boeynaems JM, Suarez Gonzalez N (2004) Involvement of multiple P2Y receptors and signaling pathways in the action of adenine nucleotides diphosphates on human monocyte-derived dendritic cells. J Leukoc Biol 76:796–803
42. Mevorach D, Mascarenhas JO, Gershov D, Elkon KB (1998) Complement-dependent clearance of apoptotic cells by human macrophages. J Exp Med 188:2313–2320
43. Mevorach D, Zhou JL, Song X, Elkon KB (1998) Systemic exposure to irradiated apoptotic cells induces autoantibody production. J Exp Med 188:387–392
44. Moudgil KD, Sercarz EE, Grewal IS (1998) Modulation of the immunogenicity of antigenic determinants by their flanking residues. Immunol Today 19:217–220
45. Moudgil KD, Southwood S, Ametani A, Kim K, Sette A, Sercarz EE (1999) The self-directed T cell repertoire against mouse lysozyme reflects the influence of the hierarchy of its own determinants and can be engaged by a foreign lysozyme. J Immunol 163:4232–4237
46. Napirei M, Karsunky H, Zevnik B, Stephan H, Mannherz HG, Moroy T (2000) Features of systemic lupus erythematosus in Dnase1-deficient mice. Nat Genet 25:177–181
47. Napirei M, Wulf S, Mannherz HG (2004) Chromatin breakdown during necrosis by serum Dnase1 and the plasminogen system. Arthritis Rheum 50:1873–1883
48. Pepys MB, Lanham JG, De Beer FC (1982) C-reactive protein in SLE. Clin Rheum Dis 8:91–103
49. Perniok A, Wedekind F, Herrmann M, Specker C, Schneider M (1998) High levels of circulating early apoptotic peripheral blood mononuclear cells in systemic lupus erythematosus. Lupus 7:113–118

50. Quartier P, Potter PK, Ehrenstein MR, Walport MJ, Botto M (2004) Predominant role of IgM-dependent activation of the classical pathway in the clearance of dying cells by murine bone marrow-derived macrophages in vitro. Eur J Immunol 35:252–260
51. Raptis L, Menard HA (1980) Quantitation and characterization of plasma DNA in normals and patients with systemic lupus erythematosus. J Clin Invest 66:1391–1399
52. Renaudineau Y, Pers JO, Bendaoud B, Jamin C, Youinou P (2004) Dysfunctional B cells in systemic lupus erythematosus. Autoimmun Rev 3: 516–523
53. Rosen A, Casciola-Rosen L, Ahearn J (1995) Novel packages of viral and self-antigens are generated during apoptosis. J Exp Med 181:1557–1561
54. Rosen A, Casciola-Rosen L (1999) Autoantigens as substrates for apoptotic proteases: implications for the pathogenesis of systemic autoimmune disease. Cell Death Differ 6:6–12
55. Rovere P, Peri G, Fazzini F, Bottazzi B, Doni A, Bondanza A, Zimmermann VS, Garlanda C, Fascio U, Sabbadini MG, Rugarli C, Mantovani A, Manfredi AA (2000) The long pentraxin PTX3 binds to apoptotic cells and regulates their clearance by antigen-presenting dendritic cells. Blood 96:4300–4306
56. Russell AI, Cunninghame Graham DS, Shepherd C, Roberton CA, Whittaker J, Meeks J, Powell RJ, Isenberg DA, Walport MJ, Vyse TJ (2004) Polymorphism at the C-reactive protein locus influences gene expression and predisposes to systemic lupus erythematosus. Hum Mol Genet 13:137–147
57. Salmon JE, Kimberly RP, Gibofsky A, Fotino M (1984) Defective mononuclear phagocyte function in systemic lupus erythematosus: dissociation of Fc receptor-ligand binding and internalization. J Immunol 133:2525–2531
58. Savill J (1997) Recognition and phagocytosis of cells undergoing apoptosis. Br Med Bull 53:491–508
59. Savill J, Dransfield I, Gregory C, Haslett C (2002) A blast from the past: clearance of apoptotic cells regulates immune responses. Nat Rev Immunol 2:965–975
60. Scaffidi P, Misteli T, Bianchi ME (2002) Release of chromatin protein HMGB1 by necrotic cells triggers inflammation. Nature 418:191–195
61. Schagat TL, Wofford JA, Wright JR (2001) Surfactant protein A enhances alveolar macrophage phagocytosis of apoptotic neutrophils. J Immunol 166:2727–2733
62. Steinman CR (1984) Circulating DNA in systemic lupus erythematosus. Isolation and characterization. J Clin Invest 73:832–841
63. Suzuki N, Harada T, Mizushima Y, Sakane T (1993) Possible pathogenic role of cationic anti-DNA autoantibodies in the development of nephritis in patients with systemic lupus erythematosus. J Immunol 151:1128–1136
64. Taylor PR, Carugati A, Fadok VA, Cook HT, Andrews M, Carroll MC, Savill JS, Henson PM, Botto M, Walport MJ (2000) A hierarchical role for classical pathway complement proteins in the clearance of apoptotic cells in vivo. J Exp Med 192:359–366
65. Vandivier RW, Ogden CA, Fadok VA, Hoffmann PR, Brown KK, Botto M, Walport MJ, Fisher JH, Henson PM, Greene KE (2002) Role of surfactant proteins A, D, and C1q in the clearance of apoptotic cells in vivo and in vitro: calreticulin and CD91 as a common collectin receptor complex. J Immunol 169:3978–3986

66. Vigushin DM, Pepys MB, Hawkins PN (1993) Metabolic and scintigraphic studies of radioiodinated human C-reactive protein in health and disease. J Clin Invest 91:1351–1357
67. Volanakis JE (2001) Human C-reactive protein: expression, structure, and function. Mol Immunol 38:189–197
68. Voll RE, Herrmann M, Roth EA, Stach C, Kalden JR, Girkontaite I (1997) Immunosuppressive effects of apoptotic cells. Nature 390:350–351
69. Walker NI, Harmon BV, Gobe GC, Kerr JF (1988) Patterns of cell death. Methods Achiev Exp Pathol 13:18–54
70. Walport MJ (2000) Lupus, DNase and defective disposal of cellular debris. Nat Genet 25:135–136
71. Winkler TH, Kalden JR (1994) Origin of anti-DNA autoantibodies in SLE. Lupus 3:75–76

The Importance of T Cell Interactions with Macrophages in Rheumatoid Cytokine Production

F. M. Brennan[1] (✉) · A. D. Foey[2] · M. Feldmann[1]

[1] Imperial College of Science, Technology and Medicine, Kennedy Institute of Rheumatology Division, Faculty of Medicine, 1 Aspenlea Road, London W6 8LH, UK
f.brennan@imperial.ac.uk

[2] School of Biological Sciences, University of Plymouth, Drake Circus, Plymouth PL4 8AA, UK

1	Introduction	178
2	Cognate-Dependent Interactions	180
2.1	The Importance of the T Cell	180
2.2	Are Rheumatoid T Cells Cytokine Activated?	182
2.3	Cell Surface Molecules of Potential Relevance	183
3	Macrophage Lineage	184
3.1	What Is the Impact of the Differentiation Status of Monocyte/Macrophage Lineage?	184
3.2	Signalling Pathways Involved in the Monocyte Lineage	184
4	Concluding Remarks	186
	References	186

Abstract The analysis of suppression of cytokines in rheumatoid synovial tissue and fluid pioneered the studies of human cytokines in diseased tissue due to the relative ease of staining samples, even at the height of the inflammatory process. These studies led to the study of synovial cytokine regulation, and the identification of TNF as a therapeutic target, which has been amply validated in clinical trials and now routine therapy. The next key question was how is TNF disregulated in synovium. Are there differences between the mechanisms of synovial TNF production compared to the production of protective TNF during an immune response? Are there differences between the induction of the pro-inflammatory TNF and the anti inflammatory IL-10? The analysis of the interaction of the two most abundant synovial cells, T lymphocytes and macrophages has provided interesting clues to new therapeutic approaches based on disrupting T-macrophage interaction.

1
Introduction

It is now well recognized that the spontaneous production of pro-inflammatory cytokines, in particular TNF, IL-1 and IL-6, produced locally in the inflamed synovial joint contribute directly to the pathogenesis of rheumatoid arthritis (RA) [1]. These observations have arisen initially from ex vivo studies with human synovial cultures, immunohistochemical and mRNA analysis of synovium and in vivo studies in animal models of arthritis. Blocking TNF ameliorated collagen type II arthritis, even after disease onset, and transgenic mice, overexpressing TNF, develop an erosive polyarthritis; these investigations have led to the development of several TNF and IL-1 inhibitors. Currently licensed are Infliximab Remicade (chimeric anti-TNF antibody) and etanercept (TNF receptor fusion protein) (adalimumab, humira human anti-TNF, anakinra (Kineret) and IL-1 receptor antagonists.

Therapies targeting TNF are useful in multiple chronic inflammatory disease including JRA, Crohn's disease, psoriasis, psoriatic arthritis and ankylosing spondylitis [2], it is also apparent that long-term blockade of a cytokine such as TNF, which is important in innate and acquired immunity, may lead to an increase in latent and/or opportunistic infections. This is now apparent, with a small but significant increase in unusual infections, as well as the re-emergence of latent TB in endemic areas, particularly in Central and Eastern Europe in about 1/2,000 anti-TNF patients [3].

It is thus important in the absence of screening or prophylaxis to understand what mechanisms lead to the production of pro-inflammatory cytokines in RA synovial tissue, and whether the molecular mechanisms differ from those generating TNF in host defence situation.

It has been observed that whilst the production of multiple pro-inflammatory cytokines and enzymes is highly increased in RA (Table 1), this activity is offset to some degree by the action of several endogenous anti-inflammatory cytokines and cytokine inhibitors. Of particular importance in this respect is IL-10, an important regulator of TNFα and IL-1β, spontaneously produced by macrophages and other cells in the rheumatoid joint [4, 5]. Thus if endogenous IL-10 is blocked in RA synovial cell cultures, the spontaneous production of both TNF and IL-1 increased 2-fold [4]. Thus there is an important need to develop therapies that block the pro-inflammatory pathways in synovium, but leave unaffected those that regulate immunoregulatory cytokines such as IL-10, and if possible leave the capacity to make TNF in infection.

Table 1 Cytokines and chemokines expressed in synovial tissue (modified and updated from [1])

Cytokine		mRNA	Protein	References
IL-1 α and β	(interleukin 1)	Yes	Yes	5, 53–60
IL-2	(interleukin 2)	Yes	+/–	61, 62
IL-3	(interleukin 3)	?	?	62
IL-6	(interleukin 6)	Yes	Yes	56, 63–68
IL-7	(interleukin 7)	Yes	Yes	68
IL-11	(interleukin 11)	Yes	Yes	63, 69
IL-12	(interleukin 12)	Yes	Yes	70
IL-15	(interleukin 15)	Yes	Yes	19
IL-17	(interleukin 17)	Yes	Yes	71
IL-18	(interleukin 18)	Yes	Yes	72
TNFα	(tumour necrosis factor)	Yes	Yes	55–58, 73–76
LT	(lymphotoxin)	Yes	+/–	74, 77
GM-CSF	(granulocyte macrophage colony-stimulating factor)	Yes	Yes	78–80
M-CSF	(macrophage colony-stimulating factor)	Yes	Yes	62
LIF	(leukocyte inhibitory factor)	Yes	Yes	63
Onco M	(oncostatin M)	Yes	Yes	63
IFNα	(interferon alpha)	Yes	Yes	75
IFNβ	(interferon beta)	?	?	
IFNγ	(interferon gamma)	Yes	+/–	56, 61, 77
IL-4	(interleukin 4)	?	No	81
IL-10	(interleukin 10)	Yes	Yes	4, 82–84
IL-13	(interleukin 13)	Yes	Yes	85
IL-16	(interleukin 16)	Yes	Yes	86, 87
TGFβ	(transforming growth factor beta)	Yes	Yes	81, 88–93
IL-8	(interleukin 8/CXCL8)	Yes	Yes	94–98
Groα	(melanoma growth stimulating activity/CXCL1)	Yes	Yes	97
MIP-1α	(macrophage inflammatory protein 1alpha/CCL3)	Yes	Yes	97, 99
MIP-1β	(macrophage inflammatory protein 1 beta/CCL4)	Yes	Yes	97
MCP-1	(monocyte chemoattractant protein 1/CCL2)	Yes	Yes	95, 97, 100–102

Table 1 (continued)

Cytokine		mRNA	Protein	References
ENA-78	(epithelial neutrophil activating peptide 78/CXCL5)	Yes	Yes	103
RANTES	(regulated upon activation t cell expressed & secreted/CCL5)	Yes	Yes	104
DC-CK1	(dendritic-cell-derived CC chemokine-1/CCL18)	Yes	?	105
MIP-3α	(macrophage inflammatory protein-3 alpha/CCL20)	?	?	106, 107
SDF-1α/β	(Stromal-cell-derived factor-1 alpha/beta/CXCL12)	?	Yes	108
MIG	(monokine induced by interferonγ/CXCL9)	Yes	?	109, 110
IP-10	(Interferon-inducible protein-10/CXCL10)	Yes	?	109
Fractalkine	(CX3CL1)	?	Yes	111
BCA-1	(B-cell-attracting chemokine-1/CXCL13)	Yes	Yes	112
VEGF	(vascular endothelial cell growth factor)	Yes	Yes	113, 114
FGF	(fibroblast growth factor)	Yes	Yes	89, 115–118
PDGF	(platelet-derived growth factor)	Yes	Yes	118–120

2 Cognate-Dependent Interactions

2.1 The Importance of the T Cell

The synovium in rheumatoid arthritis (RA) is very cellular, with several different cell types including macrophages and T cells, in close proximity [6]. This biological appearance suggests that contact signals between macrophages and T cells could be of importance in vivo in modulating macrophage function. Our prior studies have found that TNFα production in RA synovium is T cell-dependent, as removal of CD3-positive T cells from RA synovial mononuclear cells resulted in significant reduced macrophage TNFα production [7].

Direct contact-mediated interactions have been studied by several groups, initially J.-M. Dayer's, using transformed T cell and monocytic lines, and were found to play an important role in inducing the synthesis of several cytokines including IL-1β, TNFα, IL-10 as well as destructive metalloproteinases [8–12]. We have studied T cell–monocyte cognate interactions using cells isolated from the peripheral blood of normal donors and also using synovial T cells. A key observation was that the manner in which T cells were activated influenced the profile of cytokines induced in the monocytes. Thus if blood T cells were activated with cross-linked anti-CD3 (a mimic of antigen stimulation) this induced the production of both pro-inflammatory TNFα and anti-inflammatory IL-10 in monocytes [12]. However, if the T cells were stimulated with a cocktail of cytokines (TNFα, IL-2 and IL-6) for 8 days, a model of bystander activation, TNFα *but not* IL-10 production ensued [11]. This suggested to us that cytokine-stimulated T cells (Tck) may physiologically resemble a highly pro-inflammatory situation, and T cells in RA synovial tissue induce macrophage TNFα production because they could induce an unbalanced pro-inflammatory cytokine response from monocytes, and thus could be part of a vicious cycle (Fig. 1). The corresponding T cell phenotype would appear to be of importance, as a study by Dayer's group [13] sug-

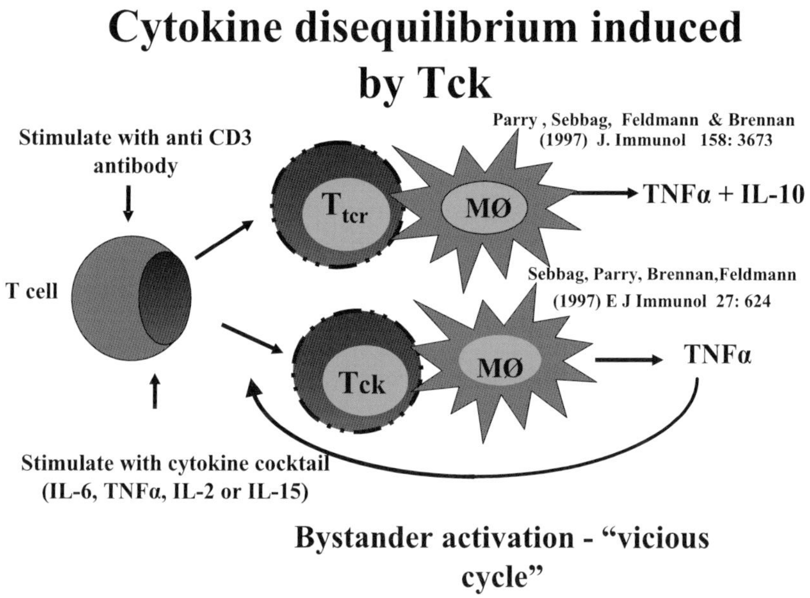

Cytokine disequilibrium induced by Tck

Fig. 1 Cytokine disequilibrium induced by Tck. Peripheral blood T cells activated with cross-linked anti-CD3 (Ttcr) for 48 h results in contact-induced production of TNFα and IL-10 in monocytes. T cells stimulated with a cocktail of cytokines (TNFα, IL-2 and IL-6) for 8 days (by-stander activation) termed Tck cells results in TNFα *but not* IL-10 production

gested a differential regulation of monocyte-derived cytokine production by Th_1-like vs Th_2-like cells. Thus $CD4^+$ Th_1 clones induced high levels of IL-1β production by THP-1 monocytes whereas Th_2 clones induced higher levels of IL-1ra, which implies that Th_1 cells are pro-inflammatory, whereas the Th_2 cells are anti-inflammatory.

2.2
Are Rheumatoid T Cells Cytokine Activated?

The hypothesis that RA T cells mimic Tck cells is attractive since T cells found in rheumatoid arthritis synovium have several unusual characteristics. They are relatively small, noncycling, but have features of activation, with over half expressing HLA class II, VLA antigens, CD25 and CD69 (reviewed in [14, 15]). T cell receptor analysis has not revealed a consistent pattern: oligoclonal and dominant clones or responses to putative auto-antigens have not been easy to reproduce (reviewed in [16]). Based on these features, and their low capacity to produce T cell derived cytokines, it has been proposed that T cells in the joint are not involved in the later stages of the disease [17]. However, our data suggests that they are involved in disease pathology through contact-dependent activation of macrophages to induce TNF. The environment of the RA synovium is conducive to the generation of Tck cells, as it is rich in the relevant cytokines. Unutmaz et al. described the generation of bystander-activated T cells from normal PBMCs with the cocktail IL-2, IL-6 and TNFα [18]; this may work via the reported upregulation of IL-2Rα (CD25) by IL-6 and TNF. We found that IL-15 could, by itself, mimic the IL-6/TNFα/IL-2 cocktail used to activate Tck [11]. This is likely to be due to the suppression of IL-15 high-affinity R in the absence of activation. IL-15 is of particular interest as it is found in RA synovium [19] and can activate peripheral blood T cells to induce TNFα synthesis in U937 cells or adherent RA synovial cells in a contact-dependent manner [20, 21].

It is likely that other cognate cell-to-cell interactions occur in the synovial joint and contribute to the disease pathology observed in RA. These interactions include the endothelial cell–T cell and the fibroblast–T cell interactions [22]. During early stages of inflammation, there is a large cellular infiltration from the blood to the synovial joint, where interactions between T cells and vascular endothelium drive further inflammation and extravasation and infiltration, mediated by the expression of cell adhesion molecules, chemokines and cytokines [22–25]. In addition, the earliest infiltrating cells, neutrophils, can be activated by contact-mediated interaction with T cells as determined by the ability of these neutrophils to be primed for respiratory burst by FMLP [26]. As the pathology of RA progresses to chronic inflammation and pannus forms at the cartilage–pannus junction (CPJ), the interactions between T cells and fibroblasts or macrophages is likely to become more important. Recently, the interaction between stimulated T cells and dermal fibroblasts or synoviocytes has been shown to induce MMP-1 (collagenase) and TIMP-1 with an imbalance in favour of the pro-inflammatory MMP-1 [27], and also inhibiting the synthesis of types I and III collagen by fibroblast cells [28].

Studies undertaken thus far have documented the potent stimulatory activity of T cells on monocyte cytokine production during the pathology of RA. However, there are abundant T cells and monocytes in the peripheral circulation, which have the potential to physically interact with each other, but this does not seem to induce cytokine production. This may be due to the serum factor, apo A-1 which acts to prevent monocyte activation [29]. The capacity of apo A-1 to inhibit T cell-mediated macrophage activation suggests that this molecule or its derivatives may have a useful anti-inflammatory therapeutic effect in chronic inflammatory diseases such as RA.

2.3
Cell Surface Molecules of Potential Relevance

As contact-dependent signals have been demonstrated to be of importance, attention has focused upon which are the important signals. There are multiple candidate molecules on the surface of cells that may be able to mediate these functions. Antibody blocking of specific surface interaction molecules has been reported to suppress the induction of monocyte cytokine synthesis. These include CD69, LFA-1 [8, 30], CD44 [31], CD45 [32], CD40 [33], membrane TNF [12], and SLAM [34]. There are technical difficulties in these experiments as blocking cell adhesion molecules on T or monocytic cells would prevent the cells interacting and would not obviously indicate that these ligation interactions were involved in monocyte activation.

Our studies have demonstrated that T cells activated through the T cell receptor complex induced monocyte IL-10 synthesis. This was partially dependent on endogenous TNFα and IL-1, and T cell membrane TNFα was an important contact-mediated signal [12, 35]. However, IL-10 synthesis still occurred when TNFα and IL-1 were neutralized, suggesting that there are TNF/IL-1-independent signals required for IL-10 synthesis, which remain to be identified.

Of particular interest are members of the TNF/TNF-R family, which include CD40, CD27, CD30, OX-40, and LTβ. The ligands of these TNF-R molecules have been described to be upregulated upon T cell activation and in addition CD40L, 4-1BB, CD27L, CD30 have been described to be released as soluble molecules after activation [36–39]. The interaction between CD40L and CD40 has been described to be of importance for inducing both IL-1 and IL-12 synthesis following T cell interaction with monocytes [33, 40] and more recently to mediate IL-10 production by human microglial cells upon interaction with anti-CD3-stimulated T cells [41]. In addition, we have shown recently that CD40L–CD40 interaction mediates cognate induction of macrophage IL-10 [42].

3
Macrophage Lineage

3.1
What Is the Impact of the Differentiation Status of Monocyte/Macrophage Lineage?

In addition to the stimulus encountered by the T cells, our data has indicated the importance of the differentiation state of the monocyte in determining cytokine profiles in response to activated T cells. We observed that CD40 signalling co-stimulates LPS-induced IL-10 production by monocytes, but also that CD40 ligation induced IL-10 production by differentiated monocytes (macrophages), even in the absence of quantifiable LPS. Indeed, the priming mechanism of the macrophage determined cytokine profile where M-CSF pre-programmed macrophages to produce both IL-10 and TNFα upon stimulation by CD40L or Tck, whereas IFNγ priming resulted predominantly in TNFα [42]. IFNγ-primed macrophages, however, can produce an endogenous IL-10 activity that is not secreted into the supernatant upon cell contact with either Tck or CD40L transfectants, as neutralization of endogenous IL-10 resulted in a marked increase in TNFα production. This observation is compatible with reports of membrane-associated IL-10 [43] and may highlight differences in the ability of these two types of macrophage-like cells to process cytokines. M-CSF is usually readily detected in the RA joint, whilst IFNγ is relatively scarce (reviewed in [44]), and this MCSF pre-programming may indicate why both TNFα and IL-10 are usually found in synovial membrane cell cultures. This pre-programming of macrophages would appear to lack an important influence irrespective of the triggering stimulus, as macrophages stimulated by Tck, CD40 ligation or LPS result in similar cytokine profiles. Thus it would appear that the route of differentiation of the monocyte is critical in the induction of IL-10 in cognate interactions between activated T cells and macrophages.

3.2
Signalling Pathways Involved in the Monocyte Lineage

Prior work has shown that TNFα synthesis in monocytes is heterogeneous in its signalling pathway's response to some stimuli, e.g. LPS but not others (zymosan or CD45 ligation). TNF production is NF-κB-dependent [32, 45, 46]. Thus it is of interest to observe that Tck- but not Ttcr-induced TNFα production in M-CSF monocytes is NF-κB-dependent. Furthermore, whereas PI3K inhibitors blocked Ttcr induction of TNFα, they paradoxically augmented TNFα in monocytes stimulated by Tck cells. We then made the important finding that RA T cells behaved like Tck cells in that the induction of TNFα in resting peripheral blood monocytes was NF-κB-dependent but super-induced if PI3K was blocked. An identical result was observed if NF-κB or PI3K was blocked in the RA synovial cell cultures.

The IL-10 production in monocytes/macrophages is equally complex. We found that in response to LPS, IL-10 production is dependent on both endogenous IL-1 and TNFα. Furthermore, there is selective utilization of mitogen-activated kinases where IL-10 production was dependent on p38 MAPK and TNFα production was dependent on both p38 and p42/44 MAPKs [47]. The involvement of p38 MAPK activity in IL-10 production subsequently led to the characterization of the downstream effector, hsp27, as an anti-inflammatory mediator [48]. Little is known however, regarding the involvement of the PI3K pathway in macrophage production of IL-10 but PI3K and its downstream substrate p70S6K mediate IL-10 induced proliferative responses but not its anti-inflammatory effects[49]. A recent study from our laboratory has described Tck-induced macrophage IL-10 production to be dependent on PI3K and p70S6K, whereas TNFα production is negatively regulated by PI3K and is p70S6K-dependent [50]. This suggests that IL-10 and TNFα share a common component, p70S6K, but differentially utilize PI3K activity. These results have been reproduced in the spontaneous cytokine production by RA-SMCs and by RA-T/macrophage co-cultures, further suggesting the relevance of this Tck/macrophage cognate co-culture system as a useful model for cytokine production occurring in the inflamed synovium of the rheumatoid joint.

Although many other studies have implicated other signalling cascades in the induction of IL-10 production, not much work exists on the signalling required in macrophages stimulated by cognate interactions with fixed activated T cells. The roles of PKC and cAMP signalling have been implicated in IL-10 and TNFα production and are currently under investigation in our group. Preliminary results would suggest that both these cascades also differentially regulate IL-10 and TNFα. Studies undertaken by other groups have reported the involvement of the cAMP/PKA pathway in the induction of IL-10 production by human PBMCs where the membrane-permeable dibutyryl cAMP was capable of elevating IL-10 mRNA and augmenting LPS induced IL-10 production but on its own was incapable of producing IL-10 protein [51]. This work also demonstrated a role for PKC in the induction of IL-10 by LPS using the PKC inhibitors calphostin C and H-7; this result contradicts our data but may reflect that this study used PBMCs, a heterogenous population, as compared to purified monocyte-derived macrophages. In addition, the selective inhibition of PDEIV by rolipram was found to augment LPS-induced IL-10 production by murine peritoneal macrophages, the mechanism of which was thought to be a consequence of LPS inducing the anti-inflammatory mediator, PGE_2, which in turn upregulates intracellular cAMP via stimulation of adenylate cyclase activity [52].

4
Concluding Remarks

The cognate activation of macrophages by T cells has focussed almost exclusively on the membrane interactions mediating macrophage effector function such as NO release, phagocytosis, B cell help, and more recently the cytokine profiles induced. The control of T cell-induced IL-10 and TNFα may discover potential therapeutic targets selectively affecting pro-inflammatory TNFα, without affecting anti-inflammatory IL-10 production. Such targets could prove to be of great benefit in the treatment of such chronic inflammatory diseases as rheumatoid arthritis.

Acknowledgements This work was funded by The Arthritis Research Campaign.

References

1. Feldmann M, Brennan FM, Maini RN (1996) Role of cytokines in rheumatoid arthritis. Annu Rev Immunol 14:397
2. Feldmann M, Maini RN (2001) Anti-TNFα therapy or rheumatoid arthritis: what have we learned? Annu Rev Immunol 19:163
3. Keane J, Gershon S, Wise RP, Mirabile-Levens E, Kasznica J, Schwieterman WD, Siegel JN, Braun MM (2001) Tuberculosis associated with infliximab, a tumor necrosis factor alpha-neutralizing agent. N Engl J Med 345:1098
4. Katsikis PD, Chu CQ, Brennan FM, Maini RN, Feldmann M (1994) Immunoregulatory role of interleukin 10 in rheumatoid arthritis. J Exp Med 179:1517
5. Chomarat P, Vannier E, Dechanet J, Rissoan MC, Banchereau J, Dinarello CA, Miossec P (1995) Balance of IL-1 receptor antagonist/IL-1 beta in rheumatoid synovium and its regulation by IL-4 and IL-10. J Immunol 154:1432
6. Duke O, Panayi GS, Janossy G, Poulter LW (1982) An immunohistological analysis of lymphocyte subpopulations and their microenvironment in the synovial membranes of patients with rheumatoid arthritis using monoclonal antibodies. Clin Exp Immunol 49:22
7. Brennan FM, Hayes AL, Ciesielski CJ, Green P, Foxwell BMJ, Feldmann M (2001) Evidence that RA synovial T cells are similar to cytokine activated T cells: involvement of PI3 kinase and NF-kB pathways in TNFa production in rheumatoid arthritis. Arthritis Rheum 46:31–41

8. Isler P, Vey E, Zhang JH, Dayer JM (1993) Cell surface glycoproteins expressed on activated human T cells induce production of interleukin-1 beta by monocytic cells: a possible role of CD69. Eur Cytokine Netw 4:15
9. Lacraz S, Isler P, Vey E, Welgus HG, Dayer JM (1994) Direct contact between T lymphocytes and monocytes is a major pathway for induction of metalloproteinase expression. J Biol Chem 269:22027
10. Suttles J, Miller RW, Tao X, Stout RD (1994) T cells which do not express membrane tumour necrosis factor-alpha activate macrophage effector function by cell contact-dependent signalling of macrophage tumour necrosis factor-alpha production. Eur J Immunol 24:1736
11. Sebbag M, Parry SL, Brennan FM, Feldmann M (1997) Cytokine stimulation of T lymphocytes regulates their capacity to induce monocyte production of tumor necrosis factor-alpha, but not interleukin-10: possible relevance to pathophysiology of rheumatoid arthritis. Eur J Immunol 27:624
12. Parry SL, Sebbag M, Feldmann M, Brennan FM (1997) Contact with T cells modulates monocyte IL-10 production: role of T cell membrane TNF-alpha. J Immunol 158:3673
13. Chizzolini C, Chicheportiche R, Burger D, Dayer JM (1997) Human Th1 cells preferentially induce interleukin (IL)-1beta while Th2 cells induce IL-1 receptor antagonist production upon cell/cell contact with monocytes. Eur J Immunol 27:171
14. Salmon M, Gaston JS (1995) The role of T-lymphocytes in rheumatoid arthritis. Br Med Bull 51:332
15. Nanki T, Lipsky PE (2000) Cytokine, activation marker, and chemokine receptor expression by individual CD4+ memory T cells in rheumatoid arthritis. Arth. Res 2:415
16. Goronzy JJ, Zettl A, Weyand CM (1998) T cell receptor repertoire in rheumatoid arthritis. Int Rev Immunol 17:339
17. Firestein GS, Zvaifler NJ (1990) How important are T cells in chronic rheumatoid synovitis? Arthritis Rheum 33:768
18. Unutmaz D, Pileri P, Abrignani S (1994) Antigen-independent activation of naive and memory resting T cells by a cytokine combination. J Exp Med 180:1159
19. McInnes IB, al-Mughales J, Field M, Leung BP, Huang FP, Dixon R, Sturrock RD, Wilkinson PC, Liew FY (1996) The role of interleukin-15 in T-cell migration and activation in rheumatoid arthritis. Nat Med 2:175
20. McInnes IB, Leung BP, Sturrock RD, Field M, Liew FY (1997) Interleukin-15 mediates T cell-dependent regulation of tumor necrosis factor-alpha production in rheumatoid arthritis. Nat Med 3:189
21. McInnes IB, Liew FY (1998) Interleukin 15: a proinflammatory role in rheumatoid arthritis synovitis. Immunol Today 19:75
22. Lou J, Dayer J-M, Grau GE, Burger D (1996) Direct cell/cell contact with stimulated T lymphocytes induces the expression of cell adhesion molecules and cytokines by human brain microvascular endothelial cells. Eur J Immunol 26:3107
23. Lou J, Ythier A, Burger D, Zheng L, Juillard P, Lucas R, Dayer J-M, Grau GE (1997) Modulation of soluble and membrane-bound TNF-induced phenotypic and functional changes of human brain microvascular endothelial cells by recombinant TNF binding protein I. J Neuroimmunol 77:107

24. Yarwood H, Mason JC, Mahiouz D, Sugars K, Haskard DO (2000) Resting and activated T cells induce expression of E-selectin and VCAM-1 by vascular endothelial cells through a contact-dependent but CD40 ligand-independent mechanism. J Leukoc Biol 68:233
25. Monaco C, Andreakos E, Young S, Feldmann M, Paleolog E (2002) T cell-mediated signalling to vascular endothelium: induction of cytokines, chemokines and tissue factor. J Leukoc Biol 71:659
26. Li JM, Isler P, Dayer J-M, Burger D (1995) Contact-dependent stimulation of monocytic cells and neutrophils by stimulated human T-cell clones. Immunology 84:571
27. Burger D, Rezzonico R, Li JM, Modoux C, Pierce RA, Welgus HG, Dayer JM (1998) Imbalance between interstitial collagenase and tissue inhibitor of metalloproteinases 1 in synoviocytes and fibroblasts upon direct contact with stimulated T lymphocytes: involvement of membrane-associated cytokines. Arthritis Rheum 41:1748
28. Rezzonico R, Burger D, Dayer JM (1998) Direct contact between T lymphocytes and human dermal fibroblasts or synoviocytes down-regulates types I and III collagen production via cell-associated cytokines. J Biol Chem 273:18720
29. Hyka N, Dayer J-M, Modoux C, Kohno T, Edwards CK, Roux-Lombard P, Burger D (2001) Apolipoprotein A-I inhibits the production of interleukin-1B and tumour necrosis factor-a by blocking contact-mediated activation of monocytes by T lymphocytes. Blood 97:2381
30. Manie S, Kubar J, Limouse M, Ferrua B, Ticchioni M, Breittmayer J-P, Peyron J-F, Schaffar L, Rossi B (1993) CD3-stimulated Jurkat T cells mediate IL-1b production in monocytic THP-1 cells. Role of LFA-1 molecule and participation of CD69 T cell antigen. Eur. Cytokine Netw 4:7
31. Zembala M, Siedlar M, Ruggiero I, Wieckiewicz J, Mytar B, Mattei M, Colizzi V (1994) The MHC class-II and CD44 molecules are involved in the induction of tumour necrosis factor (TNF) gene expression by human monocytes stimulated with tumour cells. Int J Cancer 56:269
32. Hayes AL, Smith C, Foxwell BM, Brennan FM (1999) CD45-induced tumor necrosis factor alpha production in monocytes is phosphatidylinositol 3-kinase-dependent and nuclear factor-kappaB-independent. J Biol Chem 274:33455
33. Wagner DH Jr, Stout RD, Suttles J (1994) Role of the CD40–CD40 ligand interaction in CD4+ T cell contact-dependent activation of monocyte interleukin-1 synthesis. Eur J Immunol 24:3148
34. Isomaki P, Aversa G, Cocks BG, Luukkainen R, Saario R, Toivanen P, de Vries JE, Punnonen J (1997) Increased expression of signaling lymphocytic activation molecule in patients with rheumatoid arthritis and its role in the regulation of cytokine production in rheumatoid synovium. J Immunol 159:2986
35. Wanidworanun C, Strober W (1993) Predominant role of tumor necrosis factor-alpha in human monocyte IL-10 synthesis. J Immunol 151:6853
36. Graf D, Muller S, Korthauer U, van Kooten C, Weise C, Kroczek RA (1995) A soluble form of TRAP (CD40 ligand) is rapidly released after T cell activation. Eur J Immunol 25:1749
37. Michel J, Langstein J, Hofstadter F, Schwarz H (1998) A soluble form of CD137 (ILA/4–1BB), a member of the TNF receptor family, is released by activated lymphocytes and is detectable in sera of patients with rheumatoid arthritis. Eur J Immunol 28:290

38. Pizzolo G, Vinante F, Chilosi M, Dallenbach F, Josimovic-Alasevic O, Diamantstein T, Stein H (1990) Serum levels of soluble CD30 molecule (Ki-1 antigen) in Hodgkin's disease: relationship with disease activity and clinical stage. Br J Haematol 75:282
39. Cheng J, Zhou T, Liu C, Shapiro JP, Brauer MJ, Kiefer MC, Barr PJ, Mountz JD (1994) Protection from Fas-mediated apoptosis by a soluble form of the Fas molecule. Science 263:1759
40. Shu U, Kiniwa M, Wu CY, Maliszewski C, Vezzio N, Hakimi J, Gately M, Delespesse G (1995) Activated T cells induce interleukin-12 production by monocytes via CD40-CD40 ligand interaction. Eur J Immunol 25:1125
41. Chabot S, Williams G, Hamilton M, Sutherland G, Yong VW (1999) Mechanisms of IL-10 production in human microglia–T cell interaction. J Immunol 162.6819
42. Foey AD, Feldmann M, Brennan FM (2000) Route of monocyte differentiation determines their cytokine production profile: CD40 ligation induces interleukin 10 expression. Cytokine 12:1496
43. Fleming SD, Campbell PA (1996) Macrophages have cell surface IL-10 that regulates macrophage bactericidal activity. J Immunol 156:1143
44. Brennan FM, Maini RN, Feldmann M (1995) Cytokine expression in chronic inflammatory disease. Br Med Bull 51:368
45. Foxwell BMJ, Browne K, Bondeson J, Clarke C, de Martin R, Brennan FM, Feldmann M (1998) Efficient adenoviral infection with IκBα reveals that TNFα production in rheumatoid arthritis is NF-κB dependent. Proc Natl Acad Sci U S A 95:8211
46. Bondeson J, Foxwell BMJ, Brennan FM, Feldmann M (1999) Defining therapeutic targets by using adenovirus: blocking NF-κB inhibits both inflammatory and destructive mechanisms in rheumatoid synovium but spares anti-inflammatory mediators. Proc Natl. Acad Sci U S A 96:5668
47. Foey AD, Parry SL, Williams LM, Feldmann M, Foxwell BM, Brennan FM (1998) Regulation of monocyte IL-10 synthesis by endogenous IL-1 and TNF-alpha: role of the p38 and p42/44 mitogen-activated protein kinases. J Immunol 160:920
48. De AK, Kodys KM, Yeh BS, Miller-Graziano C (2000) Exaggerated human monocyte IL-10 concomitant to minimal TNF-alpha induction by heat-shock protein 27 (Hsp27) suggests Hsp27 is primarily an antiinflammatory stimulus. J Immunol 165:3951–3958
49. Crawley JB, Williams LM, Mander T, Brennan FM, Foxwell BM (1996) Interleukin-10 stimulation of phosphatidylinositol 3-kinase and p70 S6 kinase is required for the proliferative but not the antiinflammatory effects of the cytokine. J Biol Chem 271:16357
50. Foey A, Green P, Foxwell B, Feldmann M, Brennan F (2002) Cytokine-stimulated T cells induce macrophage IL-10 production dependent on phosphatidylinositol 3-kinase and p70S6K: implications for rheumatoid arthritis. Arthritis Res 4:64
51. Meisel C, Vogt K, Platzer C, Randow F, Liebenthal C, Volk HD (1996) Differential regulation of monocytic tumor necrosis factor-alpha and interleukin-10 expression. Eur J Immunol 26:1580

52. Kambayashi T, Jacob CO, Zhou D, Mazurek N, Fong M, Strassmann G (1995) Cyclic nucleotide phosphodiesterase type IV participates in the regulation of IL-10 and in the subsequent inhibition of TNF-alpha and IL-6 release by endotoxin-stimulated macrophages. J Immunol 155:4909
53. Fontana A, Hengartner H, Weber E, Fehr K, Grob PJ, Cohen G (1982) Interleukin 1 activity in the synovial fluid of patients with rheumatoid arthritis. Rheumatol Int 2:49
54. Buchan G, Barrett K, Turner M, Chantry D, Maini RN, Feldmann M (1988) Interleukin-1 and tumour necrosis factor mRNA expression in rheumatoid arthritis: prolonged production of IL-1 alpha. Clin Exp Immunol 73:449
55. Hopkins SJ, Humphreys M, Jayson MI (1988) Cytokines in synovial fluid. I. The presence of biologically active and immunoreactive IL-1. Clin Exp Immunol 72:422
56. Firestein GS, Alvaro-Gracia JM, Maki R (1990) Quantitative analysis of cytokine gene expression in rheumatoid arthritis. J Immunol 144:3347
57. Wood NC, Dickens E, Symons JA, Duff GW (1992) In situ hybridization of interleukin-1 in CD14-positive cells in rheumatoid arthritis. Clin Immunol Immunopathol 62:295
58. Brennan FM, Chantry D, Jackson A, Maini R, Feldmann M (1989) Inhibitory effect of TNF α antibodies on synovial cell interleukin-1 production in rheumatoid arthritis. Lancet 2:244
59. Fell HB, Jubb RW (1977) The effect of synovial tissue on the breakdown of articular cartilage in organ culture. Arthritis Rheum 20:1359
60. Deleuran BW, Chu CQ, Field M, Brennan FM, Katsikis P, Feldmann M, Maini RN (1992) Localization of interleukin-1 alpha, type 1 interleukin-1 receptor and interleukin-1 receptor antagonist in the synovial membrane and cartilage/pannus junction in rheumatoid arthritis. Br J Rheumatol 31:801
61. Buchan G, Barrett K, Fujita T, Taniguchi T, Maini R, Feldmann M (1988) Detection of activated T cell products in the rheumatoid joint using cDNA probes to Interleukin-2 (IL-2) IL-2 receptor and IFN-gamma. Clin Exp Immunol 71:295
62. Firestein GS, Xu WD, Townsend K, Broide D, Alvaro-Gracia J, Glasebrook A, Zvaifler NJ (1988) Cytokines in chronic inflammatory arthritis. I. Failure to detect T cell lymphokines (interleukin 2 and interleukin 3) and presence of macrophage colony-stimulating factor (CSF-1) and a novel mast cell growth factor in rheumatoid synovitis. J Exp Med 168:1573
63. Okamoto H, Yamamura M, Morita Y, Harada S, Makino H, Ota Z (1997) The synovial expression and serum levels of interleukin-6, interleukin-11, leukemia inhibitory factor, and oncostatin M in rheumatoid arthritis. Arthritis Rheum 40:1096
64. Hirano T, Matsuda T, Turner M, Miyasaka N, Buchan G, Tang B, Sato K, Shimizu M, Maini R, Feldmann M et al (1988) Excessive production of interleukin 6/B cell stimulatory factor-2 in rheumatoid arthritis. Eur J Immunol 18:1797
65. Houssiau FA, Devogelaer JP, Van Damme J, de Deuxchaisnes CN, Van Snick J (1988) Interleukin-6 in synovial fluid and serum of patients with rheumatoid arthritis and other inflammatory arthritides. Arthritis Rheum 31:784
66. Field M, Chu C, Feldmann M, Maini RN (1991) Interleukin-6 localisation in the synovial membrane in rheumatoid arthritis. Rheumatol Int 11:45

67. Helle M, Boeije L, de Groot E, de Vos A, Aarden L (1991) Sensitive ELISA for interleukin-6. Detection of IL-6 in biological fluids: synovial fluids and sera. J Immunol Methods 138:47
68. Harada S, Yamamura M, Okamoto H, Morita Y, Kawashima M, Aita T, Makino H (1999) Production of interleukin-7 and interleukin-15 by fibroblast-like synoviocytes from patients with rheumatoid arthritis. Arthritis Rheum 42:1508
69. Hermann JA, Hall MA, Maini RN, Feldmann M, Brennan FM (1998) Important immunoregulatory role of interleukin-11 in the inflammatory process in rheumatoid arthritis. Arthritis Rheum 41:1388
70. Morita Y, Yamamura M, Nishida K, Harada S, Okamoto H, Inoue H, Ohmoto Y, Modlin RL, Makino H (1998) Expression of interleukin-12 in synovial tissue from patients with rheumatoid arthritis. Arthritis Rheum 41:306
71. Chabaud M, Durand JM, Buchs N, Fossiez F, Page G, Frappart L, Miossec P (1999) Human interleukin-17: A T cell-derived proinflammatory cytokine produced by the rheumatoid synovium. Arthritis Rheum 42:963
72. Gracie JA, Forsey RJ, Chan WL, Gilmour A, Leung BP, Greer MR, Kennedy K, Carter R, Wei XQ, Xu D, Field M, Foulis A, Liew FY, McInnes IB (1999) A proinflammatory role for IL-18 in rheumatoid arthritis. J Clin Invest 104:1393
73. Di Giovine FS, Nuki G, Duff GW (1988) Tumour necrosis factor in synovial exudates. Ann Rheum Dis 47:768
74. Saxne T, Palladino MA Jr, Heinegard D, Talal N, Wollheim FA (1988) Detection of tumor necrosis factor alpha but not tumor necrosis factor beta in rheumatoid arthritis synovial fluid and serum. Arthritis Rheum 31:1041
75. Hopkins SJ, Meager A (1988) Cytokines in synovial fluid: II. The presence of tumour necrosis factor and interferon. Clin Exp Immunol 73:88
76. Chu CQ, Field M, Feldmann M, Maini RN (1991) Localization of tumor necrosis factor α in synovial tissues and at the cartilage-pannus junction in patients with rheumatoid arthritis. Arthritis Rheum 34:1125
77. Brennan FM, Chantry D, Jackson AM, Maini RN, Feldmann M (1989) Cytokine production in culture by cells isolated from the synovial membrane. J Autoimmun 2 [Suppl]:177
78. Xu WD, Firestein GS, Taetle R, Kaushansky K, Zvaifler NJ (1989) Cytokines in chronic inflammatory arthritis. II. Granulocyte-macrophage colony-stimulating factor in rheumatoid synovial effusions. J Clin Invest 83:876
79. Haworth C, Brennan FM, Chantry D, Turner M, Maini RN, Feldmann M (1991) Expression of granulocyte-macrophage colony-stimulating factor in rheumatoid arthritis: regulation by tumor necrosis factor-α. Eur J Immunol 21:2575
80. Alvaro-Gracia JM, Zvaifler NJ, Brown CB, Kaushansky K, Firestein GS (1991) Cytokines in chronic inflammatory arthritis. VI. Analysis of the synovial cells involved in granulocyte-macrophage colony-stimulating factor production and gene expression in rheumatoid arthritis and its regulation by IL-1 and tumor necrosis factor-alpha. J Immunol 146:3365
81. Miossec P, Naviliat M, Dupuy d'Angeac A, Sany J, Bancherau J (1990) Low levels of interleukin-4 and high levels of transforming growth factor beta in rheumatoid synovitis. Arthritis Rheum 33:1180

82. Cohen SB, Katsikis PD, Chu CQ, Thomssen H, Webb LM, Maini RN, Londei M, Feldmann M (1995) High level of interleukin-10 production by the activated T cell population within the rheumatoid synovial membrane. Arthritis Rheum 38:946
83. Llorente L, Richaud-Patin Y, Fior R, Alcocer-Varela J, Wijdenes J, Fourrier BM, Galanaud P, Emilie D (1994) In vivo production of interleukin-10 by non-T cells in rheumatoid arthritis, Sjogren's syndrome, and systemic lupus erythematosus. A potential mechanism of B lymphocyte hyperactivity and autoimmunity. Arthritis Rheum 37:1647
84. Cush JJ, Splawski JB, Thomas R, McFarlin JE, Schulze-Koops H, Davis LS, Fujita K, Lipsky PE (1995) Elevated interleukin-10 levels in patients with rheumatoid arthritis. Arthritis Rheum 38:96
85. Isomaki P, Luukkainen R, Toivanen P, Punnonen J (1996) The presence of interleukin-13 in rheumatoid synovium and its antiinflammatory effects on synovial fluid macrophages from patients with rheumatoid arthritis. Arthritis Rheum 39:1693
86. Franz JK, Kolb SA, Hummel KM, Lahrtz F, Neidhart M, Aicher WK, Pap T, Gay RE, Fontana A, Gay S (1998) Interleukin-16, produced by synovial fibroblasts, mediates chemoattraction for CD4+ T lymphocytes in rheumatoid arthritis. Eur J Immunol 28:2661
87. Blaschke S, Schulz H, Schwarz G, Blaschke V, Muller GA, Reuss-Borst M (2001) Interleukin 16 expression in relation to disease activity in rheumatoid arthritis. J Rheumatol 28:12
88. Fava R, Olsen N, Keski-Oja J, Moses H, Pincus T (1989) Active and latent forms of transforming growth factor beta activity in synovial effusions. J Exp Med 169:291
89. Bucala R, Ritchlin C, Winchester R, Cerami A (1991) Constitutive production of inflammatory and mitogenic cytokines by rheumatoid synovial fibroblasts. J Exp Med 173:569
90. Lafyatis R, Thompson NL, Remmers EF, Flanders KC, Roche NS, Kim SJ, Case JP, Sporn MB, Roberts AB, Wilder RL (1989) Transforming growth factor-beta production by synovial tissues from rheumatoid patients and streptococcal cell wall arthritic rats. Studies on secretion by synovial fibroblast-like cells and immunohistologic localization. J Immunol 143:1142
91. Brennan FM, Chantry D, Turner M, Foxwell B, Maini RN, Feldmann M (1990) Transforming growth factor-β in rheumatoid arthritis synovial tissue: lack of effect on spontaneous cytokine production in joint cell cultures. Clin Exp Immunol 81:278
92. Lotz M, Kekow J, Carson DA (1990) Transforming growth factor-beta and cellular immune responses in synovial fluids. J Immunol 144:4189
93. Chu CQ, Field M, Abney E, Zheng RQ, Allard S, Feldmann M, Maini RN (1991) Transforming growth factor-beta 1 in rheumatoid synovial membrane and cartilage/pannus junction. Clin Exp Immunol 86:380
94. Brennan FM, Zachariae CO, Chantry D, Larsen CG, Turner M, Maini RN, Matsushima K, Feldmann M (1990) Detection of interleukin 8 biological activity in synovial fluids from patients with rheumatoid arthritis and production of interleukin 8 mRNA by isolated synovial cells. Eur J Immunol 20:2141

95. Koch AE, Kunkel SL, Burrows JC, Evanoff HL, Haines GK, Pope RM, Strieter RM (1991) Synovial tissue macrophage as a source of the chemotactic cytokine IL-8. J Immunol 147:2187
96. Seitz M, Dewald B, Gerber N, Baggiolini M (1991) Enhanced production of neutrophil-activating peptide-1/interleukin-8 in rheumatoid arthritis. J Clin Invest 87:463
97. Hosaka S, Akahoshi T, Wada C, Kondo H (1994) Expression of the chemokine superfamily in rheumatoid arthritis. Clin Exp Immunol 97:451
98. Deleuran B, Lemche P, Kristensen M, Chu CQ, Field M, Jensen J, Matsushima K, Stengaard-Pedersen K (1994) Localisation of interleukin 8 in the synovial membrane, cartilage-pannus junction and chondrocytes in rheumatoid arthritis. Scand J Rheumatol 23:2
99. Koch AE, Kunkel SL, Harlow LA, Mazarakis DD, Haines GK, Burdick MD, Pope RM, Strieter RM (1994) Macrophage inflammatory protein-1 alpha. A novel chemotactic cytokine for macrophages in rheumatoid arthritis. J Clin Invest 93:921
100. Villiger PM, Terkeltaub R, Lotz M (1992) Production of monocyte chemoattractant protein-1 by inflamed synovial tissue and cultured synoviocytes. J Immunol 149:722
101. Akahoshi T, Wada C, Endo H, Hirota K, Hosaka S, Takagishi K, Kondo H, Kashiwazaki S, Matsushima K (1993) Expression of monocyte chemotactic and activating factor in rheumatoid arthritis. Regulation of its production in synovial cells by interleukin-1 and tumor necrosis factor. Arthritis Rheum 36:762
102. Hachicha M, Rathanaswami P, Schall TJ, McColl SR (1993) Production of monocyte chemotactic protein-1 in human type B synoviocytes. Synergistic effect of tumor necrosis factor alpha and interferon-gamma. Arthritis Rheum 36:26
103. Koch AE, Kunkel SL, Harlow LA, Mazarakis DD, Haines GK, Burdick MD, Pope RM, Walz A, Strieter RM (1994) Epithelial neutrophil activating peptide-78: a novel chemotactic cytokine for neutrophils in arthritis. J Clin Invest 94:1012
104. Rathanaswami P, Hachicha M, Sadick M, Schall TJ, McColl SR (1993) Expression of the cytokine RANTES in human rheumatoid synovial fibroblasts. Differential regulation of RANTES and interleukin-8 genes by inflammatory cytokines. J Biol Chem 268:5834
105. Radstake TR, van der Voort R, Ten Brummelhuis M, de Waal Malefijt M, Looman M, Figdor CG, van den Berg WB, Barrera P, Adema GJ (2005) Increased expression of CCL18, CCL19, and CCL17 by dendritic cells from patients with rheumatoid arthritis, and regulation by Fc gamma receptors. Ann Rheum Dis 64:359
106. Page G, Miossec P (2004) Paired synovium and lymph nodes from rheumatoid arthritis patients differ in dendritic cell and chemokine expression. J Pathol 204:28
107. Ruth JH, Shahrara S, Park CC, Morel JC, Kumar P, Qin S, Koch AE (2003) Role of macrophage inflammatory protein-3alpha and its ligand CCR6 in rheumatoid arthritis. Lab Invest 83:579
108. Grassi F, Cristino S, Toneguzzi S, Piacentini A, Facchini A, Lisignoli G (2004) CXCL12 chemokine up-regulates bone resorption and MMP-9 release by human osteoclasts: CXCL12 levels are increased in synovial and bone tissue of rheumatoid arthritis patients. J Cell Physiol 199:244

109. Ruschpler P, Lorenz P, Eichler W, Koczan D, Hanel C, Scholz R, Melzer C, Thiesen HJ, Stiehl P (2003) High CXCR3 expression in synovial mast cells associated with CXCL9 and CXCL10 expression in inflammatory synovial tissues of patients with rheumatoid arthritis. Arthritis Res Ther 5:R241
110. Konig A, Krenn V, Toksoy A, Gerhard N, Gillitzer R (2000) Mig, GRO alpha and RANTES messenger RNA expression in lining layer, infiltrates and different leucocyte populations of synovial tissue from patients with rheumatoid arthritis, psoriatic arthritis and osteoarthritis. Virchows Arch 436:449
111. Ruth JH, Volin MV, Haines GK 3rd, Woodruff DC, Katschke KJ Jr, Woods JM, Park CC, Morel JC, Koch AE (2001) Fractalkine, a novel chemokine in rheumatoid arthritis and in rat adjuvant-induced arthritis. Arthritis Rheum 44:1568
112. Shi K, Hayashida K, Kaneko M, Hashimoto J, Tomita T, Lipsky PE, Yoshikawa H, Ochi T (2001) Lymphoid chemokine B cell-attracting chemokine-1 (CXCL13) is expressed in germinal center of ectopic lymphoid follicles within the synovium of chronic arthritis patients. J Immunol 166:650
113. Fava RA, Olsen NJ, Spencer-Green G, Yeo KT, Yeo TK, Berse B, Jackman RW, Senger DR, Dvorak HF, Brown LF (1994) Vascular permeability factor/endothelial growth factor (VPF/VEGF): accumulation and expression in human synovial fluids and rheumatoid synovial tissue. J Exp Med 180:341
114. Koch AE, Harlow LA, Haines GK, Amento EP, Unemori EN, Wong WL, Pope RM, Ferrara N (1994) Vascular endothelial growth factor. A cytokine modulating endothelial function in rheumatoid arthritis. J Immunol 152:4149
115. Goddard DH, Grossman SL, Moore ME (1990) Autocrine regulation of rheumatoid arthritis synovial cell growth in vitro. Cytokine 2:149
116. Sano H, Forough R, Maier JA, Case JP, Jackson A, Engleka K, Maciag T, Wilder RL (1990) Detection of high levels of heparin binding growth factor-1 (acidic fibroblast growth factor) in inflammatory arthritic joints. J Cell Biol 110:1417
117. Goddard DH, Grossman SL, Williams WV, Weiner DB, Gross JL, Eidsvoog K, Dasch JR (1992) Regulation of synovial cell growth. Coexpression of transforming growth factor beta and basic fibroblast growth factor by cultured synovial cells. Arthritis Rheum 35:1296
118. Sano H, Engleka K, Mathern P, Hla T, Crofford LJ, Remmers EF, Jelsema CL, Goldmuntz E, Maciag T, Wilder RL (1993) Coexpression of phosphotyrosine-containing proteins, platelet-derived growth factor-B, and fibroblast growth factor-1 in situ in synovial tissues of patients with rheumatoid arthritis and Lewis rats with adjuvant or streptococcal cell wall arthritis. J Clin Invest 91:553
119. Remmers EF, Lafyatis R, Kumkumian GK, Case JP, Roberts AB, Sporn MB, Wilder RL (1990) Cytokines and growth regulation of synoviocytes from patients with rheumatoid arthritis and rats with streptococcal cell wall arthritis. Growth Factors 2:179
120. Remmers EF, Sano H, Lafyatis R, Case JP, Kumkumian GK, Hla T, Maciag T, Wilder RL (1991) Production of platelet derived growth factor B chain (PDGF-B/c-sis) mRNA and immunoreactive PDGF B-like polypeptide by rheumatoid synovium: coexpression with heparin binding acidic fibroblast growth factor-1. J Rheumatol 18:7

T Cell Activation as Starter and Motor of Rheumatic Inflammation

A. Skapenko[1] · P. E. Lipsky[2] · H. Schulze-Koops[1] (✉)

[1]Nikolaus Fiebiger Center for Molecular Medicine, Clinical Research Group III, Department of Internal Medicine III and Institute for Clinical Immunology, University of Erlangen-Nuremberg, Glückstrasse 6, 91054 Erlangen, Germany
Schulze-Koops@med3.imed.uni-erlangen.de
[2]National Institute of Arthritis and Musculoskeletal and Skin Diseases, 9000 Rockville Pike, Bethesda, MD 20892, USA

1	T Cell Development and T Cell Subsets	196
2	CD4 T Cells in Rheumatic Inflammation	199
3	The Th1/Th2 Dichotomy	200
4	Rheumatic Inflammation Is Driven by Activated Th1 Cells	202
5	T Cell-Directed Therapies	204
6	Conclusion	207
References		208

Abstract Rheumatic inflammation is driven by sustained specific immunity against self-antigens, resulting in local inflammation and cellular infiltration and, subsequently, in tissue damage. Although the specific autoantigen(s) eliciting the detrimental immune reactions in rheumatic diseases have rarely been defined, it has become clear that the mechanisms resulting in the destruction of tissue and the loss of organ function during the course of the diseases are essentially the same as in protective immunity against invasive microorganisms. Of fundamental importance in initiating, controlling, and driving these specific immune responses are CD4 T cells. Currently available data provide compelling evidence for a major role of CD4 T cells in the initiation and perpetuation of chronic rheumatic inflammation. Consequently, T cell-directed therapies have been employed with substantial clinical success in the treatment of rheumatic diseases. Here, we review current knowledge based on which CD4 T cells can be implicated as the motor of rheumatic inflammation.

1
T Cell Development and T Cell Subsets

The peripheral T cell repertoire consists of T cells that have survived dual selection in the thymus and comprises several distinct T cell subsets that can be identified based on their characteristic cell surface molecule expression (Germain 2002; Spits 2002; Weiss 1993). All T cells express a disulfide-linked heterodimeric T cell receptor (TCR), which confers antigen specificity to the T cell. Associated with the TCR and required for its surface expression is the CD3 complex, which consists of four invariant transmembrane polypeptides (designated γδεε). The CD3 complex mediates signaling and is linked to a largely intracytoplasmic homodimer of ζ-chains, which are critical for maximal signaling (Chan et al. 1992). CD4 or CD8, co-receptors, whose expression is mutually exclusive on mature post-thymic T cells, bind to invariant sites of the major histocompatibility complex (MHC) class II or I molecules on antigen-presenting cells (APCs), respectively, stabilize the MHC/peptide/TCR complex during T cell activation, and thus increase the sensitivity of a T cell for activation by MHC-presented antigen by approximately 100-fold (Weiss 1993).

In humans, the great majority of peripheral blood T cells expresses TCRs consisting of α and β chains (αβ T cells). αβ T cells can be divided into two subgroups, characterized by the expression of either CD4 or CD8 (Table 1). CD4 αβ T cells primarily function as regulators of other immune cells either through secreted cytokines or by direct cell–cell contact. Consequently, CD4 αβ T cells mediate the classical helper T cell responses. CD8 αβ T cells, on the other hand, are programmed to become cytotoxic effector cells that kill infected target cells. CD8 T cells are therefore named cytotoxic T cells. As the αβ TCR does not bind antigen directly, T cell activation is dependent on

Table 1 Human T cell subsets

TCR	Frequency	Co-receptor	Function	Restriction	Antigen
αβ	95%–98%	CD4 helper (50–80%)	Regulators of other immune cells; cytokine secretion; cell–cell contact;	MHC class II	Exogenous peptides
		CD8 cytotoxic (20–50%)	Cytolysis of target cells	MHC class I	Endogenous peptides
γδ	2%–5%	None, CD8α		None	Unknown, peptides?

TCR, T cell receptor; MHC, major histocompatibility complex

an interaction of the TCR with MHC molecules that present small peptide fragments that have been generated from protein antigens. Whereas MHC class I molecules are virtually expressed on all nucleated cells, MHC class II expression is restricted to professional APCs, such as B cells, dendritic cells, and macrophages, and to activated T cells in humans. MHC class I molecules bind antigens that are generated by the particular cells themselves as well as antigens from intracellular pathogens that reside in the cytoplasm; they present their antigens to CD8 T cells. MHC class II molecules, in contrast, present antigens derived from ingested proteins, such as extracellular bacteria or damaged self-tissue, to CD4 T cells.

As almost all cells express MHC class I molecules and, thus, may become the targets of CD8 T cell-mediated killing, CD8 cells evidently express a great potential for tissue damage. Moreover, activated CD8 T cells can produce very high levels of tumor necrosis factor (TNF) and interferon (IFN)-γ, which may contribute directly and/or indirectly to target cell destruction in autoimmune diseases. Notwithstanding these characteristics, however, there is inconclusive evidence to suggest that CD8 T cells are key players in rheumatic inflammation and contribute to tissue damage. Although some observations imply that activated CD8 T cells are involved in aggravating pathologic responses in rheumatoid synovitis as producers of pro-inflammatory cytokines (Berner et al. 2000) and regulators of the structural integrity and functional activity of germinal center-like structures in ectopic lymphoid follicles within the synovial membrane (Kang et al. 2002; Wagner et al. 1998), studies in animals deficient for CD4 or CD8 have clearly demonstrated a limited importance for CD8 T cells in initiating and maintaining autoimmune inflammatory arthritis. For example, whereas B10.Q mice lacking CD4 are less susceptible to collagen-induced arthritis (CIA), but not completely resistant, the CD8 deficiency has no significant impact on the disease (Ehinger et al. 2001). Moreover, in mice transgenic for the RA-susceptibility gene *HLA-DQ8*, CD4-deficient mice were resistant to developing CIA, whereas CD8-deficient mice developed disease with increased incidence and greater severity (Taneja et al. 2002). These data may suggest that CD8 T cells are not only incapable of initiating CIA but may, alternatively, have a regulatory and protective effect on rheumatic inflammation.

A small group of peripheral T cells bears an alternative TCR composed of γ and δ chains (γδ T cells). γδ TCRs appear to recognize antigen directly, similar to immunoglobulins (Ig), but do not require presentation by an MHC protein or other molecules and do not depend on antigen processing (Table 1). The function of γδ T cells within the human immune system is largely unknown. In particular, the role of synovial γδ T cells, and their contribution to rheumatic inflammation is incompletely defined. In the remainder of this review, we will therefore concentrate on the role of αβ T cells in rheumatic diseases and we refer to αβ T cells when using the term "T cell" unless specifically noted otherwise.

CD4 T cells that emerge from the thymus belong to the naïve T cell pool that consists of T cells that have never encountered their specific antigen. Naïve T cells are long lived, have a restricted function (for example, naïve CD4 T cells only produce interleukin [IL]-2), but stringent requirements for activation (Table 2). In humans, naïve T cells are characterized phenotypically by the expression of the long isoform of CD45, CD45RA. Naïve T cells are restricted to recirculate between the blood and secondary lymphoid tissues, although in some autoimmune diseases they may also accumulate in chronically inflamed tissues. Upon proper activation, naïve T cells proliferate and differentiate into specialized effector cells. Differentiation of T cells is characterized by a number of phenotypic and functional alterations, such as changes in their migratory capacities, modifications in life span, and secretion of effector cytokines (for example, IL-4 and IFN-γ) (Table 1). Most activated naïve T cells become short-lived effector cells, but some enter the long-lived memory T cell pool. Memory T cells, in humans, can be characterized by the expression of the short isoform of CD45, CD45RO. Memory cells respond more rapidly to antigen challenge and express a diverse array of effector functions. In contrast to naïve T cells, memory cells do not require co-stimulation for activation. Thus, memory T cells do not depend on the interaction with professional

Table 2 Characteristics of naïve, memory and effector αβ T cells

	Naïve	Memory	Effector
Activation requirement	Stringent	Low	Low
Migration pattern	Blood; peripheral LN	Inflamed tissue; mucosal tissue	Inflamed tissue
Frequency responding to particular antigen	Very low	Low	High
Cytokine production	No	No	Yes
Cell cycling	No	No	Yes
Live span	Long	Long	Short
Surface protein expression			
CD25	Low	Low	High
Adhesion molecules	Low	High	High
CD45 isoform	CD45RA	CD45RO	CD45RO

LN, lymph node

APCs for activation, provided their specific antigen can be presented in the context of the appropriate MHC molecules by nonprofessional APCs.

2
CD4 T Cells in Rheumatic Inflammation

In contrast to the limited and partially controversial information about the role of CD8 T cells and γδ T cells in rheumatic inflammation, extensive and compelling evidence exists to suggest that CD4 T cells play a dominant role in the immunopathogenesis of autoimmune inflammatory rheumatic diseases, such as rheumatoid arthritis (RA) (Table 3). For example, activated CD4 memory T cells can be found in the inflammatory infiltrates of the rheumatoid synovium (Van Boxel and Paget 1975). Moreover, appropriate T cell-directed therapies have clearly provided clinical benefit in RA (Table 4) (Panayi and Tugwell 1994; Paulus et al. 1977; Strober et al. 1985). The most compelling data, however, implying a central role for CD4 T cells in propagating rheumatoid inflammation remain the association of aggressive forms of the disease with particular MHC class II alleles, such as subtypes of HLA-DR4, that contain similar amino acid motifs in the CDR3 region of the DRβ-chain (Calin et al. 1989; Winchester 1994). Although the exact meaning of this association has not been resolved, all interpretations imply that CD4 T cells orchestrate the local inflammation and cellular infiltration, following which a large number of subsequent inflammatory events occur. The requirement for CD4 T cells in the induction of inflammatory arthritis in a variety of animal models of rheumatic inflammation and the induction of tissue damaging autoimmunity in these models by transfer of CD4 T cells from sick animals into healthy syngeneic recipients can be regarded as further evidence of the importance of CD4 T cells in autoimmune rheumatic inflammation (Banerjee et al. 1992; Breedveld et al. 1989).

Table 3 Indications for a pathogenic role of CD4 T cells in rheumatoid inflammation

Association of rheumatoid arthritis with HLA-DR4 and DR1 subtypes (shared epitope)
Enrichment of activated CD4 memory T cells in peripheral blood, synovial membrane, and synovial fluid
Important role in disease initiation in several animal models of inflammatory arthritis
Clinical efficacy of appropriate T cell-directed therapies

Table 4 T cell-directed therapies in rheumatoid arthritis

Reduction of T cell number or function
    Total lymphoid irradiation
    Thoracic duct drainage
Immunosuppressive drugs
    Glucocorticoids
    Methotrexate
    Leflunomide
    Cyclosporine
    FK 506 (tacrolimus)
    Rapamycin (sirolimus)
Biologicals
    TCR vaccination
    mAbs to T cell surface receptors
    mAbs to surface receptors on cells interacting with T cells
    Cytokines, mAbs to cytokines
    Inhibitors of T cell/APC interactions

TCR, T cell receptor; *APC,* antigen-presenting cells

3
The Th1/Th2 Dichotomy

Whereas the specific antigen(s) recognized by the autoreactive CD4 T cells in rheumatic disease are largely still unknown, much progress has been made in defining the phenotype and function of those pathogenic CD4 T cells. In 1986, it was discovered that repeated antigen-specific stimulation of murine CD4 T cells in vitro results in the development of restricted and stereotyped patterns of cytokine secretion profiles in the resultant T cell populations (Mosmann et al. 1986). Based on these distinctive cytokine secretion pattern and concomitant effector functions, CD4 T cells can be divided into at least two major subsets (Fig. 1). Th1 cells develop preferentially during infections with intracellular bacteria. Upon activation, Th1 cells secrete the pro-inflammatory cytokines IL-2, IFN-γ, and lymphotoxin-α (LT, TNF-β). They activate macrophages to produce reactive oxygen intermediates and nitric oxide, stimulate their phagocytic functions and enhance their ability for antigen presentation by upregulation of MHC class II molecules. Moreover, Th1 cells promote the induction of complement fixing, opsonizing antibodies and of antibodies involved in antibody-dependent cell cytotoxicity, e.g., IgG1 in humans and IgG2a in mice. Consequently, Th1 cells are involved in cell-

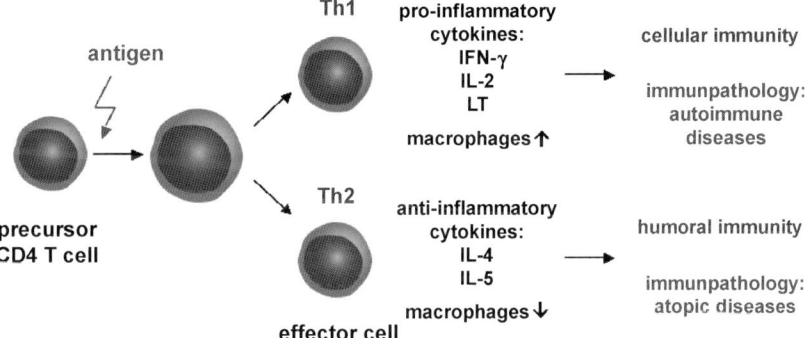

Fig. 1 Differentiation of CD4 T cells into specialized Th1 or Th2 effector cells. Upon activation with specific antigen, CD4 T cells proliferate and differentiate into either the Th1 or the Th2 subset. Th1 cells promote cellular immunity and are involved in the development of autoimmune diseases; Th2 cells mediate humoral immunity and are involved in allergic immune responses. (From Skapenko et al. 2005, with permission)

mediated immunity. Immune responses driven by Th1 cells are exemplified by the delayed type hypersensitivity (DTH) reaction (Abbas et al. 1996; Mosmann et al. 1986). Th2 cells predominate after infestations with gastrointestinal nematodes and helminths. They produce the anti-inflammatory cytokines IL-4, IL-5, and IL-13 and provide potent help for B cell activation and Ig class switching to IgE and subtypes of IgG that do not fix complement, e.g., IgG2 in humans and IgG1 in the mouse. Th2 cells mediate allergic immune responses and have been associated with downmodulation of macrophage activation, which is conferred largely by the anti-inflammatory effects of IL-4 (Abbas et al. 1996; Mosmann et al. 1986). Th2 cells can also secrete IL-6 and IL-10. However, in contrast to mice, those cytokines in humans are not confined to the Th2 subset but can also be produced by Th1 cells (Abbas et al. 1996).

The different functional T cell subsets do not derive from different pre-committed lineages but rather develop from the same uncommitted precursor cell under the influence of environmental and genetic factors (Rocken et al. 1992). Cytokines are the most important regulators of Th subset differentiation. Whereas IL-2 is required for the differentiation of naïve cells into either Th subset without imposing a functional bias, priming of naïve CD4 T cells in the presence of IL-4 induces differentiation of Th2 effector cells. In contrast, Th1 cell development occurs in the absence of IL-4 and is greatly enhanced by IL-12 (Abbas et al. 1996). Other factors that control Th subset polarization include the nature and intensity of co-stimulatory signals, in particular via CD28 and OX40, the intensity of TCR ligation during priming, the type of antigen-presenting cells, the MHC class II genotype, minor histocompatibility complex genes, and corticosteroids or endogenous hormones (Abbas et al. 1996).

Importantly, Th1 and Th2 cells antagonize each other by blocking the generation of the antipodal cell type and by blocking each other's effector functions. For instance, the generation of Th1 cells can be effectively blocked by high concentrations of IL-4, even in the presence of IL-12 (Hsieh et al. 1993). At the level of effector functions, IL-4 antagonizes much of the pro-inflammatory effects of IFN-γ and inhibits the proliferation of Th1 cells. Conversely, IFN-γ secreted by Th1 cells blocks the proliferation of Th2 cells.

Differentiation of the appropriate T cell subset is of crucial importance to the host in mounting protective immunity against exogenous microorganisms. However, it is apparent that immune responses driven preferentially by activated T cell subsets are also involved in the development of pathological immune disorders. Whereas atopic diseases result from Th2-dominated responses to environmental allergens, Th1-mediated immunity is involved in the generation of several organ-specific experimental autoimmune diseases in animals, such as experimental allergic encephalomyelitis, insulin-dependent diabetes mellitus, or CIA (Abbas et al. 1996). Although dichotomizing complex diseases such as rheumatic diseases in terms of Th1 or Th2 patterns may be an oversimplification, evidence is accumulating to suggest that human autoimmune diseases, such as rheumatoid arthritis (RA), might also be driven by preferentially activated Th1 cells without sufficient Th2 cell development to downregulate inflammation.

4
Rheumatic Inflammation Is Driven by Activated Th1 Cells

Various epidemiological and clinical observations suggest a pathogenic Th1 drive in rheumatoid inflammation. For several decades, clinical observations have highlighted the ameliorating effect of pregnancy on the course of RA (Da Silva and Spector 1992). Pregnancy improves the symptoms of RA in about 75% of women, leading to a significant resolution of inflammation and a relief of symptoms, which enables the patients to taper or even stop the use of medications. In fact, the effect of pregnancy on RA activity is greater than the effect of some of the newer therapeutic agents. Although the mechanisms for this phenomenon are still unclear, a marked decrease in Th1-mediated immunity during pregnancy has been firmly established. For example, pregnant women have a higher incidence of infections compared to nonpregnant females, in particular infections with intracellular pathogens. Most recently, a placental derived protein (placental protein 14) was identified; it inhibits

Th1 immune responses and synergizes with IL-4 to promote Th2 immunity by inhibiting the downmodulation of the Th2 specific transcription factor, GATA-3 (Mishan-Eisenberg et al. 2004). These data suggest that pregnancy induces a shift from Th1 to Th2 immune responses, thereby increasing anti-inflammatory cytokines, which may contribute to the gestational amelioration of RA. Interestingly, relapses of RA occur within 6 months postpartum in 90% of the cases. At that time, pregnancy-associated alterations in Th subset activation can no longer be found (Da Silva and Spector 1992), suggesting that the beneficial Th2 shift has resolved and has allowed the Th1 dominated autoimmune inflammation to recur.

Patients with RA have a decreased prevalence of allergic diseases (Verhoef et al. 1998). Moreover, those patients with RA who, for example, have hay fever have less severe disease compared with control patients with RA without hay fever (Verhoef et al. 1998). As expected, atopic RA patients have higher levels of serum IgE and peripheral blood eosinophils, but their T cells produce less IFN-γ after maximum in vitro stimulation (Verhoef et al. 1998). As allergy is the prototype Th2 disease and activated Th2 cells are able to inhibit the generation and the function of Th1 effectors, these studies support the contention that the occurrence of a Th2-mediated immune response might be beneficial in RA by inhibiting Th1-driven immunity.

In addition to these clinical observations, various experimental approaches have also emphasized the dominance of activated Th1 effector cells in rheumatoid inflammation. For example, the vast majority of T cell clones from the human rheumatoid synovial membrane functionally represent the Th1 subset, producing large amounts of IFN-γ but no IL-4 upon challenge with their specific antigens (Miltenburg et al. 1992; Quayle et al. 1993). In the majority of synovial biopsies, IFN-γ, as assessed by different techniques, prevails, whereas IL-4 is rarely found (Canete et al. 2000; Kusaba et al. 1998). Importantly, synovial fluid- and synovial tissue-derived T cells express activation markers on their surface, indicating that these IFN-γ expressing cells are actively engaged in driving synovial inflammation. The frequency of IFN-γ producing CD4 T cells is significantly increased in the synovial fluid compared to the peripheral blood (Davis et al. 2001), resulting in a markedly elevated Th1/Th2 ratio in the synovial fluid that correlates with disease activity (van der Graaff et al. 1999). Likewise, drastically reduced synthesis of IL-4 and IL-10 mRNA by synovial fluid mononuclear cells of RA patients correlates with disease activity (Miyata et al. 2000). Together, these data strongly suggest that CD4 T cells from the inflamed rheumatoid synovium represent activated Th1 cells, secreting IFN-γ, which, in turn, orchestrates synovial inflammation.

Activated CD4 T cells expressing elevated mRNA levels for IL-2 and/or for IFN-γ can also be detected in the peripheral blood of patients with active RA

(Schulze-Koops et al. 1995). Most interestingly, when re-entry of circulating T cells into sites of inflammation in vivo was blocked by administration of a monoclonal antibody (mAb) to intercellular adhesion molecule (ICAM)-1 (CD54), a significant increase in IFN-γ mRNA levels in the peripheral blood occurred that might reflect a redistribution of activated Th1 cells from sites of inflammation into the peripheral circulation (Schulze-Koops et al. 1995). Moreover, the frequencies of IFN-γ secreting peripheral blood T cells in patients with new onset synovitis (<1 year duration) correlate well with disease activity, emphasizing the role of Th1 cells in the initiation of the disease (Kanik et al. 1998).

The arguments depicted here in detail demonstrate that Th1 cells and their cytokines are not only present in RA but contribute to the perpetuation of chronic inflammation. However, the data do not yet allow a conclusion about whether Th1 cells are the initiators of rheumatoid inflammation or rather appear as a consequence of it. In order to delineate the mechanisms underlying the dominant Th1 drive in RA, studies were carried out to assess the functional capability of T cells in RA patients. Isolated memory CD4 T cells from the majority of patients with early RA manifested a profound inability to mount Th2 responses (Skapenko et al. 1999). Thus, those patients cannot generate immunoregulatory Th2 cells that might downmodulate ongoing Th1-mediated inflammation. Failure to downregulate activated Th1 cells might allow Th1 inflammation to persist and evolve into chronic inflammation, characterized by the continuous activation of T cells, macrophages, fibroblasts, and osteoclasts and, subsequently, the destruction of tissue. As this functional abnormality of CD4 T cells in RA is evident at the time of initial clinical symptoms of arthritis (Skapenko et al. 1999), the data strongly suggest that the Th1 dominated immunity is the basis of rheumatoid inflammation and is not merely its consequence.

Together, these data indicate that Th1 cells and their cytokines promote many aspects of synovial inflammation. Moreover, evidence is accumulating that dysregulated T cell differentiation with impaired Th2 cell generation is instrumental in allowing the initial Th1-driven autoimmune response in RA to evolve into chronic inflammation. Interference with the activation and generation of Th1 cells and with the activity of their secreted cytokines might, therefore, be beneficial in the treatment of RA.

5
T Cell-Directed Therapies

Based on the concept that activated T cells are the key mediators of chronic autoimmune inflammation, various T cell-directed therapeutic interventions have been introduced for the treatment of RA. Comprehensive reviews have discussed the concepts and the clinical efficacy of T cell-directed therapy in RA (Panayi 1999; Schulze-Koops and Lipsky 2000; Schulze-Koops and Kalden 2003; Yocum 1999). Here, we will review those approaches that target the pathogenetically important alterations of CD4 T cell functions as outlined above.

As RA is driven by pro-inflammatory Th1 cells with impaired differentiation of immunoregulatory Th2 cells, a shift in the balance of Th1/Th2 effector cells toward anti-inflammatory Th2 cells would be expected to be clinically beneficial. The concept of modulating the Th1/Th2 balance as a treatment for chronic autoimmunity has been successfully applied in a number of animal models of autoimmune diseases (Bessis et al. 1996; Joosten et al. 1999). It is therefore of interest to note that several recent studies have indicated that DMARDs appear to be able to modulate the Th1/Th2 balance. For example, leflunomide, a potent nontoxic inhibitor of the rate-limiting enzyme of the de novo synthesis of pyrimidines, dihydroorotate dehydrogenase (Bruneau et al. 1998), selectively decreases the activation of pro-inflammatory Th1 cells while promoting Th2 cell differentiation from naïve precursors (Dimitrova et al. 2002). Sulfasalazine potently inhibits the production of IL-12 in a dose-dependent manner in mouse macrophages stimulated with LPS. Importantly, pretreatment of macrophages with sulfasalazine either in vitro or in vivo reduces their ability to induce the Th1 cytokine IFN-γ and increases the ability to induce the Th2 cytokine IL-4 in antigen-primed CD4 T cells (Kang et al. 1999). Methotrexate significantly decreases the production of IFN-γ and IL-2 by in vitro stimulated peripheral blood mononuclear cells while increasing the concentration of IL-4 and IL-10 (Constantin et al. 1998). Likewise, clinical efficacy of cyclosporine is associated with decreased serum levels of IFN-γ, IL-2 and IL-12 and with significant increases in IL-10 (de Groot and Gross 1998). Bucillamine decreases the frequency of IFN-γ-producing CD4 T cells generated after a priming culture of mononuclear cells from the peripheral blood (Morinobu et al. 2000). Finally, reports have suggested that glucocorticoids inhibit cytokine expression indirectly through promotion of a Th2 cytokine secretion profile, presumably by their action on monocyte activation (Almawi et al. 1999). Together, the data suggest that the anti-inflammatory effect of a number of current treatment modalities in RA is characterized by an inhibition of Th1 cell activation and effector cell generation and by favoring Th2 differentiation, thereby shifting the Th1/Th2 balance toward the Th2 direction.

In an attempt to target only those cells perpetuating the chronic inflammation specifically, with minimal effects on other aspects of the immune or inflammatory systems, therapeutic tools ("biologicals") with defined targets and effector functions have been designed and tested in clinical applications. As CD4 T cells are central in initiating and perpetuating the chronic autoimmune response in rheumatic diseases, a large number of biologicals has aimed to interfere with T cell activation and/or migration.

A major advance in the understanding of T cell activation has been the identification of the critical co-stimulatory molecules on T cells, such as CD28, LFA-1, CD2, CD4, CD30, CD44, and CD154 (CD40L), and their interacting ligands on APCs or B cells. Although these molecules act through different mechanisms, some delivering co-stimulatory biochemical signals to the T cell, some enhancing adhesion to target tissues, they all have the ability to augment the T cell proliferative responses to antigenic stimuli. Biologicals designed to interfere with co-stimulation via inhibiting engagement of co-stimulatory ligands have been used in several animal models of inflammatory arthritis and in treatment trials in RA. In experimental autoimmune diseases in animals, mAbs to CD4 have been used to prevent the induction of the disease (Ranges et al. 1985; Waldor et al. 1985). Of relevance to human disease, mAbs to CD4 were also able to inhibit further progression when given after the initial inflammation has already become manifest (Waldor et al. 1985; Wofsy and Seaman 1987), although, with one notable exception (Schulze-Koops et al. 1998), controlled human trials have largely failed to demonstrate favorable results to date (Schulze-Koops and Lipsky 2000). Interaction of CD2 with its ligand, CD58 has been blocked by application of a soluble fully human recombinant fusion protein comprising the first extracellular domain of CD58 and the hinge, CH2 and CH3 sequences of human IgG1 (LFA-3-IgG1, alefacept). Alefacept has been employed in patients with psoriasis with substantial clinical response (Ellis and Krueger 2001). Inhibition of CD28-mediated co-stimulatory signals is a potent means of immunosuppression that can be achieved by blocking either CD28 or CD80 and CD86, for example by coating CD80 and CD86 with a soluble Ig fusion protein of the extracellular domain of CTLA-4 (CD152). CTLA-4 is a homolog to CD28 and is expressed by activated T cells. It can bind both CD80 and CD86 with higher affinity than CD28. Because CD152 has a high affinity for CD80 and CD86, soluble forms of CTLA-4 inhibit the interaction of CD28 with its ligands. In clinical trials, CTLA4-Ig (CTLA-4-IgG1, abatacept) demonstrated favorable effects in patients with psoriasis vulgaris (Abrams et al. 1999) and in patients with rheumatoid arthritis (Kremer et al. 2003; Moreland et al. 2002). The adhesion receptor/counter-receptor pair, LFA-1 (CD11α/CD18) and ICAM-1, is critical for transendothelial migration of T cells and their subsequent activation (Kavanaugh et al. 1991). Therefore, mAbs to LFA-1 and ICAM-1 have been employed in autoimmune diseases in an attempt to block migration of T cells into sites of inflammation and their subsequent stimulation by locally expressed antigenic peptides in vivo (Kavanaugh et al. 1994; Schulze-Koops et al. 1995). Significant clinical benefit was achieved with the mAb to ICAM-1 in patients with active RA (Kavanaugh et al. 1994). It is of interest that clinical benefit was restricted to those patients who showed a marked increase in the levels of Th1 cytokine-producing T cells in their circulation immediately following the administration of the mAb (Schulze-Koops et al. 1995). Thus, it can be reasoned that in the responding patients the circulatory pattern of activated Th1 cells was altered by inhibiting their migration into the inflamed synovium. These data emphasize the pathogenic Th1 drive in those patients responding to therapy.

Together, T cell-directed therapy in RA is based on the idea that CD4 T cells initiate and continuously drive systemic rheumatoid inflammation. T cell-directed DMARDs and some of the recently employed mAbs have been successful in ameliorating signs and symptoms of the diseases and some also seem to be able to slow disease progression. Thus, although sustained clinical improvement has not been achieved with a short course of the biologicals, the idea that targeting the CD4 T cells as the motor of rheumatoid inflammation will interrupt chronic autoimmune inflammation and subsequent tissue destruction has been strongly supported.

6
Conclusion

Strong evidence has been provided for a central role of T cells in the pathogenesis of rheumatoid inflammation. Whereas clinical and epidemiological observations have indicated that T cell-mediated cellular immunity is involved in several aspects of RA, experimental data have revealed phenotypic and functional alterations of T cells in the peripheral circulation and the synovial infiltrates that are sufficient to mediate continuous upregulation of pro-inflammatory effector functions. The data suggest that T cells play an important role in initiating the autoimmune disease and maintaining inflammation by activating synovial macrophages to produce inflammatory mediators. Alterations in the activity and frequency of pro-inflammatory T cells are associated with the clinical course of the disease, further emphasizing the role of T cells in RA. Finally, T cell directed therapies that modulate T cell function or activity have been successfully employed in modern therapy of RA. The clinical efficacy of T cell-directed therapies have firmly established the central role of T cells in autoimmune rheumatic inflammation.

Acknowledgements This work was supported in part by the Deutsche Forschungsgemeinschaft (Schu 786/2-3 and 2-4) and the Interdisciplinary Center for Clinical Research in Erlangen (Projects B3 and A18).

References

Abbas AK, Murphy KM, Sher A (1996) Functional diversity of helper T lymphocytes. Nature 383:787–793

Abrams JR, Lebwohl MG, Guzzo CA, Jegasothy BV, Goldfarb MT, Goffe BS, Menter A, Lowe NJ, Krueger G, Brown MJ, Weiner RS, Birkhofer MJ, Warner GL, Berry KK, Linsley PS, Krueger JG, Ochs HD, Kelley SL, Kang S (1999) CTLA4Ig-mediated blockade of T-cell costimulation in patients with psoriasis vulgaris. J Clin Invest 103:1243–1252

Almawi WY, Melemedjian OK, Rieder MJ (1999) An alternate mechanism of glucocorticoid anti-proliferative effect: promotion of a Th2 cytokine-secreting profile. Clin Transplant 13:365–374

Banerjee S, Webber C, Poole AR (1992) The induction of arthritis in mice by the cartilage proteoglycan aggrecan: roles of CD4+ and CD8+ T cells. Cell Immunol 144:347–357

Berner B, Akca D, Jung T, Muller GA, Reuss-Borst MA (2000) Analysis of Th1 and Th2 cytokines expressing CD4+ and CD8+ T cells in rheumatoid arthritis by flow cytometry. J Rheumatol 27:1128–1135

Bessis N, Boissier MC, Ferrara P, Blankenstein T, Fradelizi D, Fournier C (1996) Attenuation of collagen-induced arthritis in mice by treatment with vector cells engineered to secrete interleukin-13. Eur J Immunol 26:2399–2403

Breedveld FC, Dynesius-Trentham R, de Sousa M, Trentham DE (1989) Collagen arthritis in the rat is initiated by CD4+ T cells and can be amplified by iron. Cell Immunol 121:1–12

Bruneau JM, Yea CM, Spinella-Jaegle S, Fudali C, Woodward K, Robson PA, Sautes C, Westwood R, Kuo EA, Williamson RA, Ruuth E (1998) Purification of human dihydro-orotate dehydrogenase and its inhibition by A77:1726, the active metabolite of leflunomide. Biochem J 336:299–303

Calin A, Elswood J, Klouda PT (1989) Destructive arthritis, rheumatoid factor, HLA-DR4. Susceptibility versus severity, a case-control study. Arthritis Rheum 32:1221–1225

Canete JD, Martinez SE, Farres J, Sanmarti R, Blay M, Gomez A, Salvador G, Munoz-Gomez J (2000) Differential Th1/Th2 cytokine patterns in chronic arthritis: interferon gamma is highly expressed in synovium of rheumatoid arthritis compared with seronegative spondyloarthropathies. Ann Rheum Dis 59:263–268

Chan AC, Iwashima M, Turck CW, Weiss A (1992) ZAP-70: a 70 kd protein-tyrosine kinase that associates with the TCR zeta chain. Cell 71:649–662

Constantin A, Loubet-Lescoulie P, Lambert N, Yassine-Diab B, Abbal M, Mazieres B, de Preval C, Cantagrel A (1998) Antiinflammatory and immunoregulatory action of methotrexate in the treatment of rheumatoid arthritis: evidence of increased interleukin-4 and interleukin-10 gene expression demonstrated in vitro by competitive reverse transcriptase-polymerase chain reaction. Arthritis Rheum 41:48–57

Da Silva JA, Spector TD (1992) The role of pregnancy in the course and aetiology of rheumatoid arthritis. Clin Rheumatol 11:189–194

Davis LS, Cush JJ, Schulze-Koops H, Lipsky PE (2001) Rheumatoid synovial CD4+ T cells exhibit a reduced capacity to differentiate into IL-4-producing T-helper-2 effector cells. Arthritis Res 3:54–64

De Groot K, Gross WL (1998) Wegener's granulomatosis: disease course, assessment of activity and extent and treatment. Lupus 7:285–291

Dimitrova P, Skapenko A, Herrmann ML, Schleyerbach R, Kalden JR, Schulze-Koops H (2002) Restriction of de novo pyrimidine biosynthesis inhibits Th1 cell activation and promotes Th2 cell differentiation. J Immunol 169:3392–3399

Ehinger M, Vestberg M, Johansson AC, Johannesson M, Svensson A, Holmdahl R (2001) Influence of CD4 or CD8 deficiency on collagen-induced arthritis. Immunology 103:291–300

Ellis CN, Krueger GG (2001) Treatment of chronic plaque psoriasis by selective targeting of memory effector T lymphocytes. N Engl J Med 345:248–255

Germain RN (2002) T-cell development and the CD4-CD8 lineage decision. Nat Rev Immunol 2:309–322

Hsieh CS, Macatonia SE, Tripp CS, Wolf SF, O'Garra A, Murphy KM (1993) Development of TH1 CD4+ T cells through IL-12 produced by Listeria-induced macrophages. Science 260:547–549

Joosten LA, Lubberts E, Helsen MM, Saxne T, Coenen-de Roo CJ, Heinegard D, and van den Berg WB (1999) Protection against cartilage and bone destruction by systemic interleukin-4 treatment in established murine type II collagen-induced arthritis. Arthritis Res 1:81–91

Kang BY, Chung SW, Im SY, Choe YK, Kim TS (1999) Sulfasalazine prevents T-helper 1 immune response by suppressing interleukin-12 production in macrophages. Immunology 98:98–103

Kang YM, Zhang X, Wagner UG, Yang H, Beckenbaugh RD, Kurtin PJ, Goronzy JJ, Weyand CM (2002) CD8 T cells are required for the formation of ectopic germinal centers in rheumatoid synovitis. J Exp Med 195:1325–1336

Kanik KS, Hagiwara E, Yarboro CH, Schumacher HR, Wilder RL, Klinman DM (1998) Distinct patterns of cytokine secretion characterize new onset synovitis versus chronic rheumatoid arthritis. J Rheumatol 25:16–22

Kavanaugh AF, Lightfoot E, Lipsky PE, Oppenheimer-Marks N (1991) The role of CD11/CD18 in adhesion and transendothelial migration of T cells: analysis utilizing CD18-deficient T cell clones. J Immunol 146:4149–4156

Kavanaugh AF, Davis LS, Nichols LA, Norris SH, Rothlein R, Scharschmidt LA, Lipsky PE (1994) Treatment of refractory rheumatoid arthritis with a monoclonal antibody to intercellular adhesion molecule 1. Arthritis Rheum 37:992–999

Kremer JM, Westhovens R, Leon M, Di Giorgio E, Alten R, Steinfeld S, Russell A, Dougados M, Emery P, Nuamah IF, Williams GR, Becker JC, Hagerty DT, Moreland LW (2003) Treatment of rheumatoid arthritis by selective inhibition of T-cell activation with fusion protein CTLA4Ig. N Engl J Med 349:1907–1915

Kusaba M, Honda J, Fukuda T, Oizumi K (1998) Analysis of type 1 and type 2 T cells in synovial fluid and peripheral blood of patients with rheumatoid arthritis. J Rheumatol 25:1466–1471

Miltenburg AM, van Laar JM, de Kuiper R, Daha MR, Breedveld FC (1992) T cells cloned from human rheumatoid synovial membrane functionally represent the Th1 subset. Scand J Immunol 35:603–610

Mishan-Eisenberg G, Borovsky Z, Weber MC, Gazit R, Tykocinski ML, Rachmilewitz J (2004) Differential regulation of Th1/Th2 cytokine responses by placental protein 14. J Immunol 173:5524–5530

Miyata M, Ohira H, Sasajima T, Suzuki S, Ito M, Sato Y, Kasukawa R (2000) Significance of low mRNA levels of interleukin-4 and -10 in mononuclear cells of the synovial fluid of patients with rheumatoid arthritis. Clin Rheumatol 19:365–370

Moreland LW, Alten R, Van Den Bosch F, Appelboom T, Leon M, Emery P, Cohen S, Luggen M, Shergy W, Nuamah I, Becker JC (2002) Costimulatory blockade in patients with rheumatoid arthritis: a pilot, dose-finding, double-blind, placebo-controlled clinical trial evaluating CTLA-4Ig and LEA29Y eighty-five days after the first infusion. Arthritis Rheum 46:1470–1479

Morinobu A, Wang Z, Kumagai S (2000) Bucillamine suppresses human Th1 cell development by a hydrogen peroxide-independent mechanism. J Rheumatol 27:851–858

Mosmann TR, Cherwinski H, Bond MW, Giedlin MA, Coffman RL (1986) Two types of murine helper T cell clone. I. Definition according to profiles of lymphokine activities and secreted proteins. J Immunol 136:2348–2357

Panayi GS (1999) Targeting of cells involved in the pathogenesis of rheumatoid arthritis. Rheumatology 38 [Suppl 2]:8–10

Panayi GS, Tugwell P (1994) The use of cyclosporine A in rheumatoid arthritis: conclusions of an international review. Br J Rheumatol 33:967–969

Paulus HE, Machleder HI, Levine S, Yu DT, MacDonald NS (1977) Lymphocyte involvement in rheumatoid arthritis. Studies during thoracic duct drainage. Arthritis Rheum 20:1249–1262

Quayle AJ, Chomarat P, Miossec P, Kjeldsen-Kragh J, Forre O, Natvig JB (1993) Rheumatoid inflammatory T-cell clones express mostly Th1 but also Th2 and mixed (Th0) cytokine patterns. Scand J Immunol 38:75–82

Ranges GE, Sriram S, Cooper SM (1985) Prevention of type II collagen-induced arthritis by in vivo treatment with anti-L3T4. J Exp Med 162:1105–1110

Rocken M, Saurat JH, Hauser C (1992) A common precursor for CD4+ T cells producing IL-2 or IL-4. J Immunol 148:1031–1036

Schulze-Koops H, Kalden JR (2003) Targeting T cells in rheumatic diseases. In: Smolen JS, Lipsky PE (eds) Biological therapy in rheumatology. Martin Dunitz, London, pp 3–24

Schulze-Koops H, Lipsky PE (2000) Anti-CD4 monoclonal antibody therapy in human autoimmune diseases. Curr Dir Autoimmun 2:24–49

Schulze-Koops H, Lipsky PE, Kavanaugh AF, Davis LS (1995) Elevated Th1- or Th0-like cytokine mRNA in peripheral circulation of patients with rheumatoid arthritis: modulation by treatment with anti-ICAM-1 correlates with clinical benefit. J Immunol 155:5029–5037

Schulze-Koops H, Davis LS, Haverty TP, Wacholtz MC, Lipsky PE (1998) Reduction of Th1 cell activity in the peripheral circulation of patients with rheumatoid arthritis after treatment with a non-depleting humanized monoclonal antibody to CD4. J Rheumatol 25:2065–2076

Skapenko A, Wendler J, Lipsky PE, Kalden JR, Schulze-Koops H (1999) Altered memory T cell differentiation in patients with early rheumatoid arthritis. J Immunol 163:491–499

Skapenko A, Leipe J, Lipsky PE, Schulze-Koops H et al (2005) The role of the T cell in autoimmune inflammation. Arthritis Res Ther 7 [Suppl 2]:S4–S14

Spits H (2002) Development of alphabeta T cells in the human thymus. Nat Rev Immunol 2:760–772

Strober S, Tanay A, Field E, Hoppe RT, Calin A, Engleman EG, Kotzin B, Brown BW, Kaplan HS (1985) Efficacy of total lymphoid irradiation in intractable rheumatoid arthritis. A double-blind, randomized trial. Ann Intern Med 102:441–449

Taneja V, Taneja N, Paisansinsup T, Behrens M, Griffiths M, Luthra H, David CS (2002) CD4 and CD8 T cells in susceptibility/protection to collagen-induced arthritis in HLA-DQ8-transgenic mice: implications for rheumatoid arthritis. J Immunol 168:5867–5875

Van Boxel JA, Paget SA (1975) Predominantly T-cell infiltrate in rheumatoid synovial membranes. N Engl J Med 293:517–520

Van der Graaff WL, Prins AP, Niers TM, Dijkmans BA, van Lier RA (1999) Quantitation of interferon gamma- and interleukin-4-producing T cells in synovial fluid and peripheral blood of arthritis patients. Rheumatology 38:214–220

Verhoef CM, van Roon JA, Vianen ME, Bruijnzeel-Koomen CA, Lafeber FP, Bijlsma JW (1998) Mutual antagonism of rheumatoid arthritis and hay fever; a role for type 1/type 2 T cell balance. Ann Rheum Dis 57:275–280

Wagner UG, Kurtin PJ, Wahner A, Brackertz M, Berry DJ, Goronzy JJ, Weyand CM (1998) The role of CD8+ CD40L+ T cells in the formation of germinal centers in rheumatoid synovitis. J Immunol 161:6390–6397

Waldor MK, Sriram S, Hardy R, Herzenberg LA, Lanier L, Lim M, Steinman L (1985) Reversal of experimental allergic encephalomyelitis with monoclonal antibody to a T-cell subset marker. Science 227:415–417

Weiss A (1993) T cell antigen receptor signal transduction: a tale of tails and cytoplasmic protein-tyrosine kinases. Cell 73:209–212

Winchester R (1994) The molecular basis of susceptibility to rheumatoid arthritis. Adv Immunol 56:389–466

Wofsy D and Seaman WE (1987) Reversal of advanced murine lupus in NZB/NZW F1 mice by treatment with monoclonal antibody to L3T4. J Immunol 138:3247–3253

Yocum DE (1999) T cells: pathogenic cells and therapeutic targets in rheumatoid arthritis. Semin Arthritis Rheum 29:27–35

Signalling Pathways in B Cells: Implications for Autoimmunity

T. Dörner[1] (✉) · P. E. Lipsky[2]

[1] Institute of Transfusion Medicine, Charite University Medicine Berlin, Campus Mitte, Coagulation Unit, Schumannstr. 20/21 , 10098 Berlin, Germany
thomas.doerner@charite.de

[2] National Institutes of Health, NIAMS, Bethesda, MD, USA

1	Introduction	214
2	Disturbed Homeostasis of Peripheral B Cells in Autoimmune Diseases	216
3	B Cellular Signal Transduction Pathways and Their Implications for Autoimmunity	218
3.1	Normal B Cell Function Results from Balanced Agonistic and Antagonistic Signals	218
3.1.1	Disturbances That Alter B Cell Survival and Lead to Autoimmunity	219
3.1.2	Altered Thresholds for B Cellular Activation Can Lead to Autoimmunity	223
3.1.3	Inhibitory Receptors of B Cells	225
4	Inhibitory Receptor Pathways and Autoimmunity	228
5	Activated B Cells May Bridge the Innate and Adaptive Immune System	230
6	Rationales of B Cell-Targeted Therapy in Autoimmune Diseases	231
References		234

Abstract Following investigations of the pathogenic role of autoantibodies in rheumatic diseases, preclinical and clinical studies suggest a more central role of B cells in the maintenance of the disease process beyond just being precursors of (auto)antibody-producing plasma cells. Detailed analyses have implicated a number of surface molecules and subsequent downstream signalling pathways in the regulation of the events induced by BCR engagement. In this review, we discuss the potential role of molecules involved in altered B cell longevity, especially molecules involved in apoptosis (bcl-2, bcl-x, mutations in the Fas/Fas-L pathway), as well as molecules that might alter activation thresholds of B cells (CD19, CD21, CD22, lyn, SHP, SHIP-1) in the development of autoimmunity. Although focused on intrinsic B cell abnormalities, the complexity of interactions of B cells with other immune cells also makes it possible that increased B cell activation can be induced by distortions in the interaction with other cells. Further delineation of these alterations of B cell function in autoimmune conditions will allow development of more precise B cell-directed therapies beyond drastic B cell depletion, with the potential to improve the risk–benefit ratio of the treatments of autoimmune diseases.

1
Introduction

Autoantibodies is among the most striking evidence of a break in immune tolerance and they occur in most systemic autoimmune diseases. Whereas some autoantibodies are pathogenic and can be used to classify specific autoimmune diseases, autoreactivity also occurs in a variety of other circumstances, such as during infections, immunizations and following certain traumatic accidents. The precise cellular and/or molecular mechanisms resulting in the development of pathogenic vs nonpathogenic antibodies remains elusive. Although pathogenic autoantibodies are usually of post-switched Ig classes and carry somatically mutated IgV genes as indications of extensive T cell help, it has not been clearly shown that the production of these autoantibodies has been initiated by specific autoantigens or whether they occur as a result of abnormalities in the control of B cell responses to exogenous antigens. Very recent evidence from B cell depletion studies using rituximab (anti-CD20) indicate that clinical improvement, decline in circulating B cells and decrease of antibody titres can all occur but do not correlate with each other, and therefore autoantibodies as products of differentiated plasma cells may not be the essential pathogenic element in a number of autoimmune disease. However, intrinsic abnormalities of B cell function (Table 1) and/or their interaction with other immune cells appear to be of central importance in these diseases. Here we discuss mechanisms, including extrinsic and intrinsic influences on B cell function and potential candidate molecules that could drive B cell dysfunction in autoimmune disease and might, therefore, serve as targets of therapeutic intervention.

The importance of precise immune regulation becomes evident when the characteristics of some immune deficiency and autoimmune disorders are compared. In the humoral immune system, B cells and their descendants, plasma cells, produce protective antibodies and thereby maintain the unique serological memory and a considerable part of cellular memory. Besides these well-known activities, a number of other immune functions of B cells have been identified in the last several years (Table 2), which need consideration not only for understanding their function in health but also under disease conditions. It is apparent that disturbances in the tightly regulated circuits of these cellular components with their products can lead to clinically important disorders. Analyses of inherited immune deficiencies have provided insights

Table 1 Potential B cell abnormalities leading to autoimmunity

a. V(D)J recombination
b. Entry of B cells into the immune repertoire
c. Survival of B cells by altered apoptosis
d. Selection
e. Somatic hypermutation
f. Receptor editing/revision
g. Differentiation of plasma cells
h. Extrinsic
   - T cells, cytokines, APC, autoantigens
i. Altered activation threshold

Table 2 Immune functions of B cells

1. Precursors of (auto)antibody-secreting plasma cells
2. Essential functions of B cells in regulating immune responses
   i. Antigen-presenting cells
   ii. Differentiation of follicular dendritic cells in secondary lymphoid organs
   iii. Essential role in lymphoid organogenesis as well as in the initiation and regulation of T and B cell responses
   iv. Development of effective lymphoid architecture (antigen-presenting M cells)
   v. Activated B cells express costimulatory molecules and may differentiate into polarized cytokine-producing effector cells that can be essential for the evolution of T effector cells
   vi. Differentiation of T effector cells
   vii. Immunoregulatory functions by IL-10 positive B cells
   viii. Cytokine production by activated B cells may influence the function of antigen-presenting dendritic cells

into the function of certain surface receptors as well as extracellular and subcellular components. For example, it is well accepted that inherited deficiencies of the complement system are associated with an increased incidence of SLE, glomerulonephritis, and vasculitis. Several antibody deficiencies are also associated with autoimmune disease. In this regard, autoimmune cytopenias are commonly observed in individuals with selective IgA deficiency and common variable immune deficiency. Polyarthritis can also be seen in patients with X-linked agammaglobulinemia. Combined cellular and antibody deficiencies, such as Wiskott-Aldrich syndrome also carry an increased risk for juvenile rheumatoid arthritis and autoimmune hemolytic anemia. Recent advances in understanding the subcellular regulation of immune activation may allow further insights into the mechanisms of autoimmunity.

Abnormalities in certain receptors involved in B cell differentiation and Ig production can also be involved in a broad variety of disorders ranging between immune deficiency and autoimmunity. In this regard, loss of function mutations of the inducible co-stimulatory molecule (ICOS) expressed on T cells has been shown to be involved in adult onset common variable deficiency (Grimbacher et al. 2003). On the other hand, in murine (Iwai et al. 2003) as well in human lupus (Hutloff et al. 2004; Iwai et al. 2003), overexpression of ICOS on T cells and an overall downmodulation of ICOS-L on B cells (Hutloff et al. 2004; Iwai et al. 2003) were identified. Similarly, CD40L and Fas mutations have also been shown to be critically involved in both immunodeficiency as well as autoimmunity. Thus, loss of precise regulatory influences stabilizing B cell homeostasis can result in autoimmunity or immune deficiency or sometimes both.

2
Disturbed Homeostasis of Peripheral B Cells in Autoimmune Diseases

Immunophenotyping of circulating B cells in patients with systemic autoimmune diseases has identified a number of specific abnormalities and may provide novel approaches in diagnosis as well as analysis of the response to therapeutic interventions (Odendahl et al. 2000a, b 2003; Hansen et al. 2002b; Jacobi et al. 2003; Anolik et al. 2004; Looney et al. 2004a, b; Cappione et al. 2002; Potter et al. 2002; Bohnhorst et al. 2001, 2002). Since B cells at many stages of development circulate in the blood and the stages of B cell development can be assessed using a number of phenotypic markers (Fig. 1), analysis of the expression profile of circulating B cells permits the detection of B cell differentiation status in health and disease. In the peripheral blood of healthy controls, approximately 60%–65% of B cells have the phenotype of CD27-naïve cells, and 30%–40% have that of memory B cells (CD27+). Typically, in such healthy donors, less than 2% of the peripheral B cells are plasma cells (CD19^{dim}, CD20$^-$, CD38^{++}, and CD27^{high}). In an analyses of SLE patients, Odendahl et al. first identified that plasma cells highly express CD27, and this population appears to be expanded in lupus (Odendahl et al. 2000b) and is usually not found in normals. By contrast, patients with Sjögren's syndrome are characterized by a different peripheral B cell composition than SLE patients. In SLE, a marked reduction of CD19$^+$/CD27$^-$ naïve B cells, enhanced frequencies of CD19$^+$/CD27$^+$ memory B cells and increased numbers

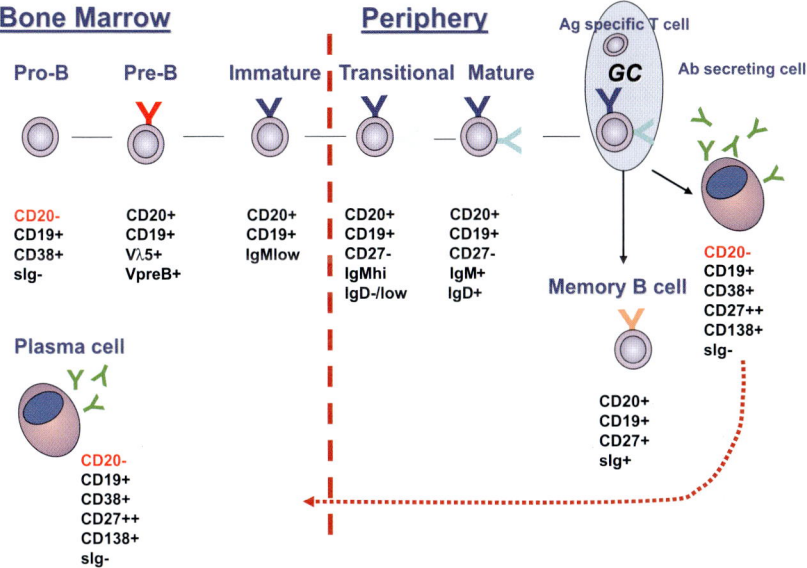

Fig. 1 Schematic development of B cells in the bone marrow as well as in the periphery based on the expression of a number of activation/differentiation markers

of $CD19^{dim}/CD27^{high}$ plasma cells were found, whereas a predominance of naïve B cells and reduced memory B cells were identified in Sjögren's patients (Bohnhorst et al. 2001a, b; Hansen et al. 2002a, b, 2004). Molecular analysis of IgV genes in one SLE patient showed that these B cell subpopulations differed in their V_H gene usage. With regard to individual genes, the V_H3–23 gene was found most often in $CD27^-/IgD^+$ naïve (6/14) and $CD27^+/IgD^+$ memory B cells (4/15), whereas V_H4–34 and V_H4–59 were frequently found in $CD27^{high}/IgD^-$ plasma cells (Bohnhorst et al. 2001a, b; Jacobi et al. 1999; Odendahl et al. 2000b). Importantly, the V_H4–34 and V_H4–59 genes in SLE plasma cells were heavily mutated. Preferential usage of V_H4 genes by post-switch cells has been reported in patients with RA (Bohnhorst et al. 2001a, b; Jacobi et al. 1999; Kim et al. 1999; Voswinkel et al. 1996). By contrast, V_H3 was most frequently found in naïve B cells or unfractionated peripheral B cells of normals (Brezinschek et al. 1995a, b; Huang et al. 1996; Jacobi et al. 1999; Kim et al. 1999; Kraj et al. 1997). Moreover, the gene V_H4–34 frequently used in clonally unrelated $CD27^{high}$ plasma cells in SLE has been reported to be involved in the formation of anti-dsDNA antibodies (van Vollenhoven et al. 1999; Voswinkel et al. 1996) and to be expanded in patients with active disease (Isenberg et al. 1998; Mockridge et al. 1998; Odendahl et al. 2000b; Rahman et al. 1998). In normals, this particular gene occurred at a frequency of 3.5% among peripheral CD5⁺ and 3.9% among CD5⁻ B cells (Brezinschek et al. 1996). VH4–34 was found to be negatively selected in an analysis of CD19⁺ peripheral cells in normals (Brezinschek et al. 1995a) and was excluded from post-switch tonsil plasma cells (Yavuz et al. 2002). In normals, B cells expressing VH4–34 are excluded from germinal centres, whereas they enter germinal cells in patients with SLE (Pugh-Bernard et al. 2001). These results are all consistent with the conclusion that there is fundamental abnormality in SLE that results in the production of plasma cells expressing heavily mutated V_H4 family genes that may encode for autoantibodies. The mechanisms underlying this abnormality is uncertain, but suggests an abnormality in the regulation of B cell differentiation.

3
B Cellular Signal Transduction Pathways and Their Implications for Autoimmunity

The immune system is maintained by a fine balance between activation and inhibition (Fig. 2). On the one hand, it must possess adequate reactivity to generate an effective immune response to target non-self molecules, while avoiding the emergence of autoimmunity on the other hand. Essential to this process is the ability to control the timing and site of B cell activation and to limit the extent of activation precisely. All of this is sufficiently regulated by a number of extrinsic and intrinsic mechanisms in a normal immune system to avoid pathogenic autoimmunity. It is currently believed that failure to maintain this balance of activating and inhibiting factors, receptors and pathways could result in either immunodeficiency or autoimmunity.

Since B cells represent a unique crossroad between the innate and adaptive immune systems, especially since they can be directly activated via toll-like receptors (TLRs), it becomes important that simple structures, such as methylated bacterial DNA, are able to activate B cells, resulting in the production of autoantibodies, such as rheumatoid factor (Leadbetter et al. 2002).

3.1
Normal B Cell Function Results from Balanced Agonistic and Antagonistic Signals

B cells undergo a tightly regulated developmental pathway from early progenitors to terminally differentiated plasma cells (Fig. 1). Many of these developmental steps are dependent on signals mediated through soluble factors and receptor-ligand interactions. In addition, multiple checkpoints permit both positive and negative selection of B cells, both centrally in the bone

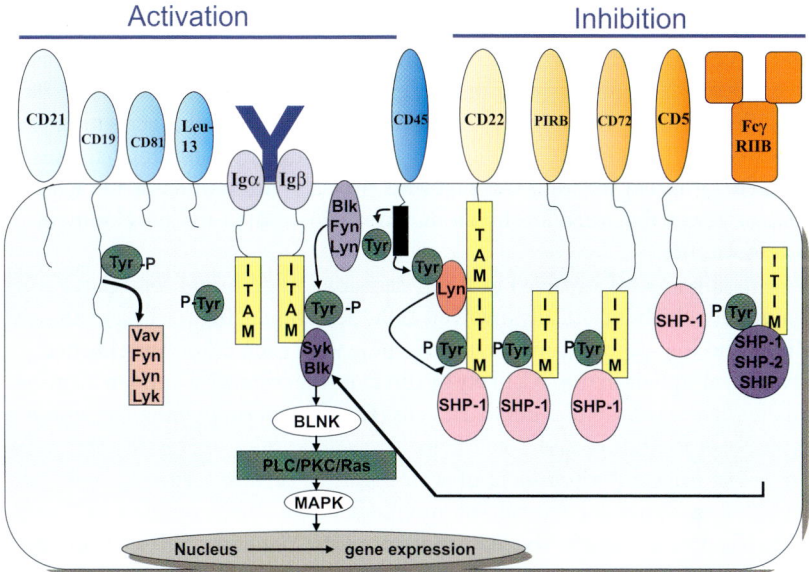

Fig. 2 Activation and inhibitory surface molecules and subsequent signalling pathways of B cells that modulate the strength of the BCR signal

marrow and in the peripheral lymphoid tissues, such as the spleen and lymph nodes. These checkpoints are necessary to produce a diverse population of B cells capable of generating high-affinity effector antibodies in the absence of pathologic autoreactivity. Transgenic mice with perturbations in selective regulatory pathways that affect B cell development often develop autoimmune disease. By genetic manipulation in murine models, it has become clear that two general defects in B cell function can lead to humoral autoimmunity:

1. Alterations in B cell survival
2. Alterations in the threshold for B cellular activation

Both confirm that intrinsic B cell defects may account for the emergence of autoimmunity, and apparently autoimmunity can develop without specific immunization to autoantigens or without abnormalities in T cells.

3.1.1
Disturbances That Alter B Cell Survival and Lead to Autoimmunity

During B cell generation in the bone marrow, the process of negative selection eliminates the majority of immature B cells before entry into peripheral lymphoid tissues. Subsequently, resident peripheral B cells undergo a second screening process for reactivity with peripheral self-antigens that results in apoptosis, receptor editing or anergy depending on the strength of BCR signalling (Fig. 3). Autoreactive B cells that have survived this screening process have apparently received sufficient growth and anti-apoptotic signals in order to progress through this rigorous process. Alterations in the expression of genes that regulate B cell survival can lead to the development of autoimmunity.

A major process involved in B cell decisions in germinal centres (GCs) is apoptosis, which is centrally involved in the selection of high-affinity variants. High- and low-affinity centrocytes compete with each other for a limited set of survival signals in the GC, likely by direct interaction with antigen localized on the surface of follicular dendritic cells (FDCs) or perhaps enhanced antigen capture, presentation and T cell help. Transgenic mice expressing the genes *bcl-2* and *bcl-x_L*, the products of which inhibit certain forms of apoptosis, provided evidence for the role of apoptosis in GC differentiation of B cells. A classical example of a dysregulated apoptotic regulatory genes leading to autoimmunity was identified in a bcl-2 transgenic mouse model. Enhanced bcl-2 expression allows inappropriate survival of autoreactive B cell clones (Strasser et al. 1991). Bcl-2 transgenic mice develop antinuclear antibodies and glomerulonephritis caused by immune complex deposition. Primary im-

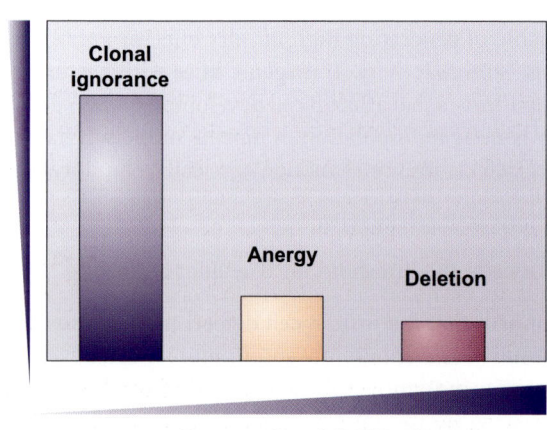

Fig. 3 Basic mechanisms known to be involved in the prevention of B cell autoreactivity and dependent on the BCR signal strength. A further mechanism known as receptor revision/editing may also prevent autoimmunity but apparently is not strictly dependent on the BCR signal

munization of *bcl*-2-transgenic mice resulted in 20-fold more memory B cells than controls. Furthermore, a high proportion of these *bcl*-2-transgenic memory B cells, despite having a typical memory phenotype, retained their V_H genes in a low-affinity configuration. Thus, these memory B cells showed no evidence of having undergone affinity maturation, as the low-affinity B cells would have been expected to lose the competition for antigen in the GC and die by apoptosis. An additional *bcl*-x_L transgenic mouse also preserved low-affinity cells in the GC, although in this case the low-affinity cells were not germline variants of the dominant clonotype, but rather were B cells using V_H genes that usually appear only during the early stages of the response (Takahashi et al. 1999). In both cases, blocking apoptosis in the GC had the effect of promoting the survival of low-affinity variants, which, in the case of the *bcl*-2-transgenic mice, entered the memory compartment. This demonstrates the role of apoptosis in selecting B cells that enter the memory compartment, including a certain frequency of autoreactive cells. In contrast with the alterations of the memory compartment, *bcl*-2-transgenic mice showed no perturbation of selection of bone marrow antibody-secreting cells. This compartment remained predominantly composed of high-affinity antibody producers. These findings suggest that resistance to apoptosis in the GC is an important prerequisite to allow differentiation of a GC cell into a memory cell, whereas the differentiation to long-lived plasma cells requires a more stringent affinity-based signal. How this translates into human autoimmunity is still a matter of debate.

Another example of autoimmunity developing as a result of alterations in lymphocyte apoptosis is provided by MRL mice homozygous for mutations in the Fas gene, a death-inducing receptor required for normal regulation of B cell and T cell survival. MRL$^{lpr/lpr}$ mice develop a spectrum of autoreactivity resembling that found in human SLE and other autoimmune diseases. Thus, inappropriate survival can be caused by inappropriate expression of apoptotic and/or anti-apoptotic signals, allowing the emergence of autoimmunity.

In addition to intrinsic defects that can lead to increased B cell survival, external signals permit autoreactive B cells to escape deletion. An important signal that is particularly important in B cell growth, differentiation, and survival is BAFF (also known as BlyS, TALL-1, THANK and zTNF4) (Dörner and Putterman 2001). BAFF is a member of the TNF family of cytokines that is produced by myeloid cells, such as dendritic cells, monocytes and macrophages in inflamed tissue. It has remote effects and induces immature B cell survival as well as growth of mature B cells within peripheral lymphoid tissues. BAFF binds three receptors: BCMA (B cell maturation antigen), TACI (transmembrane activator and calcium-modulator and cyclophilin ligand interactor) and BAFF receptor. Through these receptors, BAFF acts as a potent co-stimulator for B cell survival when coupled with B cell antigen receptor ligation. In this regard, it was reported that BAFF ligation increased bcl-2 expression and increased activation of NF-κb, both of which increase B cell survival (Mackay and Browning 2002). BCMA or BAFF transgenic mice display mature B cell hyperplasia and develop an SLE-like disease, with anti-DNA antibodies, elevated serum IgM, vasculitis and glomerulonephritis (Mackay and Mackay 2002). Moreover, BAFF expression is elevated in MRL$^{lpr/lpr}$ mice and lupus-prone (NZW×NZB)F1 hybrid mice and correlates with disease progression (Mackay and Browning 2002; Mackay and Mackay 2002). In this regard, elevated BAFF levels were found in the serum of some patients with SLE, Sjögren's and idiopathic thrombocytopenic purpura patients (Mackay and Browning 2002; Mackay and Mackay 2002) as well as in the synovial fluid of rheumatoid arthritis patients. Conversely, BAFF-deficient mice show a complete loss of follicular and marginal-zone B lymphocytes (Gross et al. 2000).

Experiments aiming at determining the role of BAFF in autoimmune disease developed and applied BCMA-immunoglobulin (Ig) and TACI-Ig fusion proteins as decoy BAFF receptors. It is noteworthy that administration of BMCA-Ig or TACI-Ig to (NZW×NZB)F1 mice led to increased survival, decreased proteinuria and delayed disease progression (Mackay et al. 1999; Mackay and Browning 2002; Mackay and Mackay 2002), suggesting that BAFF plays a crucial role in longevity of autoimmune B cells and inhibiting this molecule may be an important approach to limit humoral autoimmunity.

Studies of knockout mice have shown that BCMA, TACI and BAFF-R are not directly equivalent in function (Thompson et al. 2001; Xu and Lam 2001). Mice lacking BCMA show normal B cell development and antibody responses (von Bulow et al. 2001; Yan et al. 2001), whereas TACI-deficient mice were shown to be deficient only in T cell-independent antibody responses (Carsetti et al. 1995; O'Connor et al. 2004). Paradoxically, mice lacking TACI show increased B cell proliferation and accumulation, suggesting an inhibitory role for TACI in B cell homeostasis. Recently, BCMA has been identified as being involved in the generation of long-lived plasma cells (Schiemann et al. 2001). Thus far, gene-targeted mice lacking BAFF-R have not been reported, but the natural mouse mutant, A/WySnJ, has a disruption of the intracellular domain of BAFF-R. A/WySnJ mice display a phenotype that is similar to BAFF$^{-/-}$ mice, although follicular and marginal-zone B cells are not completely abolished (Benschop and Cambier 1999). A/WySnJ mice are impaired only in T cell-dependent antibody responses, in contrast to the comprehensive defect of BAFF-deficient mice. These results suggest that, while BAFF-R may be the major receptor of BAFF-mediated signals for B cell survival, redundancy in function may be provided by the other two receptors, especially by TACI.

An interesting role for BAFF was recently shown when it was reported that BAFF regulated the survival of both marginal zone and follicular B cells in mice treated with anti-CD20 antibody (Gong et al. 2005). The increased levels of BAFF found in some subjects with SLE or Sjögren's syndrome may limit the therapeutic potential of this B cell-depleting antibody.

3.1.2
Altered Thresholds for B Cellular Activation Can Lead to Autoimmunity

As noted above, signals generated through the B cell antigen receptor (BCR) are critical for B cell development and survival (Maruyama et al. 2000) as well as responses to antigen. The BCR is noncovalently associated with the signal transduction elements, Igα (CD79a) and Igβ (CD79b) (Fig. 2). The cytoplasmic domains of Igα and β contain highly conserved motifs that are the sites of Src family kinase docking and tyrosine phosphorylation, termed the immunoreceptor tyrosine-based activation motifs (ITAM). Phosphorylation of tyrosines within these motifs is mediated by Src family kinases, including Lyn, Fyn or Blk. This phosphorylation cascade promotes BCR recruitment of another tyrosine kinase, Syk, which facilitates receptor phosphorylation and initiates downstream signalling cascades that promote B cell activation (Tedder et al. 1997).

The generation and maintenance of self-reactive B cells is regulated by autoantigen signalling through the BCR complex. These responses are further influenced by other cell surface signal transduction molecules, including CD19, CD21 and CD22, which function as response regulators to amplify or inhibit BCR signalling. CD19, CD21 and CD22 modulate BCR-mediated signals by altering intrinsic intracellular signal transduction thresholds and thereby adjusting the strength of signal needed to initiate BCR-mediated activation (Cornall et al. 1998). Intracellular regulatory molecules that also control the BCR signalling intensity include Lyn, Btk, Vav and the SHP1 protein tyrosine phosphatase (Inaoki et al. 1997; Tedder 1998). Notably, CD19, CD21, CD22, Lyn, Vav and SHP1 are functionally linked in a common signalling pathway, as summarized in Fig. 2.

CD19 Recent evidence indicates that the expression of CD19 is involved in regulating autoimmunity. Mice with altered CD19, CD21, CD22, Lyn or SHP1 expression produce autoantibodies and develop a spectrum of autoimmunity. Peripheral tolerance was found to be disrupted in mice that overexpress CD19 with resultant B cell hyperactivity and the spontaneous production of IgG subclass autoantibodies (Chan et al. 1999). Mice that have only a 15%–30% increase in CD19 expression have a phenotype distinct from normal controls and also develop SLE-like manifestations (Saito et al. 2002).

Although multiple molecules involved in a common CD19 signal transduction pathway influence autoimmunity in mice, similar examples in humans are very limited. In systemic sclerosis, autoantibodies are detected in more than 90% of patients and are considered to play a critical role in the pathogenesis of the disease. Interestingly, CD19 and CD21 expression levels is 20% higher on B cells from patients with systemic sclerosis compared with healthy individuals, whereas the expression of other cell surface markers, such as CD20, CD22, and CD40, is normal. Notably, CD19 overexpression by 20% induced autoantibody production in a nonautoimmune strain of mice (Prodeus et al. 1998). Antinuclear antibodies and rheumatoid factor were induced in these mice, but not wild type controls. Like mice that overexpress CD19, the tight-skin mouse, a genetic model for human systemic sclerosis, also contains spontaneously activated B cells and autoantibodies against systemic sclerosis-specific autoantigens. Tight-skin mice also develop cutaneous fibrosis. In contrast to mice that overexpress CD19, mice that are CD19$^{-/-}$ have a markedly elevated BCR signalling threshold as compared to wild type mice. CD19 deficiency in tight-skin mice results in quiescent B cells, with significantly reduced autoantibody production and skin fibrosis. Overall, modest alterations in CD19 expression could contribute to the development of autoantibodies in humans, as reported for systemic sclerosis (Doody et al. 1995). Distinct alterations in expression or function in B cell response-regulators, such as CD19, may, therefore, play a role in autoimmune diseases. The explanation for the apparent tendency of CD19 to predispose to the development of systemic sclerosis-associated autoantibodies is not known.

A very recent analysis in CD19$^{-/-}$ mice (Diamant et al. 2005) demonstrated that lack of this surface molecule resulted in enhanced tonic signalling, impaired B cell maturation and, importantly, intensive receptor editing, which has been suggested to be impaired in autoimmunity (Dörner et al. 1998).

CD21 CD19 physically interacts with CD21, a complement receptor expressed on the surface of B cells. Thereby, CD19 transduces signals generated by the interaction of CD21 with complement fragment C3d. This may amplify signals generated by simultaneous BCR ligation, as might occur with a complement-containing immune complex. Multiple studies have suggested that altered CD21 function associates with autoimmunity in animal models. In addition, self-reactive B cells with 60% reduced CD21 expression are not anergized by soluble self-antigen in mouse models of tolerance (Smith et al. 1998). Although these studies suggest a direct role for CD21 in regulating B cell function and autoantibody production, this may actually reflect a role for CD21 in regulating cell surface CD19 expression.

3.1.3
Inhibitory Receptors of B Cells

Currently, two major classes of inhibitory receptors have been described that share a number of structural and functional similarities. Each inhibitory receptor contains one or more immunoreceptor tyrosine-based inhibitory motifs (ITIMs) within its cytoplasmic domain essential for generation and transduction of inhibitory signals. Ligation of the inhibitory receptor to an immunoreceptor tyrosine-based activating motif (ITAM) -containing activating molecule results in tyrosine kinase phosphorylation of the tyrosine residue within the ITIM (Tamir et al. 2000) by lyn (Daeron 1997), which allows it to bind and activate phosphatases containing an src homology 2 (SH2) domain. Two classes of SH2-containing inhibitory phosphatases have been identified: (a) the protein tyrosine phosphatases SHP-1 and SHP-2, and (b) the phosphoinositol phosphatases SHIP and SHIP2. These classes have separate downstream signalling pathways through which they modulate cellular inhibition. In general, each class of phosphatase interacts with the ITIMs of different inhibitory receptors, but each inhibitory receptor acts predominantly through only one class of phosphatase (Malbec et al. 1999).

The surface molecules FcγRII, CD22, and PDγ1 are inhibitory surface receptors and experimental evidence suggests that defective regulation by B cell inhibitory receptors may be of importance in autoimmunity.

Fc Receptors FcγRIIb   Three classes of FcγR have been described in humans, FcγRI, FcγRII and FcγRIII. FcγRII and III are further divided into an a and b form. FcγRI, IIa and IIIa are activating receptors, whereas FcγRIIb is considered as an inhibitory receptor. The function of FcγRIIIb, which lacks an intracellular domain, is still unknown. Coordinate expression of FcγR has been implicated in various diseases involving immune complexes, such as insulin-dependent diabetes mellitus, SLE, rheumatoid arthritis, multiple sclerosis and autoimmune anemia. FcγRIIb is a member of the Ig superfamily and represents a single-chain, low-affinity receptor for the Fc portion of IgG. It is a 40-kDa protein that consists of two extracellular Ig-like domains, a transmembrane domain and an intracytoplasmic domain that contains a single ITIM. It binds IgG either complexed to multivalent soluble antigens as immune complexes or bound to cell membranes (Latour et al. 1996). The isoform on B cells is unique in containing an intracytoplasmic motif that prevents its internalization (Pritchard and Smith 2003).

In B cells, which do not express any Fc receptors other than FcγRIIb, it acts to inhibit signalling through the B cell receptor (BCR), whereas in myeloid cells FcγRIIb inhibits activation through activating Fc receptors. Co-ligation of FcγRIIb to the BCR leads to tyrosine phosphorylation of the ITIM by the tyrosine kinase lyn, recruitment of SHIP and inhibition of Ca^{2+} flux and proliferation. The precise mechanism by which SHIP prevents B cell proliferation is uncertain (Bolland and Ravetch 2000).

FcγRIIb also induces apoptosis upon aggregation of the receptor in the absence of BCR signalling. In this circumstance, an apoptotic signal is generated through Btk and Jnk independent of the ITIM, which is abrogated when FcγRIIb is cross-linked with the BCR. Co-ligation of FcγRIIb is thought to provide feedback control of the B cell immune response, shutting off or preventing a response if sufficient antigen-specific IgG is present.

Evidence of a role for defective FcγRIIb inhibition in the pathogenesis of autoimmunity is provided by studies of FcγRII-deficient mice, murine models of autoimmune disease and human SLE as well as rheumatoid arthritis. FcγRIIb deficiency renders normally resistant strains of mice susceptible to collagen-induced arthritis and Goodpasture's syndrome (Boackle et al. 2001). FcγRIIb$^{-/-}$ mice derived on a C57BL/6 but not a Balb/c background produce autoantibodies and develop immune complex-mediated autoimmune disease resembling SLE, including immune complex-mediated glomerulonephritis and renal failure.

Genetic studies of polygenic murine models of human autoimmune diseases further implicate FcγRIIb in SLE pathogenesis. A number of independent linkage studies in murine models of SLE and RA have identified disease susceptibility loci that contain *fcgr2*. It should be emphasized that the region on chromosome 1 containing *fcgr2* also contains a number of other candidate genes, for example complement receptor 2 and SLE-1 (Shai et al. 1999). Genetic studies in human autoimmune diseases, such as SLE and insulin-dependent diabetes mellitus (IDDM) have demonstrated significant linkage to the region of chromosome 1 (1q23) containing the low-affinity Fc receptors (both activating and inhibitory) (Gaffney et al. 1998; Harley et al. 1998; Wakeland et al. 2001). A number of studies have also found a correlation between specific polymorphisms in FcγRIIA, FcγRIIIA and FcγRIIIB and the development of a number of different autoimmune diseases (Kyogoku et al. 2002), although this has not been a consistent finding (Fujimoto et al. 1999). Further genetic studies identifying a linkage of polymorphisms in FcγRIIB to disease pathogenesis in humans found a single nucleotide polymorphism in the *Fcgr2b* gene that results in an Ile232Thr substitution (Smith and Fearon 2000). In that study, the 232T/T genotype was found at a significantly higher frequency in Japanese SLE patients as compared to controls. Although the precise effect of this mutation is unknown, it encodes part of the *trans*-membrane region of the molecule and it is known that an intact transmembrane region is required for induction of apoptotic signals through FcγRIIB in the mouse. Thus, *Fcgr2b* and its polymorphisms represent a candidate gene of an inhibitory receptor that is likely to be involved in human autoimmune disease.

CD22 CD22 is a B cell-specific glycoprotein that first appears intracellularly during the late pro-B cell stage of ontogeny. Subsequently, CD22 shifts to the plasma membrane with B cell maturation until plasma cell differentiation. Plasma cells do not express the molecule. CD22 has seven extracytoplasmic Ig-like domains and belongs to the Ig superfamily. It serves as a receptor for carbohydrate determinants on a wide variety of cell surface and soluble molecules in vivo. In contrast to CD19, CD22 can act as an antagonist to B cell activation most likely by enhancing the threshold of BCR-induced signals. Following BCR engagement, CD22 is predominantly phosphorylated within ITIMs present in its cytoplasmic domain. Phosphorylation is predominantly mediated by Lyn, downstream of the CD19-dependent Lyn kinase amplification loop. If phosphorylated by Lyn, CD22 recruits the SHP-1 and SHIP phosphatases, leading to activation of a CD22/SHP-1/SHIP regulatory pathway that downregulates CD19 phosphorylation and BCR-mediated signal transduction. Thus, CD19 and CD22 together define signalling thresholds critical for expansion of the peripheral B cell pool (Smith and Fearon 2000). Ligation of CD22 to the BCR, and subsequent SHP-1 activation inhibits B cell activation by inhibiting the MAP kinases ERK2, JNK and p38 and dephosphorylating molecules involved in the early events of BCR-mediated activation. These include the BCR itself, tyrosine kinases activated by phosphorylation of Igαβ (such as syk) and the targets of these kinases (including the adaptor protein BLNK and PLCγ). Since co-ligation of CD22 to the BCR reduces B cell activation, the interaction of CD22 with its ligand may be involved in downregulating B cell activation (O'Keefe et al. 1999).

CD22 has been linked genetically to autoimmune disease, indicating a possible role for defects in CD22 and subsequent signalling pathways in the development of autoimmunity. It has been shown that CD22-deficient mice have an expanded B1 cell population and develop increased serum IgM. The B cells of these mice are hyper-responsive to stimulation through the BCR (Okazaki et al. 2001), suggesting that CD22 is an important inhibitory receptor in BCR-dependent B cell activation. Importantly, these mice develop high-affinity autoantibodies to dsDNA, myeloperoxidase and cardiolipin, although they do not develop autoimmune disease (Nishimura and Honjo 2001). Interestingly, CD22 has been successfully used as target of biological therapies in patients with non-Hodgkin lymphomas as well as in SLE (J. Kaufmann et al., personal communication) by employing a humanized monoclonal antibody to CD22. To which extent this monoclonal exerts its effects by depletion, inducing apoptosis or by inhibition of B cell activation via CD22, remains to be shown.

PD-1 PD-1 is a 55-kDa highly conserved inhibitory receptor of the Ig superfamily (Nishimura and Honjo 2001). It is expressed on resting B cells, T cells and macrophages and is induced on activation of these cells (Nishimura and Honjo 2001; Okazaki et al. 2001). PD-1 is composed of a single extracellular Ig-like domain, a transmembrane region and has two tyrosine residues in the cytoplasmic tail, one of which forms part of an ITIM. Two PD-1 ligands (PD-Ls) have been identified and are constitutively expressed on dendritic cells and on heart, lung, thymus and kidney and also on monocytes after IFN-γ stimulation. In vitro studies on a B cell lymphoma line using a chimaeric molecule with the FcγRII extracellular domain and the PD-1 cytoplasmic domain have shown that ligation of the PD-1 cytoplasmic domain to the BCR can inhibit BCR mediated signalling. This inhibition prevented BCR-mediated proliferation, Ca^{2+} mobilization and tyrosine phosphorylation of molecules, including CD79beta, syk, PLCγ2 and ERK1/2. The physiological role of PD-1 in B cells remains unclear, but it may play a role in maintaining peripheral tolerance by limiting activation of autoreactive B cells by cross-linking PD-1 during interactions with PD-L-expressing cells.

From an epidemiologic perspective, linkage studies in human autoimmune diseases have identified susceptibility loci for both SLE and insulin-dependent diabetes mellitus that lie close to the gene encoding PD-1 (Pritchard and Smith 2003). However, no direct evidence for abnormal PD-1 function in human disease has been identified so far. A role in the development of autoimmunity, however, is suggested by the observation that PD-1 knockout mice develop autoantibodies and autoimmune disease.

Collectively, preclinical studies in animal models, genetic analysis as well as linkage studies indicate the three inhibitory receptors PD-1, CD22 and FcγRIIb candidate as being involved in autoimmunity. Whether these potential defects are involved in initiation or the maintenance of autoimmunity needs to be addressed. If so, additional analyses will be needed to assess whether the defect lies in the molecules or their ligand or intracellular signalling pathways.

4
Inhibitory Receptor Pathways and Autoimmunity

It must be emphasized that the large number of inhibitory receptors on the surface of B cells are subserved by remarkably similar signalling pathways. To date, Lyn is the only tyrosine kinase that has been identified as phosphorylating ITIMs on the B cell inhibitory receptors. Most of these ITIMs then associate with SHP-1 or SHIP (Fig. 2).

Inhibitory receptors control the activation threshold of many immune cells, including B cells. There are many similarities in the signalling pathways of these inhibitory receptors. Inhibitory receptors also have specific effects, as they bind different ligands, and signal through different phosphatases. Consistent with a role of defects in inhibitory receptor function in autoimmunity is the finding that B cells from inhibitory receptor-deficient mice have similarities in phenotype and lowered thresholds for activation to those reported for B cells from SLE patients.

SHP-1 SHP-1 is a protein tyrosine phosphatase and is similar in structure to SHP-2. SHP-1 is the phosphatase that is utilized most widely in the inhibitory receptor signalling pathways. SHP-1 plays the predominant role in regulating through ITIMs, whereas increasing evidence suggests that SHP-2 may well have an additional activating role. Obviously, these molecules have an important role in regulation of a normal immune system.

Consistent with its role in mediating inhibitory receptor function, SHP-1 deficiency results in the development of spontaneous autoimmune disease. SHP-1 also associates with BCR, Fc, growth factor, complement and cytokine receptors (Shultz et al. 1984). SHP-1 knockout mice have a phenotype consistent with a prominent role of this tyrosine phosphatase in inhibitory receptor pathways (Sidman et al. 1986; Yu et al. 1996). These mice have B cells that are hyper-responsive to BCR stimulation, raised levels of serum immunoglobulin, develop autoantibodies and manifest severe autoimmune disease with immune complex deposition in skin, lung and kidney (Lioubin et al. 1996; Sidman et al. 1986; Yu et al. 1996) and a number of other inflammatory changes.

So far, there are no clear data that show linkage between SHP-1 and the development of autoimmune disease in human subjects. However, defects in SHP-1 expression have been associated with SLE in humans; reduced levels of SHP-1 and Lyn are found in the lymphocytes of patients with inactive SLE, suggesting a potential role in pathogenesis.

SHIP SHIP is an highly conserved SH2-containing inositol phosphatase related to SHIP-2 (Helgason et al. 1998). Both share a conserved N-terminal SH2 catalytic domain. SHIP acts predominantly on the FcγRIIb signalling pathway. The molecule is expressed in myeloid and lymphoid lineages, including B cells.

The pattern of B cell abnormalities seen in the SHIP-deficient mouse indicates its inhibitory role in B cell signalling. Splenic B cells have an activated phenotype with lower surface levels of IgM and higher levels of IgD and are hyper-responsive to BCR-mediated stimulation measured by expression of the activation markers CD69 and CD86 (Helgason et al. 1998).

Genetic studies in humans have identified susceptibility loci for both diabetes and SLE mapping to the region of the genome containing SHIP, although direct evidence for abnormal SHIP function in human disease is lacking.

The phenotype of most murine models of SLE suggests impaired inhibitory receptor function, with hyperactive B cells and a similar pattern of autoantibody production and glomerular disease to that seen in inhibitory receptor knockout mice. Nonetheless, at almost every genetic susceptibility locus containing an inhibitory receptor implicated in SLE, there are large numbers of genes encoding other immunologically relevant molecules, which may also play a role in disease pathogenesis. The role of inhibitory receptors in spontaneous disease has therefore yet to be established firmly, but nonetheless the evidence favours contributions by defective inhibitory receptor function to the pathogenesis of B cell-mediated autoimmune disease.

5
Activated B Cells May Bridge the Innate and Adaptive Immune System

The cross-talk between the innate and adaptive immune systems in general as well as in rheumatoid arthritis has regained significant attention (Corr and Firestein 2002) with the "one-way" concept of activation of the adaptive by the innate path less likely. In this regard, there is a general perception of three stages in the course of rheumatoid arthritis: disease initiation, perpetuation and a terminal destructive process (Corr and Firestein 2002; Firestein and Zvaifler 2002; Kouskoff et al. 1996; Mangialaio et al. 1999). However, the distinct role of antigen-specific lymphocytes remains a matter of debate. Recent concepts (Mangialaio et al. 1999) repostulated that the initiation of RA may be antigen-independent by involving joint constituents. Secondly, the inflammatory phase appears to be driven by specific antigens—either foreign or native and either integral to the joint or presented in the periphery. In the third stage, however, destruction of the synovium seems to be again antigen-independent. Although it is not clear to which extent B cells are involved in each stage of the disease, their role appears to be significant either as a link to other immune cells, potentially bridging the innate and the adaptive immune systems, or as directing cellular components in inflammation. Nevertheless, B cells can be considered as an "enhancing element" of rheumatoid arthritis severity by taking into account that patients producing autoantibodies usually have a more severe disease course.

Recently, the K/BxN mouse has generated particular interest. In this model, spontaneous arthritis occurs in mice that express both the transgene encoded KRN T cell receptor and the IAg^7 MHC class II allele (Kouskoff et al. 1996;

Maccioni et al. 1999; Matsumoto et al. 1999). The transgenic T cells have a specificity for glucose-6-phosphate isomerase (G6PI) and are able to break tolerance in the B cell compartment, resulting in the production of autoantibodies to G6PI. Affinity-purified anti-G6PI Ig from these mice can transfer joint-specific inflammation to healthy recipients (Korganow et al. 1999). A mechanism for joint-specific disease arising from autoimmunity to G6PI has been suggested recently. G6PI bound to the surface of cartilage serves as the target for anti-G6PI binding and subsequent complement-mediated damage. In this model, the inciting event is the expression of an autoreactive T cell receptor in the periphery. However, joint destruction is delegated by the adaptive response to innate immune mechanisms and can be transferred to animals that lack B and T cells (Korganow et al. 1999; Kouskoff et al. 1996). Whereas these animal studies are very compelling, anti-G6PI antibodies do not frequently occur in the serum of RA patients (Kassahn et al. 2002; Schubert et al. 2002).

6
Rationales of B Cell-Targeted Therapy in Autoimmune Diseases

Although identification of the central antigens in a number of rheumatic diseases is still lacking, formation of T cell/B cell aggregates and the formation of germinal centre-like structures can be correlated with increasing disease activity, including the production of autoantibodies (Leadbetter et al. 2002; Shlomchik et al. 2001). It needs to be shown whether apparent differences in the underlying pathologic process, with the disease activity likely escalating from 1) non-organized infiltrate to 2) T/B aggregates through 3) ectopic germinal centre formation. Such distinctions might indicate differences in the course of the disease correlating with the degree of B cell activity and may provide the benefit of tuning therapeutic strategies.

Despite the role of T cell help in the differentiation of B cells, recent studies suggest that B cells not only play an interactive role between the innate and adaptive immune system, but can also be activated without additional T cell help using either TLR- or BAFF-dependent activation pathways. This emphasizes the central role of B cells in immune responses and the need for B cell-directed therapies. A recent study (Leadbetter et al. 2002) showed that effective activation of rheumatoid factor-positive B cells can be mediated by IgG2a-chromatin immune complexes via engagement of the B cell receptor and TLR9, a member of the MyD88-dependent toll-like receptor (TLR) family. Bacterial and vertebrate DNAs differ by the absence of CpG methylation in bacteria and therefore TLR9 can detect unmethylated CpG dinucleotides as a signal of infection initiating B cell activation. In humans, the expression of TLR9 appears to be relatively restricted to B cells and $CD123^+$ dendritic cells. After ligation of CpG motifs to TLR9, B cells are induced to proliferate and secrete Ig, and DCs secrete a wide array of cytokines, interferons and chemokines that activate T_H1 cells. Bacterial DNA or CpG motifs co-stimulate B cell activation through cell membrane Ig and thereby promote an early antigen-specific response. This study (Leadbetter et al. 2002) found that immune complexes containing self-DNA activate rheumatoid factor-specific B cells as a result of two distinct signals: (a) engagement of the B cell antigen receptor (BCR) and (b) activation of TLR9 through the histone/DNA portion of the immune complex. Although the implications of these findings for certain autoimmune diseases need further studies, the evidence that TLR9 activation co-stimulates autoreactive B cells provides a mechanism of action for an established therapy for systemic autoimmune diseases. Decades ago, it was found that chloroquine is an effective therapy for systemic autoimmunity, but the mechanism of its activity was not identified. Chloroquine and other compounds that interfere with endosomal acidification and maturation specifically block all the CpG-mediated signals (Yin et al. 1998). The established efficacy of chloroquine and related compounds in treating autoimmune diseases could be related to a requirement for continuous co-stimulation of the BCR and TLR9 pathways in sustaining disease activity. Chloroquine also blocks antigen presentation, interleukin-6 production and directly binds DNA, which could contribute to its effectiveness. Moreover, it has been shown that sulfasalazine also has effects on reducing B cell activity, which further indicates that known disease-modifying antirheumatic drugs may have the capacity to influence the biologic activity of these cells (Cambridge et al. 2003). Moreover, other TLRs can also be considered as candidates in rheumatoid arthritis pathogenesis, i.e. TLR4 recognizing LPS, but this needs further investigation.

Therapy for severe autoimmune disease has primarily relied on broadly immunosuppressive agents such as cyclophosphamide, methotrexate, cyclosporine, leflunomide, mycophenolate mofetil and corticosteroids (Hirohata et al. 2002). Although survival rates have improved dramatically, none of these therapies offers a cure and most have significant toxicity. With the advent of monoclonal antibody and specific small-molecule-based therapies, more specific and effective therapies are possible. Therapy directed at specifically reducing B cell numbers has recently gained attention and enthusiasm (Cambridge et al. 2002; Dörner and Burmester 2003). Based on the ability of the chimerized anti-CD20 monoclonal antibody (rituximab) to reduce B cell numbers without significant toxicity, it is also being evaluated in human clinical trials for patients with a number of autoimmune diseases (Cambridge et al. 2002; De Vita et al. 2002; Edwards et al. 2000, 2004; Leandro et al. 2001, 2002a, b; Leandro, 2003). Rituximab functions by binding the membrane-embedded CD20 surface molecule on B cells, leading to B cell elimination by host immune effector mechanisms such as ADCC, inducing apoptosis and cell-mediated cytotoxicity.

A further humanized antibody directed to CD22 previously applied in non-Hodgkin's patients is also under evaluation in early clinical studies of patients with autoimmune disease (J. Kaufmann et al., personal communication).

Considering our current understanding of the role of B cells in the pathogenesis of autoimmune disease, the potential specificity of monoclonal antibodies with minimal toxicity, and the encouraging preliminary results in human clinical trials, one can expect to see a significant expansion in the use of B cell-directed therapy. Notably, however, most autoimmune patients that have benefited from rituximab therapy have not manifested remarkable decreases in measurable Ig levels, but have been associated with some—but not uniform—decreases in autoantibody titres, such as rheumatoid factor, antineutrophil cytoplasmic antigen, cryoglobulins. These data suggest that the therapeutic effect may not simply rely on deleting precursors of autoantibody-producing cells, but possibly also by interfering with the life-cycle of specific antigen-presenting B cells.

Beyond overall B cell depletion allowing common targeting of T cell-dependent and -independent B cell activation, future therapies need to identify the most important common pathways of B cell activation that provide similar efficiency but avoid complete loss of B cells. Other potential targets for treating B cell-mediated human autoimmune diseases include BAFF antagonists and decoy receptors utilizing BMCA-Ig or TACI-Ig. Recent trials of CTLA-4-lg fusion proteins that disrupt T–B cell interactions (Kremer et al. 2003) and T cell activation have been promising in the treatment of rheumatoid arthritis, showing moderate efficacy with no evidence of significant toxicity. The development of therapeutic monoclonal antibodies that block certain ligand engagement or intracellular pathways may have considerable benefit for the treatment of autoimmunity, without the risk of eliminating bulk B cell populations, as with anti-CD20-directed therapies. Since CD19 deficiency ameliorates autoimmunity in mice, a further understanding of the molecular aspects of CD19–Src-family kinase interactions may lead to the identification of target molecules for therapeutic intervention during human autoimmunity.

Rapidly advancing molecular understanding of regular and disturbed immune responses will provide abundant targets appropriate for drug development. It is expected and likely that many of these drugs will target B cell function directly since it is becoming more obvious that abnormally activated B cells contribute substantially to many human autoimmune diseases.

Acknowledgements Supported by Sonderforschungsbereich 421 and 650, and DFG grants 491/4-7, 5-3, 4.

References

Anolik JH, Barnard J, Cappione A, Pugh-Bernard AE, Felgar RE, Looney RJ, Sanz I (2004) Rituximab improves peripheral B cell abnormalities in human systemic lupus erythematosus. Arthritis Rheum 50:3580–3590

Benschop RJ, Cambier JC (1999) B cell development: signal transduction by antigen receptors and their surrogates. CurrOpin Immunol11:143–151

Boackle SA, Holers VM, Chen XJ, Szakonyi G, Karp DR, Wakeland EK, Morel L (2001) Cr2, a candidate gene in the murine Sle1c lupus susceptibility locus, encodes a dysfunctional protein. Immunity 15:775–785

Bohnhorst JO, Bjorgan MB, Thoen JE, Natvig JB, Thompson KM (2001a) Bm1-Bm5 classification of peripheral blood B cells reveals circulating germinal center founder cells in healthy individuals and disturbance in the B cell subpopulations in patients with primary Sjogren's syndrome. J Immunol 167:3610–3618

Bohnhorst JO, Thoen JE, Natvig JB, Thompson KM (2001b) Significantly depressed percentage of CD27+(memory) B cells among peripheral blood B cells in patients with primary Sjogren's syndrome. Scan J Immunol 54:421–427

Bohnhorst JO, Bjorgan MB, Thoen JE, Jonsson R, Natvig JB, Thompson KM (2002) Abnormal B cell differentiation in primary Sjogren's syndrome results in a depressed percentage of circulating memory B cells and elevated levels of soluble CD27 that correlate with serum IgG concentration. Clin Immunol 103:79–88

Bolland S, Ravetch JV (2000) Spontaneous autoimmune disease in Fc gamma RIIB-deficient mice results from strain-specific epistasis. Immunity 13:277–285

Brezinschek HP, Brezinschek RI, Lipsky PE (1995a) Analysis of the heavy-chain repertoire of human peripheral B-cells using single-cell polymerase chain reaction. JImmunol 155:190–202

Brezinschek HP, Foster SJ, Brezinschek RI, Lipsky PE (1995b) The human-immunoglobulin variable heavy-chain repertoire. Arthritis Rheum 38:1007

Brezinschek HP, Brezinschek RI, Foster SJ, Dörner T, Lipsky PE (1996) Analysis of the immunoglobulin repertoire of human B-1 (CD5+) B cells. Arthritis Rheum 39:102

Cambridge G, Leandro MJ, Edwards JCW, Ehrenstein MR, Salden M, Webster D (2002) B lymphocyte depletion in patients with rheumatoid arthritis: serial studies of immunological parameters. Arthritis Rheum 46:S506

Cambridge G, Leandro MJ, Edwards JCW, Ehrenstein MR, Salden M, Bodman-Smith M, Webster ADB (2003) Serologic changes following B lymphocyte depletion therapy for rheumatoid arthritis. Arthritis Rheum 48:2146–2154

Cappione A, Anolik J, Pugh-Bernard A, Silverman G, Sanz I (2002) Human autoreactive VH4.34 B-cells are compartmentalized in the spleen marginal zone. Arthritis Rheum 46:S416

Carsetti R, Kohler G, Lamers MC (1995) Transitional B-cells are the target of negative selection in the B-cell compartment. J Exp Med 181:2129–2140

Chan OTM, Madaio MP, Shlomchik MJ (1999) The central and multiple roles of B cells in lupus pathogenesis. Immunol Rev 169:107–121

Cornall RJ, Cyster JG, Hibbs ML, Dunn AR, Otipoby KL, Clark EA, Goodnow CC (1998) Polygenic autoimmune traits: Lyn, CD22, and SHP-1 are limiting elements of a biochemical pathway regulating BCR signaling and selection. Immunity 8:497–508

Corr M, Firestein GS (2002) Commentary—innate immunity as a hired gun: but is it rheumatoid arthritis? J Exp Med 195:F33–F35

Daeron M (1997) Fc receptor biology. Ann Rev Immunol 15:203–234

De Vita S, Zaja F, Sacco S, De Candia A, Fanin R, Ferraccioli G (2002) Efficacy of selective B cell blockade in the treatment of rheumatoid arthritis—evidence for a pathogenetic role of B cells. Arthritis Rheum 46:2029–2033

Doody GM, Justement LB, Delibrias CC, Matthews RJ, Lin JJ, Thomas ML, Fearon DT (1995) A role in B-cell activation for Cd22 and the protein-tyrosine-phosphatase Shp. Science 269:242–244

Dörner T, Burmester GR (2003) The role of B cells in rheumatoid arthritis: mechanisms and therapeutic targets. Curr Opin Rheumatol 15:246–252

Dörner T, Putterman C (2001) B cells, BAFF/zTNF4, TACl, and systemic lupus erythematosus. Arthritis Res 3:197–199

Dörner T, Foster SJ, Farner NL, Lipsky PE (1998) Immunoglobulin kappa chain receptor editing in systemic lupus erythematosus. J Clin Invest 102:688–694

Edwards JC, Cambridge G, Leandro MJ (2000) Sustained improvement in rheumatoid arthritis following B lymphocyte depletion. Arthritis Rheum 43:S391

Edwards JCW, Szczepanski L, Szechinski J, Filipowicz-Sosnowska A, Emery P, Close DR, Stevens RM, Shaw T (2004) Efficacy of B-cell-targeted therapy with rituximab in patients with rheumatoid arthritis. N Eng J Med 350:2572–2581

Firestein GS, Zvaifler NJ (2002) How important are T cells in chronic rheumatoid synovitis? II. T cell-independent mechanisms from beginning to end. Arthritis Rheum 46:298–308

Fujimoto M, Bradney AP, Poe JC, Steeber DA, Tedder TF (1999) Modulation of B lymphocyte antigen receptor signal transduction by a CD19/CD22 regulatory loop. Immunity 11:191–200

Gaffney PM, Kearns GM, Shark KB, Ortmann WA, Selby SA, Malmgren ML, Rohlf KE, Ockenden TC, Messner RP, King RA, Rich SS, Behrens TW (1998) A genome-wide search for susceptibility genes in human systemic lupus erythematosus sib-pair families. Proc Natl Acad Sci U S A 95:14875–14879

Grimbacher B, Hutloff A, Schlesier M, Glocker E, Warnatz K, Drager R, Eibel H, Fischer B, Schaffer AA, Mages HW, Kroczek RA, Peter HH (2003) Homozygous loss of ICOS is associated with adult-onset common variable immunodeficiency. Nat Immunol 4:261–268

Gross JA, Johnston J, Mudri S, Enselman R, Dillon SR, Madden K, Xu WF, Parrish-Novak J, Foster D, Lofton-Day C, Moore M, Littau A, Grossman A, Haugen H, Foley K, Blumberg H, Harrison K, Kindsvogel W, Clegg CH (2000) TACI and BCMA are receptors for a TNF homologue implicated in B-cell autoimmune disease. Nature 404:995–999

Hansen A, Odendahl M, Reiter K, Jacobi A, Burmester GR, Lipsky PE, Dörner T (2002a) Disturbances in peripheral B cell subsets in patients with primary Sjogren's syndrome with a markedly diminished peripheral CD5+/CD27+ memory population. Arthritis Rheum 46:S597

Hansen A, Odendahl M, Reiter K, Jacobi AM, Feist E, Scholze J, Burmester GR, Lipsky PE, Dörner T (2002b) Diminished peripheral blood memory B cells and accumulation of memory B cells in the salivary glands of patients with Sjogren's syndrome. Arthritis Rheum 46:2160–2171

Hansen A, Gosemann M, Pruss A, Reiter K, Ruzickova S, Lipsky PE, Dörner T (2004) Abnormalities in peripheral B cell memory of patients with primary Sjogren's syndrome. Arthritis Rheum 50:1897–1908

Harley JB, Moser KL, Gaffney PM, Behrens TW (1998) The genetics of human systemic lupus erythematosus. Curr Opin Immunol 10:690–696

Helgason CD, Damen JE, Rosten P, Grewal R, Sorensen P, Chappel SM, Borowski A, Jirik F, Krystal G, Humphries RK (1998) Targeted disruption of SHIP leads to hemopoietic perturbations lung pathology, and a shortened life span. Genes Dev 12:1610–1620

Hirohata S, Ohshima N, Yanagida T, Aramaki K (2002) Regulation of human B cell function by sulfasalazine and its metabolites. Int Immunopharmacol 2:631–640

Huang SC, Jiang RH, Glas AM, Milner ECB (1996) Non-stochastic utilization of Ig V region genes in unselected human peripheral B cells. Mol Immunol 33:553–560

Hutloff A, Buchner K, Reiter K, Baelde HJ, Odendahl M, Jacobi A, Dörner T, Kroczek RA (2004) Involvement of inducible costimulator in the exaggerated memory B cell and plasma cell generation in systemic lupus erythematosus. Arthritis Rheum 50:3211–3220

Inaoki M, Sato S, Weintraub BC, Goodnow CC, Tedder TF (1997) CD19-regulated signaling thresholds control peripheral tolerance and autoantibody production in B lymphocytes. J Exp Med 186:1923–1931

Isenberg DA, McClure C, Farewell V, Spellerberg M, Williams W, Cambridge G, Stevenson F (1998) Correlation of 9G4 idiotope with disease activity in patients with systemic lupus erythematosus. Ann Rheum Dis 57:566–570

Iwai H, Abe M, Hirose S, Tsushima F, Tezuka K, Akiba H, Yagita H, Okumura K, Kohsaka H, Miyasaka N, Azuma M (2003) Involvement of inducible costimulator-B7 homologous protein costimulatory pathway in murine lupus nephritis. J Immunol 171:2848–2854

Jacobi A, Dörner T, Hansen A, Lipsky PE (1999) Identification of enhanced mutational activity and disturbed selection mechanisms on V-H gene rearrangements in systemic lupus erythematosus (SLE). Arthritis Rheum 42:S54

Jacobi AM, Odendahl M, Reiter K, Bruns A, Burmester GR, Radbruch A, Valet G, Lipsky PE, Dörner T (2003) Correlation between circulating CD27 (high) plasma cells and disease activity in patients with systemic lupus erythematosus. Arthritis Rheum 48:1332–1342

Kassahn D, Kolb C, Solomon S, Bochtler P, Illges H (2002) Few human autoimmune sera detect GPI. Nat Immunol 3:411–412

Kim HJ, Krenn V, Steinhauser G, Berek C (1999) Plasma cell development in synovial germinal centers in patients with rheumatoid and reactive arthritis. J Immunol 162:3053–3062

Korganow AS, Ji H, Mangialaio S, Duchatelle V, Pelanda R, Martin T, Degott C, Kikutani H, Rajewsky K, Pasquali JL, Benoist C, Mathis D (1999) From systemic T cell self-reactivity to organ-specific autoimmune disease via immunoglobulins. Immunity 10:451–461

Kouskoff V, Korganow AS, Duchatelle V, Degott C, Benoist C, Mathis D (1996) Organ-specific disease provoked by systemic autoimmunity. Cell 87:811–822

Kraj P, Rao SP, Glas AM, Hardy RR, Milner ECB, Silberstein LE (1997) The human heavy chain Ig V region gene repertoire is biased at all stages of B cell ontogeny, including early pre-B cells. J Immunol 158:5824–5832

Kremer JM, Westhovens R, Leon M, Di Giorgio E, Alten R, Steinfeld S, Russell A, Dougados M, Emery P, Nuamah IF, Williams GR, Becker JC, Hagerty DT, Moreland LW (2003) Treatment of rheumatoid arthritis by selective inhibition of T-cell activation with fusion protein CTLA4Ig. N Eng J Med 349:1907–1915

Kyogoku C, Dijstelbloem HM, Tsuchiya N, Hatta Y, Kato H, Yamaguchi A, Fukazawa T, Jansen MD, Hashimoto H, van de Winkel JGJ, Kallenberg CGM, Tokunaga K (2002) Fc gamma receptor gene polymorphisms in Japanese patients with systemic lupus erythematosus—contribution of FCGR2B to genetic susceptibility. Arthritis Rheum 46:1242–1254

Latour S, Fridman WH, Daeron M (1996) Identification, molecular cloning, biologic properties, and tissue distribution of a novel isoform of murine low-affinity IgG receptor homologous to human Fc gamma RIIB1. J Immunol 157:189–197

Leadbetter EA, Rifkin IR, Hohlbaum AM, Beaudette BC, Shlomchik MJ, Marshak-Rothstein A (2002) Chromatin-IgG complexes activate B cells by dual engagement of IgM and Toll-like receptors. Nature 416:603–607

Leandro MJ, Edwards JCW, Cambridge G (2001) B lymphocyte depletion in rheumatoid arthritis. Early evidence for safety, efficacy, and dose response. Arthritis Rheum 44: S370

Leandro MJ, Edwards JC, Cambridge G, Ehrenstein MR, Isenberg DA (2002a) An open study of B lymphocyte depletion in systemic lupus erythematosus. Arthritis Rheum 46:2673–2677

Leandro MJ, Edwards JCW, Cambridge G (2002b) Clinical outcome in 22 patients with rheumatoid arthritis treated with B lymphocyte depletion. Ann Rheum Dis 61:883–888

Leandro MJ, Ehrenstein MR, Edwards JCW, Manson J, Cambridge G, Isenberg DA (2003) Treatment of refractory lupus nephritis with B lymphocyte depletion. Arthritis Rheum 48:S378

Lioubin MN, Algate PA, Tsai S, Carlberg K, Aebersold R, Rohrschneider LR (1996) p150(Ship), a signal transduction molecule with inositol polyphosphate-5-phosphatase activity. Genes Dev 10:1084–1095

Looney RJ, Anolik J, Sanz I (2004a) B cells as therapeutic targets for rheumatic diseases. Curr Opin Rheumatol 16:180–185

Looney RJ, Anolik J, Sanz I (2004b) B lymphocytes in systemic lupus erythematosus: lessons from therapy targeting B cells. Lupus 13:381–390

Maccioni M, Zeder-Lutz G, Huang HC, Ebel C, Gerber P, Hergueux J, Marchal P, Duchatelle V, Degott C, van Regenmortel M, Benoist C, Mathis D (2002) Arthritogenic monoclonal antibodies from K/BxN mice. J Exp Med 195:1071–1077

Mackay F, Browning JL (2002) BAFF: a fundamental survival factor for B cells. Nature Rev Immunol 2:465–475

Mackay F, Mackay CR (2002) The role of BAFF in B-cell maturation, T-cell activation and autoimmunity. Trends Immunol 23:113–115

Mackay F, Woodcock SA, Lawton P, Ambrose C, Baetscher M, Schneider P, Tschopp J, Browning JL (1999) Mice transgenic for BAFF develop lymphocytic disorders along with autoimmune manifestations. J Exp Med 190:1697–1710

Malbec O, Fridman WH, Daeron M (1999) Negative regulation of hematopoietic cell activation and proliferation by Fc gamma RIIB. Curr Top Microbiol Immunol 244:13–27

Mangialaio S, Ji H, Korganow AS, Kouskoff V, Benoist C, Mathis D (1999) The arthritogenic T cell receptor and its ligand in a model of spontaneous arthritis. Arthritis Rheum 42:2517–2523

Maruyama M, Lam KP, Rajewsky K (2000) Memory B-cell persistence is independent of persisting immunizing antigen. Nature 407:636–642

Matsumoto I, Staub A, Benoist C, Mathis D (1999) Arthritis provoked by linked T and B cell recognition of a glycolytic enzyme. Science 286:1732–1735

Mockridge CI, Chapman CJ, Spellerberg MB, Sheth B, Fleming TP, Isenberg DA, Stevenson FK (1998) Sequence analysis of V4-34-encoded antibodies from single B cells of two patients with systemic lupus erythematosus (SLE). Clin Exp Immunol 114:129–136

Nishimura H, Honjo T (2001) PD-1: an inhibitory immunoreceptor involved in peripheral tolerance. Trends Immunol 22:265–268

O'Connor BP, Raman VS, Erickson LD, Cook WJ, Weaver LK, Ahonen C, Lin LL, Mantchev GT, Bram RJ, Noelle RJ (2004) BCMA is essential for the survival of long-lived bone marrow plasma cells. J Exp Med 199:91–97

O'Keefe TL, Williams GT, Batista FD, Neuberger MS (1999) Deficiency in CD22, a B cell-specific inhibitory receptor, is sufficient to predispose to development of high affinity autoantibodies. J Exp Med 189:1307–1313

Odendahl M, Jacobi A, Hansen A, Feist E, Hiepe F, Burmester GR, Lipsky PE, Radbruch A, Dörner T (2000a) Disturbed peripheral B cell hemeostasis in SLE. Arthritis Rheum 43:S234

Odendahl M, Jacobi A, Hansen A, Feist E, Hiepe F, Burmester GR, Lipsky PE, Radbruch A, Dörner T (2000b) Disturbed peripheral B lymphocyte homeostasis in systemic lupus erythematosus. J Immunol 165:5970–5979

Odendahl M, Keitzer R, Wahn U, Hiepe F, Radbruch A, Dörner T, Bunikowski R (2003) Perturbations of peripheral B lymphocyte homoeostasis in children with systemic lupus erythematosus. Ann Rheum Dis 62:851–858

Okazaki T, Maeda A, Nishimura H, Kurosaki T, Honjo T (2001) PD-1 immunoreceptor inhibits B cell receptor-mediated signaling by recruiting src homology 2-domain-containing tyrosine phosphatase 2 to phosphotyrosine. Proc Natl Acad Sci U S A 98:13866–13871

Potter KN, Mockridge CI, Rahman A, Buchan S, Hamblin T, Davidson B, Isenberg DA, Stevenson FK (2002) Disturbances in peripheral blood B cell subpopulations in autoimmune patients. Lupus 11:872–877

Pritchard NR, Smith KGC (2003) B cell inhibitory receptors and autoimmunity. Immunology 108:263–273

Prodeus AP, Goerg S, Shen LM, Pozdnyakova OO, Chu L, Alicot EM, Goodnow CC, Carroll MC (1998) A critical role for complement in maintenance of self-tolerance. Immunity 9:721–731

Pugh-Bernard AE, Silverman GJ, Cappione AJ, Villano ME, Ryan DH, Insel RA, Sanz I (2001) Regulation of inherently autoreactive VH4–34B cells in the maintenance of human B cell tolerance. J Clin Invest 108:1061–1070

Rahman A, Latchman DS, Isenberg DA (1998) Immunoglobulin variable region sequences of human monoclonal anti-DNA antibodies. Semin Arthritis Rheum 28:141–154

Saito E, Fujimoto M, Hasegawa M, Komura K, Hamaguchi Y, Koburagi Y, Nagaoka T, Takehara K, Tedder TF, Sato S (2002) CD19-dependent B lymphocyte signaling thresholds influence skin fibrosis and autoimmunity in the tight-skin mouse. J Clin Invest 109:1453–1462

Schiemann B, Gommerman JL, Vora K, Cachero TG, Shulga-Morskaya S, Dobles M, Frew E, Scott ML (2001) An essential role for BAFF in the normal development of B cells through a BCMA-independent pathway. Science 293:2111–2114

Schubert D, Schmidt M, Zaiss D, Jungblut PR, Kamradt T (2002) Autoantibodies to GPI and creatine kinase in RA. Nature Immunol 3:411

Shai R, Quismorio FP, Li LL, Kwon OJ, Morrison J, Wallace DJ, Neuwelt CM, Brautbar C, Gauderman WJ, Jacob CO (1999) Genome-wide screen for systemic lupus erythematosus susceptibility genes in multiplex families. Human Mol Genet 8:639–644

Shlomchik MJ, Craft JE, Mamula MJ (2001) From T to B and back again: positive feedback in systemic autoimmune disease. Nature Rev Immunol 1:147–153

Shultz LD, Coman DR, Bailey CL, Beamer WG, Sidman CL (1984) Viable motheaten, a new allele at the motheaten locus .1. Pathology. Am J Pathol 116:179–192

Sidman CL, Shultz LD, Hardy RR, Hayakawa K, Herzenberg LA (1986) Production of immunoglobulin isotypes by Ly-1+ B cells in viable moth-eaten and normal mice. Science 232:1423–1425

Smith KGC, Fearon DT (2000) Receptor modulators of B-cell receptor signalling—CD19/CD22. Signal transduction and the coordination of B lymphocyte development and function I. Curr Top Microbiol Immunol 245:195–212

Smith KGC, Tarlinton DM, Doody GM, Hibbs ML, Fearon DT (1998) Inhibition of the B cell by CD22: a requirement for Lyn. J Exp Med 187:807–811

Strasser A, Whittingham S, Vaux DL, Bath ML, Adams JM, Cory S, Harris AW (1991) Enforced Bcl2 expression in B-lymphoid cells prolongs antibody-responses and elicits autoimmune-disease. Proc Natl Acad Sci U S A 88:8661–8665

Takahashi Y, Cerasoli DM, Dal Porto JM, Shimoda M, Freund R, Fang W, Telander DG, Malvey EN, Mueller DL, Behrens TW, Kelsoe G (1999) Relaxed negative selection in germinal centers and impaired affinity maturation in bcl-x(L) transgenic mice. J Exp Med 190:399–409

Tamir I, Dal Porto JM, Cambier JC (2000) Cytoplasmic protein tyrosine phosphatases SHP-1 and SHP-2: regulators of B cell signal transduction. CurrOpin Immunol 12:307–315

Tedder TF (1998) Introduction: response-regulators of B lymphocyte signaling thresholds provide a context for antigen receptor signal transduction. Semin Immunol 10:259–265

Tedder TF, Tuscano J, Sato S, Kehrl JH (1997) CD22, a B lymphocyte-specific adhesion molecule that regulates antigen receptor signaling. Ann Rev Immunol 15:481–504

Thompson JS, Bixler SA, Qian F, Vora K, Scott ML, Cachero TG, Hession C, Schneider P, Sizing ID, Mullen C, Strauch K, Zafari M, Benjamin CD, Tschopp J, Browning JL, Ambrose C (2001) BAFF-R, a newly identified TNF receptor that specifically interacts with BAFF. Science 293:2108–2111

Van Vollenhoven RF, Bieber MM, Powell MJ, Gupta PK, Bhat NM, Richards KL, Albano SA, Teng NNH (1999) VH4-34 encoded antibodies in systemic lupus erythematosus: a specific diagnostic marker that correlates with clinical disease characteristics. J Rheumatol 26:1727–1733

Von Bulow GU, van Deursen JM, Bram RJ (2001) Regulation of the T-independent humoral response by TACI. Immunity 14:573–582

Voswinkel J, Trumper L, Carbon G, Hopf T, Pfreundschuh M, Gause A (1996) Evidence for a selected humoral immune response encoded by V(H)4 family genes in the synovial membrane of a patient with rheumatoid arthritis (RA). Clin Exp Immunol 106:5–12

Wakeland EK, Liu K, Graham RR, Behrens TW (2001) Delineating the genetic basis of systemic lupus erythematosus. Immunity 15:397–408

Xu SL, Lam KP (2001) B-cell maturation protein, which binds the tumor necrosis factor family members BAFF and APRIL, is dispensable for humoral immune responses. Mol Cell Biol 21:4067–4074

Yan MH, Wang M, Chan B, Roose-Girma M, Erickson S, Baker T, Tumas D, Grewal IS, Dixit VM (2001) Activation and accumulation of B cells in TACI-deficient mice. Nature Immunol 2:638–643

Yavuz AS, Monson NL, Yavuz S, Grammer AC, Longo N, Girschick HJ, Lipsky PE (2002) Different patterns of bcl-6 and p53 gene mutations in tonsillar B cells indicate separate mutational mechanisms. Mol Immunol 39:485–493

Yi AK, Tuetken R, Redford T, Waldschmidt M, Kirsch J, Krieg AM (1998) CpG motifs in bacterial DNA activate leukocytes through the pH-dependent generation of reactive oxygen species. J Immunol 160:4755–4761

Yu CCK, Tsui HW, Ngan BY, Shulman MJ, Wu GE, Tsui FWL (1996) B and T cells are not required for the viable motheaten phenotype. J Exp Med 183:371–380

Immunological Memory Stabilizing Autoreactivity

R. A. Manz[1,2] (✉) · K. Moser[1] · G.-R. Burmester[2] · A. Radbruch[1] · F. Hiepe[1]

[1] Deutsches Rheumaforschungszentrum Berlin (DRFZ), Schumannstrasse 21/22, 10117 Berlin, Germany
manz@drfz.de

[2] Charite, Humboldt University, Berlin, Germany

1	Mechanisms Contributing to Autoimmune Diseases	242
2	Immunological Memory and Chronic Autoimmune Diseases	243
2.1	Chronicity	243
2.2	B Cell Memory	245
2.3	T Cell Memory	246
2.4	Humoral Memory	247
2.4.1	Autoantibody-Mediated Pathological Mechanisms	248
3	Autoreactive Memory and Chronic Inflammation	249
	References	251

Abstract The etiopathologies of autoimmune diseases are complex. A broad variety of cell types and gene products are involved. However, clinical and experimental evidence suggests that the importance of an individual factor changes during the course of the disease. Factors and cell types that induce acute autoreactivity and initiate an autoimmune disease could be distinct from those that drive a chronic course of that disease. Autoreactive immunological memory, in particular B cell and plasma cell memory, contributes to chronicity through several mechanisms. Formation of autoreactive memory B cells leads to an increase in the numbers of autoreactive cells. In comparison to naïve B cells, these memory B cells show a decreased threshold for activation. Additionally, a fraction of memory B cells express the chemokine receptor CXCR3, which supports their accumulation within chronically inflamed tissues. This may allow their escape from mechanisms for induction of peripheral tolerance. Within the inflamed tissue, inflammatory cytokines and autoantigens provide activation signals that promote plasma cell differentiation and survival. The autoantibodies produced locally by these plasma cells contribute to the severity of inflammation. Together, an autoreactive loop of autoantibody-induced inflammation is formed. Another integral part of immunological memory are long-lived plasma cells. These cells provide persistent humoral antibody memory. Though not all autoantibodies are produced by long-lived plasma cells, these cells have a special impact on immune pathology. Long-lived plasma cells are relatively resistant to existing therapies of immunosuppression and continuously secrete antibodies, without need for restimulation. Long-lived plasma cells provide titers of autoantibodies even during clinically quiescent phases and after immunosuppression. These persisting autoantibody titers, though often low and not causing acute clinical symptoms, are likely to maintain a low level of chronic inflammation and progressive tissue destruction, which reduces the threshold for another break of immunological tolerance.

Abbreviations

CXCL	C-X-C motif chemokine ligand
CXCR	C-X-C motif chemokine receptor
EAE	Experimental autoimmune encephalomyelitis
IFN	Interferon
MS	Multiple sclerosis
RA	Rheumatoid arthritis
SLE	Systemic lupus erythematosus
SS	Sjögren's syndrome

1
Mechanisms Contributing to Autoimmune Diseases

In the course of autoimmune diseases, the immune system, upon reacting to bacteria, viruses, and other exogenous pathogens, also can attack self-antigens and tissues. Numerous autoimmune diseases are known, each of them exhibiting a distinct general etiopathology and affecting a limited number of defined self-antigens and tissues. Some autoimmune diseases are clinically heterogeneous and merely defined by common clinical criteria. These diseases may resemble a collection of genuinely distinct autoimmune disorders that share only distinct features. Examples include such widespread autoimmune disorders as rheumatoid arthritis (RA) and systemic lupus erythematosus (SLE). Frequently, these diseases initially present with mild symptoms but then become chronic and progressive, eventually resulting in severe and irreversible obstructions.

Autoimmune diseases affecting humans and animals are genetically complex [1, 2]. Multiple gene defects contributing to the development of lupus in the NZB/W mouse model and the development of pristane-induced arthritis in particular rat strains have been identified [3–5]. Due to the complexity of factors influencing autoimmunity, the pathomechanisms of autoimmune diseases are diverse. Often, effector mechanisms of the innate immune system as well as of the adapted immune system are involved [6–10]. Autoreactive B cells, autoantibodies, and autoreactive effector T cells targeting specific self-antigens mediate the tissue specificity observed for particular autoimmune diseases. Complement, macrophages, and a self-sustaining chronic inflammatory environment substantially contribute to the local pathogenesis [11–13]. Though in some animal models either autoreactive B cells or autoreactive T cells alone can be sufficient to induce an autoimmune disease, usually several mechanisms and cell types contribute to the development and/or maintenance of immunopathology in a cooperative manner [5, 14–16]. However, the factors initiating an autoimmune disease or promoting acute autoreactivity could be different from those driving the chronic course of that very same disease [17]. Here, we will discuss pathological mechanisms involved in autoimmune diseases and their contribution to maintaining a chronic course of disease, with a special focus on the role of the immunological memory in that process.

2
Immunological Memory and Chronic Autoimmune Diseases

2.1
Chronicity

Though most autoimmune diseases become chronic, spontaneous remission occurs in a small, but considerable proportion of patients suffering from various autoimmune diseases [18, 19]. Complete remission is common among autoimmune diseases that had been induced by an exogenous stimulus in individuals bearing an otherwise intact immune system. This applies for most animal models, where autoreactivity is induced in animals that otherwise would not develop that autoimmune disorder such as experimental autoimmune encephalomyelitis (EAE) [20]. Similarly, drug-induced human SLE usually undergoes remission in patients no longer receiving this drug [21]. These observations suggest that the factors that induce acute autoreactivity and autoimmune tissue destruction are not necessarily sufficient to make immunopathology and inflammation chronic.

Clear evidence that induction and chronicity of an autoimmune disease could be driven by distinct mechanisms is provided by genetic approaches in animal models [5]. Genetic dissection shows that the gene loci involved in the onset of pristane-induced arthritis are different from those involved in the chronic phase of that disease [17, 22]. It seems likely that following the initial loss of immunological self-tolerance, additional factors are required to maintain inflammation. Such considerations are well in accordance with clinical observations and experimental results obtained in animal models. Some of these observations even suggest that those factors that had induced the disease initially are of minor importance at later stages of the disease. For example, in the K/BxN mouse model, the presence of both T cells and B cells is required to induce pathogenic autoantibody production and induction of arthritis [14, 23]. Accordingly, depletion of T cells in vivo by therapeutic antibodies efficiently prevents the production of autoantibodies and the onset of inflammation, when applied early. However, when T cells are depleted once the disease has started, it inhibits neither the production of autoantibodies nor the progression of arthritis. When transferred into immunodeficient recipients, antibodies from arthritic K/BxN mice are sufficient to induce and maintain inflammation, in the complete absence of T cells [14]. Thus, in this model, T cells are of prime importance for the initial generation of autoreactive antibodies, but they are of minor importance for the maintenance of inflammation. Despite their potential to induce autoreactivity, therapeutic targeting of T cells does not suffice to cure the established disease. For several human autoimmune diseases, similar principles are likely to apply. There is good evidence for a critical participation of T cells in the pathogenesis of RA, SLE, and many other autoimmune diseases [24–26]. Nevertheless, disease activity in RA patients usually remains unaltered upon T cell depletion [27]. Instead, recent clinical trials show that the therapeutic depletion of B cells expressing CD20 with rituximab results in remarkable clinical improvement in many patients with RA [28, 29] or SLE [30]. This is in agreement with the speculation that T cells are involved in the initiation of rheumatic inflammation, but B cells are more relevant for maintenance of inflammation.

In understanding autoimmune inflammation, most attention so far has been directed to the mechanisms of breaking tolerance and developing tissue-specific autoreactivity, i.e., the initiation of inflammation. Predominantly, it is anticipated that inflammation is maintained by chronic autoimmune reactions. This view, already challenged by the apparent lack of efficacy of immunosuppressive therapies in many chronic inflammatory situations, has been challenged further by the recent development of new concepts of immunological memory. These concepts introduce the "memory plasma cell" as a new cellular entity [31, 32] and reveal a considerable epigenetic and transcriptional imprinting of distinct pro- and anti-inflammatory effector functions of memory T lymphocytes, including cytokine expression and expression of particular receptors for chemokines and adhesion molecules [33–35]. In addition, it becomes clear that memory T and B lymphocytes, unlike their naïve precursors, can be reactivated independent of antigen, by pro-inflammatory cytokines and pathogen-associated molecular patterns [36, 37]. In addition to these qualitative differences, quantitative differences between naïve and memory lymphocytes may contribute to the chronic course of most autoimmune diseases. These include the presence of increased numbers of

B and T lymphocytes specific for the recall antigen, higher affinities of the antibodies produced, a reduced threshold for activation of responding memory cells compared to naïve cells and an accelerated production of effector cytokines.

2.2
B Cell Memory

B cells that express autoantibodies with hypermutated antigen-binding sites are frequently found in patients suffering from RA, SLE, and other autoimmune diseases in which B cells or autoantibodies are likely to play key roles in the pathogenesis [38–40]. Memory B cells accumulate within inflamed salivary glands and within joints of patients suffering from Sjögren's syndrome (SS) or RA, respectively. This is due to immigration of memory B cells into inflamed tissues and their local clonal expansion there [41–43]. It had been assumed that this expansion might be autoantigen-driven and that the responding autoreactive cells might be directly involved in local pathogenesis [43]. Interestingly enough, in individuals suffering from autoimmune diseases, somatic mutation of the genes coding for the antibody binding sites can take place in lymphoid tissues outside of classical germinal centers [44–46] (Table 1). Such mutations also can occur in germinal center-like structures of inflamed synovial tissue of RA patients, and in B cells of the marginal sinus-bridging channels of MRL/lpr mice [47]. In MRL/lpr mice, the mutation rates of autoreactive B cells found in extrafollicular sites are similar to those of B cells of germinal centers, activated by an alloantigen [48].

The generation of an autoreactive B cell memory could contribute in several ways to autoimmune inflammation. Memory B cells are increased in numbers and show a reduced threshold for reactivation. Plasma cells derived from memory B cells will secrete autoantibodies of increased affinities and switched isotypes, which may switch them from harmless to pathogenic. Probably most importantly, memory B cells can be reactivated independent of antigen-receptor signaling, by pathogen-associated molecular patterns and cytokines. Such signals will drive memory B cells into differentiation to antibody-secreting cells [36]. Reactivation of memory B cells can occur also independent of T cell help [49]. Thus even in a situation when T cell tolerance is (re-)established, autoreactive memory B cells, when reactivated by pathogenic insult, may start an inflammatory autoreactive flare, or entertain chronic autoimmune inflammation, by differentiating into potent autoantigen-presenting cells [50] and into cells secreting potentially pathogenic autoantibodies.

Table 1 B cell and humoral memory origin and persistence

Protective immunity	Autoimmune diseases
Formation of memory B cells in germinal centers within secondary lymphoid tissues [44, 45]	Spontaneous formation of splenic germinal centers in murine models [66, 94]
Persistence of long-lived plasma cells providing humoral antibody-memory mainly in the bone marrow [61, 62], and to a lower extent in spleen [64]	Persistence of long-lived plasma cells providing humoral autoreactive antibody memory in the spleen [65] and most likely the inflamed kidneys of NZB/W mice [66]
	Somatic hypermutation of autoreactive B cells (indicating memory B cell formation) in extrafollicular areas within secondary lymphoid tissues demonstrated in Fas-deficient MRL/lpr mice [47]
	Ectopic germinal center-like structures (indicating memory B cell formation) within chronically inflamed joints of RA patients [95–97]

2.3
T Cell Memory

Like memory B cells, memory T cells, compared to naïve T cells, have a reduced threshold for reactivation by antigen and can also be reactivated independent of antigen, e.g., by ligands for TLR2 [37] and cytokines, such as type I interferons [51]. Autoreactive T cells have been found in patients suffering from various autoimmune diseases. Upon restimulation in vitro, many of these cells express effector cytokines and show the phenotype of memory cells [52, 53]. It is controversial whether the frequencies of autoreactive T cells are higher in autoimmune patients than in normal controls, with some reports finding no differences [54, 55], while others do [56]. In an attempt to determine the frequencies of autoreactive T cells with high functional avidity to myelin in patients and controls, Bilekova and colleagues have used low amounts of the autoantigen myelin for the ex vivo restimulation of T cells from patients with multiple sclerosis (MS) and found the frequencies of autoreactive T cells about four times as high in patients compared to controls [57]. This increase, though small, is in accordance with the idea that an autoreactive T cell memory is formed in MS patients. Many autoreactive T cells isolated from patients also show a cytokine memory [33], e.g., for IFN-γ [58].

The contribution of autoreactive T cell memory to the pathology of murine models for autoimmune diseases is poorly understood. T cells are considered to be of prime relevance for the development of MS and its murine model EAE. However, the presence of autoreactive memory T cells might not be required for the chronic phase of the disease [59], but rather for the development of chronicity [60]. A single immunization with self-antigen leads to acute EAE inflammation, followed by stable remission. Induction of autoreactive immunological memory to neuronal antigens leads to a chronic relapsing-remitting form of EAE, more closely resembling MS [60]. While the detailed mechanisms behind these observations are not completely understood, they suggest that the formation of autoreactive immunological memory might be a prerequisite for chronicity in EAE. Whether or not T cell memory is crucial in this process remains speculative. Autoreactive T cells have a great potential to contribute to autoreactive pathogenicity and definitively can induce autoimmune diseases in animal models, but experiments and clinical observations demonstrating a crucial role for T cell memory in causing chronicity of autoimmune diseases are still lacking.

2.4
Humoral Memory

Immunological memory is characterized by increased numbers of clonally expanded B and T cells specific for an antigen previously encountered, along with an increase in the affinity of the antibody response. Long-lived plasma cells provide humoral memory in terms of specific antibodies [61–64]. These plasma cells have a lifespan comparable to that of memory B cells and maintain antibody secretion for months and years, without need for restimulation. They are a major source of long-term persisting serum antibody titers in protective immunity. Recently, it has been demonstrated that long-lived plasma cells also contribute to the production of autoantibodies in lupus-prone NZB/W mice [65]. In these mice, total plasma cell numbers are significantly increased in the spleen, as compared to healthy mice [66]. The splenic plasma cell population of NZB/W mice consists of about 60% short-lived cells, and about 40% nondividing, long-lived plasma cells with half-lives of several months, at least. Cells secreting autoantibodies binding to DNA are present in the short-lived and in the long-lived plasma cell population [65]. Treatment with the immunosuppressive drug cyclophosphamide readily depletes the short-lived, but not the long-lived plasma cells in NZB/W mice. Whether autoreactive long-lived plasma cells are also found in other tissues of NZB/W mice remains to be established. Chronically inflamed tissues are potential candidates to harbor long-lived plasma cells. Plasma cells accumulate at these sites in large numbers, and many factors supporting plasma cell survival belong to the family of inflammatory cytokines [67]. Interestingly, the bone marrow plasma cell compartment that contains the largest numbers of long-lived plasma cells in nonautoimmune individuals is not increased in NZB/W mice.

In humans, the lifetime of individual plasma cells cannot be measured directly, for ethical reasons. Indirect evidence suggests, however, that also in humans long-lived plasma cells contribute to the pathogenesis of autoimmune diseases. Long-lived plasma cells will produce antibodies in the absence of an acute reactive immune flare, i.e., during disease remission, and will survive conventional immunosuppressive therapy [32]. This is exactly the observation for many patients with autoimmune diseases, which maintain expression of autoantibodies during clinical quiescent phases [32, 68–70] and despite immunosuppressive or B cell- or T cell-depleting therapy [28, 71–73]. The autoantibodies produced in the remitting phases, although obviously not leading to acute clinical symptoms, may well contribute essentially to the maintenance of chronic inflammation and set the stage for the next relapse.

2.4.1
Autoantibody-Mediated Pathological Mechanisms

In mice, and probably also in humans, long-lived plasma cells can maintain a relevant level of autoantibody titers during clinically quiescent states, even in face of immunosuppressive therapy. Though some autoantibodies may have no pathogenetic potential, others fuel chronic inflammation and accelerate relapses of acute pathology by a variety of mechanisms (Table 2). Autoantibodies directed to targets on cell surfaces can damage or destroy these cells by classical immune effector mechanisms, such as complement lysis or antibody-dependent cell-mediated immunity (ADCC), e.g., autoantibodies binding to erythrocytes and thrombocytes can cause autoimmune hemolytic anemia and thrombocytopenia, respectively. Autoantibodies reacting with cell surface receptors can modify cell activity by modulation, blockage, or stimulation [74]. Autoantibody-induced cross-linking of cell surface receptors may result in aggregation and redistribution of the receptors and their internalization, mimicking the respective signals or making the cell refractory to them. By this mechanism, anti-acetylcholine receptor antibodies impair neuromuscular function in myasthenia gravis [75]. Type 1 anti-intrinsic factor antibodies block the cobalamin binding site of the gastric protein intrinsic factor, required for the uptake of cobalamin, causing pernicious anemia [76]. In Graves' disease, thyroid-stimulating autoantibodies mimic the action of the thyroid-stimulating hormone. The resulting stimulation of thyroid cells leads to hyperthyroidism and overproduction of thyroid hormone [77].

Table 2 Antibody mediated pathological mechanisms

Mechanism	Syndrome	References
Autoantibodies to cell surface and matrix antigens	Autoimmune anemia, thrombocytopenia	[74]
Blockade or stimulation of proteins/receptors	Myasthenia gravis, pernicious anemia; Graves' disease	[74, 76, 77]
Immune complex-mediated	Nephritis, vasculitis, etc.	[84–87]

Antibodies to intracellular autoantigens can also be pathogenetic. Several studies have demonstrated binding of such autoantibodies to the outside of the cell membrane. The reason for this extracellular binding is less clear. Membrane proteins may show cross-reactive epitopes to intracellular proteins, and/or under certain conditions intracellular antigens may be exposed at the cell surface, e.g., in cells undergoing apoptosis [78]. It has also been reported that autoantibodies specific for intracellular antigens penetrate into living cells [79–81], although this idea is controversially discussed [81].

DNA–anti-DNA antibody complexes directly induce production of type I interferon by plasmacytoid dendritic cells [82, 83]. Deposits of immune complexes can mediate vasculitis, cryoglobulinemia, nephritis, and other syndromes [84–87]. The significant contribution of secreted autoantibodies to pathogenesis of autoimmune diseases and the resistance of long-lived plasma cells to conventional immunosuppression underlines the necessity of developing novel therapeutic approaches for the elimination of long-lived plasma cells.

3
Autoreactive Memory and Chronic Inflammation

In addition to autoreactive immunological memory, other factors may contribute to or stabilize chronic autoreactive inflammation, either on their own or in concert with autoreactive cellular and/or humoral memory. Inflammation as such may cause a break in immunological tolerance, particularly if present in an individual bearing autoreactive memory cells or persistent autoantibody titers. It has been shown that fibroblastoid cells isolated from chronically inflamed tissue are able to sustain the production of pro-inflammatory cytokines in the absence of lymphocytes for several weeks or longer in vitro [13]. In RA synovial tissue, fibroblastoid cells are a major source of inflammatory cytokines [88, 89]. In any case, antigen-presenting cells (APCs) emigrating from the site of ongoing inflammation are likely to stimulate the production of pro-inflammatory cytokines such as interferon (IFN) -γ in the adjacent lymph nodes and modulate the immune reactions going on there accordingly. It has been demonstrated that this cytokine induces the expression of the C-X-C motif chemokine receptor (CXCR) 3 on activated B cells [90]. CXCR3 is absent from naïve B cells. Once its expression is induced in memory B cells, these cells remain CXCR3-positive. On T cells, CXCR3 is

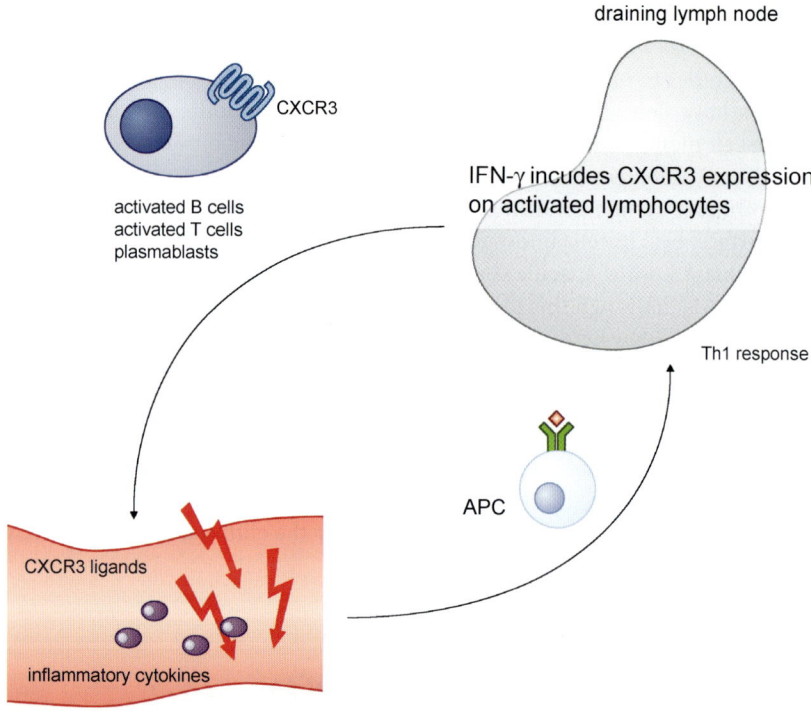

Fig. 1 A possible mechanism of how CXCR3-mediated recruitment of autoreactive lymphocytes into inflamed tissues contributes to a break in self-tolerance. Inflammatory cytokines induce the production of CXCR3 ligands within inflamed tissues. APCs leaving the site of inflammation are likely to induce Th1 responses within draining lymph nodes. Local production of Th1 cytokines, particularly IFN-γ, induces the expression of CXCR3 on activated B cells, plasma cell precursors, and likely also on T cells. CXCR3 expression is stable on memory B cells and allows accumulation within the inflamed tissue where they may escape effective mechanisms controlling self-tolerance

expressed preferentially on Th1 cells [91]. The corresponding chemokines CXC ligand (CXCL) 9, CXCL10, and CXCL11 are induced by IFN-γ at the site of inflammation and attract CXCR3-expressing lymphocytes [92]. Activated B cells and migratory plasmablasts accumulate within chronically inflamed tissues independent of their antigenic specificity [66, 93]; for example in patients with established autoimmune memory, autoreactive memory cells with decreased activation thresholds are found in relatively large numbers (Fig. 1) [90]. At these sites, inflammatory cytokines, bacterial products, and autoantigen may stimulate these cells to become plasma cells or form ectopic germinal centers to increase the numbers of autoreactive memory cells.

References

1. Mathis D, Benoist C (2004) Back to central tolerance. Immunity 20:509–516
2. Jirholt J, Lindqvist AB, Holmdahl R (2001) The genetics of rheumatoid arthritis and the need for animal models to find and understand the underlying genes. Arthritis Res 3:87–97
3. Wakui M, Kim J, Butfiloski EJ, Morel L, Sobel ES (2004) Genetic dissection of lupus pathogenesis: Sle3/5 impacts IgH CDR3 sequences, somatic mutations, and receptor editing. J Immunol 173:7368–7376
4. Wakeland EK, Wandstrat AE, Liu K, Morel L (1999) Genetic dissection of systemic lupus erythematosus. Curr Opin Immunol 11:701–707
5. Holmdahl R (2003) Dissection of the genetic complexity of arthritis using animal models. J Autoimmun 21:99–103
6. Viau M, Zouali M (2005) B-lymphocytes, innate immunity, and autoimmunity. Clin Immunol 114:17–26
7. Toubi E, Shoenfeld Y (2004) Toll-like receptors and their role in the development of autoimmune diseases. Autoimmunity 37:183–188
8. Carroll MC (2004) A protective role for innate immunity in systemic lupus erythematosus. Nat Rev Immunol 4:825–831
9. Benoist C, Mathis D (2002) Mast cells in autoimmune disease. Nature 420:875–878
10. Pritchard NR, Cutler AJ, Uribe S, Chadban SJ, Morley BJ, Smith KG (2000) Autoimmune-prone mice share a promoter haplotype associated with reduced expression and function of the Fc receptor FcgammaRII. Curr Biol 10:227–230
11. Manderson AP, Botto M, Walport MJ (2004) The role of complement in the development of systemic lupus erythematosus. Annu Rev Immunol 22:431–456
12. Calandra T, Roger T (2003) Macrophage migration inhibitory factor: a regulator of innate immunity. Nat Rev Immunol 3:791–800
13. Bucala R, Ritchlin C, Winchester R, Cerami A (1991) Constitutive production of inflammatory and mitogenic cytokines by rheumatoid synovial fibroblasts. J Exp Med 173:569–574

14. Ji H, Korganow AS, Mangialaio S, Hoglund P, Andre I, Luhder F, Gonzalez A, Poirot L, Benoist C, Mathis D (1999) Different modes of pathogenesis in T-cell-dependent autoimmunity: clues from two TCR transgenic systems. Immunol Rev 169:139–146
15. Benoist C, Mathis D (2000) A revival of the B cell paradigm for rheumatoid arthritis pathogenesis? Arthritis Res 2:90–94
16. Chan OT, Madaio MP, Shlomchik MJ (1999) The central and multiple roles of B cells in lupus pathogenesis. Immunol Rev 169:107–121
17. Holmdahl R, Lorentzen JC, Lu S, Olofsson P, Wester L, Holmberg J, Pettersson U (2001) Arthritis induced in rats with nonimmunogenic adjuvants as models for rheumatoid arthritis. Immunol Rev 184:184–202
18. Patel B, Haddad R, Saxena I, Gossain VV (2003) Spontaneous long-term remission in a patient with premature ovarian failure. Endocr Pract 9:380–383
19. Heine G, Sester U, Sester M, Scherberich JE, Girndt M, Kohler H (2002) A shift in the Th(1)/Th(2) ratio accompanies the clinical remission of systemic lupus erythematosus in patients with end-stage renal disease. Nephrol Dial Transplant 17:1790–1794
20. Swanborg RH (2001) Experimental autoimmune encephalomyelitis in the rat: lessons in T-cell immunology and autoreactivity. Immunol Rev 184:129–135
21. Rubin RL (2005) Drug-induced lupus. Toxicology 209:135–147
22. Wester L, Olofsson P, Ibrahim SM, Holmdahl R (2003) Chronicity of pristane-induced arthritis in rats is controlled by genes on chromosome 14. J Autoimmun 21:305–313
23. Korganow AS, Ji H, Mangialaio S, Duchatelle V, Pelanda R, Martin T, Degott C, Kikutani H, Rajewsky K, Pasquali JL, Benoist C, Mathis D (1999) From systemic T cell self-reactivity to organ-specific autoimmune disease via immunoglobulins. Immunity 10:451–461
24. Riemekasten G, Langnickel D, Ebling FM, Karpouzas G, Kalsi J, Herberth G, Tsao BP, Henklein P, Langer S, Burmester GR, Radbruch A, Hiepe F, Hahn BH (2003) Identification and characterization of SmD183–119-reactive T cells that provide T cell help for pathogenic anti-double-stranded DNA antibodies. Arthritis Rheum 48:475–485
25. Goronzy JJ, Weyand CM (2004) T-cell regulation in rheumatoid arthritis. Curr Opin Rheumatol 16:212–217
26. Cope AP (2002) Studies of T-cell activation in chronic inflammation. Arthritis Res 4 [Suppl 3]:S197–S211
27. Burmester GR, Emmrich F (1993) Anti-CD4 therapy in rheumatoid arthritis. Clin Exp Rheumatol 11 [Suppl 8]:S139–S145
28. Cambridge G, Leandro MJ, Edwards JC, Ehrenstein MR, Salden M, Bodman-Smith M, Webster AD (2003) Serologic changes following B lymphocyte depletion therapy for rheumatoid arthritis. Arthritis Rheum 48:2146–2154
29. De Vita S, Zaja F, Sacco S, De Candia A, Fanin R, Ferraccioli G (2002) Efficacy of selective B cell blockade in the treatment of rheumatoid arthritis: evidence for a pathogenetic role of B cells. Arthritis Rheum 46:2029–2033
30. Looney RJ, Anolik J, Sanz I (2005) Treatment of SLE with anti-CD20 monoclonal antibody. Curr Dir Autoimmun 8:193–205

31. Manz RA, Hauser AE, Hiepe F, Radbruch A (2004) Maintenance of serum antibody levels. Annu Rev Immunol 23:367–386
32. Manz RA, Arce S, Cassese G, Hauser AE, Hiepe F, Radbruch A (2002) Humoral immunity and long-lived plasma cells. Curr Opin Immunol 14:517–521
33. Lohning M, Richter A, Radbruch A (2002) Cytokine memory of T helper lymphocytes. Adv Immunol 80:115–181
34. Syrbe U, Jennrich S, Schottelius A, Richter A, Radbruch A, Hamann A (2004) Differential regulation of P-selectin ligand expression in naive versus memory CD4+ T cells: evidence for epigenetic regulation of involved glycosyltransferase genes. Blood 104:3243–3248
35. Huehn J, Siegmund K, Lehmann JC, Siewert C, Haubold U, Feuerer M, Debes GF, Lauber J, Frey O, Przybylski GK, Niesner U, de la Rosa M, Schmidt CA, Brauer R, Buer J, Scheffold A, Hamann A (2004) Developmental stage, phenotype, and migration distinguish naive- and effector/memory-like CD4+ regulatory T cells. J Exp Med 199:303–313
36. Bernasconi NL, Onai N, Lanzavecchia A (2003) A role for toll-like receptors in acquired immunity: up-regulation of TLR9 by BCR triggering in naive B cells and constitutive expression in memory B cells. Blood 101:4500–4504
37. Xu D, Komai-Koma M, Liew FY (2005) Expression and function of Toll-like receptor on T cells. Cell Immunol 233:85–89
38. Shlomchik MJ, Aucoin AH, Pisetsky DS, Weigert MG (1987) Structure and function of anti-DNA autoantibodies derived from a single autoimmune mouse. Proc Natl Acad Sci U S A 84:9150–9154
39. McIntosh RS, Asghar MS, Watson PF, Kemp EH, Weetman AP (1996) Cloning and analysis of IgG kappa and IgG lambda anti-thyroglobulin autoantibodies from a patient with Hashimoto's thyroiditis: evidence for in vivo antigen-driven repertoire selection. J Immunol 157:927–935
40. McIntosh R, Watson P, Weetman A (1998) Somatic hypermutation in autoimmune thyroid disease. Immunol Rev 162:219–231
41. Schroder AE, Greiner A, Seyfert C, Berek C (1996) Differentiation of B cells in the nonlymphoid tissue of the synovial membrane of patients with rheumatoid arthritis. Proc Natl Acad Sci U S A 93:221–225
42. Jacobi AM, Hansen A, Burmester GR, Dorner T, Lipsky PE (2000) Enhanced mutational activity and disturbed selection of mutations in V(H) gene rearrangements in a patient with systemic lupus erythematosus. Autoimmunity 33:61–76
43. Jacobi AM, Hansen A, Kaufmann O, Pruss A, Burmester GR, Lipsky PE, Dorner T (2002) Analysis of immunoglobulin light chain rearrangements in the salivary gland and blood of a patient with Sjogren's syndrome. Arthritis Res 4:R4
44. Berek C, Berger A, Apel M (1991) Maturation of the immune response in germinal centers. Cell 67:1121–1129
45. MacLennan IC, Liu YJ, Johnson GD (1992) Maturation and dispersal of B-cell clones during T cell-dependent antibody responses. Immunol Rev 126:143–161
46. Tarlinton D (1998) Germinal centers: form and function. Curr Opin Immunol 10:245–251
47. William J, Euler C, Christensen S, Shlomchik MJ (2002) Evolution of autoantibody responses via somatic hypermutation outside of germinal centers. Science 297:2066–2070

48. Shlomchik MJ, Euler CW, Christensen SC, William J (2003) Activation of rheumatoid factor (RF) B cells and somatic hypermutation outside of germinal centers in autoimmune-prone MRL/lpr mice. Ann N Y Acad Sci 987:38–50
49. Hebeis BJ, Klenovsek K, Rohwer P, Ritter U, Schneider A, Mach M, Winkler TH (2004) Activation of virus-specific memory B cells in the absence of T cell help. J Exp Med 199:593–602
50. Liu YJ, Barthelemy C, de Bouteiller O, Arpin C, Durand I, Banchereau J (1995) Memory B cells from human tonsils colonize mucosal epithelium and directly present antigen to T cells by rapid up-regulation of B7-1 and B7-2. Immunity 2:239–248
51. Tough DF, Borrow P, Sprent J (1996) Induction of bystander T cell proliferation by viruses and type I interferon in vivo. Science 272:1947–1950
52. Hacker-Foegen MK, Zillikens D, Giudice GJ, Lin MS (2004) T cell receptor gene usage of BP180-specific T lymphocytes from patients with bullous pemphigoid and pemphigoid gestationis. Clin Immunol 113:179–186
53. Lin MS, Fu CL, Aoki V, Hans-Filho G, Rivitti EA, Moraes JR, Moraes ME, Lazaro AM, Giudice GJ, Stastny P, Diaz LA (2000) Desmoglein-1-specific T lymphocytes from patients with endemic pemphigus foliaceus (fogo selvagem). J Clin Invest 105:207–213
54. Muraro PA, Vergelli M, Kalbus M, Banks DE, Nagle JW, Tranquill LR, Nepom GT, Biddison WE, McFarland HF, Martin R (1997) Immunodominance of a low-affinity major histocompatibility complex-binding myelin basic protein epitope (residues 111–129) in HLA-DR4 (B1*0401) subjects is associated with a restricted T cell receptor repertoire. J Clin Invest 100:339–349
55. Martin R, Jaraquemada D, Flerlage M, Richert J, Whitaker J, Long EO, McFarlin DE, McFarland HF (1990) Fine specificity and HLA restriction of myelin basic protein-specific cytotoxic T cell lines from multiple sclerosis patients and healthy individuals. J Immunol 145:540–548
56. Ott PA, Dittrich MT, Herzog BA, Guerkov R, Gottlieb PA, Putnam AL, Durinovic-Bello I, Boehm BO, Tary-Lehmann M, Lehmann PV (2004) T cells recognize multiple GAD65 and proinsulin epitopes in human type 1 diabetes, suggesting determinant spreading. J Clin Immunol 24:327–339
57. Bielekova B, Sung MH, Kadom N, Simon R, McFarland H, Martin R (2004) Expansion and functional relevance of high-avidity myelin-specific CD4+ T cells in multiple sclerosis. J Immunol 172:3893–3904
58. Van der Aa A, Hellings N, Bernard CC, Raus J, Stinissen P (2003) Functional properties of myelin oligodendrocyte glycoprotein-reactive T cells in multiple sclerosis patients and controls. J Neuroimmunol 137:164–176
59. Hofstetter HH, Targoni OS, Karulin AY, Forsthuber TG, Tary-Lehmann M, Lehmann PV (2005) Does the frequency and avidity spectrum of the neuroantigen-specific T cells in the blood mirror the autoimmune process in the central nervous system of mice undergoing experimental allergic encephalomyelitis? J Immunol 174:4598–4605
60. Yang J, Kubera M, Zelek-Molik A, Nalepa I, Hukkanen V, Lindsberg PJ, Meri S, Seljelid R (2000) Splenectomy and adoptive cell transfer reveal a prominent role for splenic memory lymphocytes in the development of chronic relapsing experimental autoimmune encephalomyelitis. Scand J Immunol 52:356–361

61. Slifka MK, Antia R, Whitmire JK, Ahmed R (1998) Humoral immunity due to long-lived plasma cells. Immunity 8:363–372
62. Manz RA, Thiel A, Radbruch A (1997) Lifetime of plasma cells in the bone marrow. Nature 388:133–134
63. Manz RA, Lohning M, Cassese G, Thiel A, Radbruch A (1998) Survival of long-lived plasma cells is independent of antigen. Int Immunol 10:1703–1711
64. Sze DM, Toellner KM, Garcia de Vinuesa C, Taylor DR, MacLennan IC (2000) Intrinsic constraint on plasmablast growth and extrinsic limits of plasma cell survival. J Exp Med 192:813–821
65. Hoyer BF, Moser K, Hauser AE, Peddinghaus A, Voigt C, Eilat D, Radbruch A, Hiepe F, Manz RA (2004) Short-lived plasmablasts and long-lived plasma cells contribute to chronic humoral autoimmunity in NZB/W mice. J Exp Med 199:1577–1584
66. Cassese G, Lindenau S, de Boer B, Arce S, Hauser A, Riemekasten G, Berek C, Hiepe F, Krenn V, Radbruch A, Manz RA (2001) Inflamed kidneys of NZB / W mice are a major site for the homeostasis of plasma cells. Eur J Immunol 31:2726–2732
67. Cassese G, Arce S, Hauser AE, Lehnert K, Moewes B, Mostarac M, Muehlinghaus G, Szyska M, Radbruch A, Manz RA (2003) Plasma cell survival is mediated by synergistic effects of cytokines and adhesion-dependent signals. J Immunol 171:1684–1690
68. Traynor AE, Schroeder J, Rosa RM, Cheng D, Stefka J, Mujais S, Baker S, Burt RK (2000) Treatment of severe systemic lupus erythematosus with high-dose chemotherapy and haemopoietic stem-cell transplantation: a phase I study. Lancet 356:701–707
69. Izumi N, Fuse I, Furukawa T, Uesugi Y, Tsuchiyama J, Toba K, Togashi K, Yamada K, Ohtake S, Saitoh Y, Yanagisawa N, Aizawa Y (2003) Long-term production of pre-existing alloantibodies to E and c after allogenic BMT in a patient with aplastic anemia resulting in delayed hemolytic anemia. Transfusion 43:241–245
70. Rosen O, Thiel A, Massenkeil G, Hiepe F, Haupl T, Radtke H, Burmester GR, Gromnica-Ihle E, Radbruch A, Arnold R (2000) Autologous stem-cell transplantation in refractory autoimmune diseases after in vivo immunoablation and ex vivo depletion of mononuclear cells. Arthritis Res 2:327–336
71. Edwards JC, Szczepanski L, Szechinski J, Filipowicz-Sosnowska A, Emery P, Close DR, Stevens RM, Shaw T (2004) Efficacy of B-cell-targeted therapy with rituximab in patients with rheumatoid arthritis. N Engl J Med 350:2572–2581
72. Edwards JC, Leandro MJ, Cambridge G (2005) B lymphocyte depletion in rheumatoid arthritis: targeting of CD20. Curr Dir Autoimmun 8:175–192
73. Leandro MJ, Edwards JC, Cambridge G, Ehrenstein MR, Isenberg DA (2002) An open study of B lymphocyte depletion in systemic lupus erythematosus. Arthritis Rheum 46:2673–2677
74. Cervera J, Shoenfeld Y (1996) Pathogenic mechanisms. In: Peter JB, Shoenfeld Y (eds) Autoantibodies. Elsevier, pp 607–17
75. Drachman DB (1994) Myasthenia gravis. N Engl J Med 330:1797–1810

76. Gueant JL, Safi A, Aimone-Gastin I, Rabesona H, Bronowicki JP, Plenat F, Bigard MA, Haertle T (1997) Autoantibodies in pernicious anemia type I patients recognize sequence 251–256 in human intrinsic factor. Proc Assoc Am Physicians 109:462–469
77. Chistiakov DA (2003) Thyroid-stimulating hormone receptor and its role in Graves' disease. Mol Genet Metab 80:377–388
78. Casciola-Rosen LA, Anhalt G, Rosen A (1994) Autoantigens targeted in systemic lupus erythematosus are clustered in two populations of surface structures on apoptotic keratinocytes. J Exp Med 179:1317–1330
79. Tan EM, Kunkel HG (1966) An immunofluorescent study of the skin lesions in systemic lupus erythematosus. Arthritis Rheum 9:37–46
80. Alarcon-Segovia D, Ruiz-Arguelles A, Fishbein E (1978) Antibody to nuclear ribonucleoprotein penetrates live human mononuclear cells through Fc receptors. Nature 271:67–69
81. Ruiz-Arguelles A, Rivadeneyra-Espinoza L, Alarcon-Segovia D (2003) Antibody penetration into living cells: pathogenic, preventive and immuno-therapeutic implications. Curr Pharm Des 9:1881–1887
82. Ronnblom L, Alm GV (2001) A pivotal role for the natural interferon alpha-producing cells (plasmacytoid dendritic cells) in the pathogenesis of lupus. J Exp Med 194: F59–F63
83. Dzionek A, Sohma Y, Nagafune J, Cella M, Colonna M, Facchetti F, Gunther G, Johnston I, Lanzavecchia A, Nagasaka T, Okada T, Vermi W, Winkels G, Yamamoto T, Zysk M, Yamaguchi Y, Schmitz J (2001) BDCA-2, a novel plasmacytoid dendritic cell-specific type II C-type lectin, mediates antigen capture and is a potent inhibitor of interferon alpha/beta induction. J Exp Med 194:1823–1834
84. Traustadottir KH, Sigfusson A, Steinsson K, Erlendsson K (2002) C4A deficiency and elevated level of immune complexes: the mechanism behind increased susceptibility to systemic lupus erythematosus. J Rheumatol 29:2359–2366
85. Oates JC, Gilkeson GS (2002) Mediators of injury in lupus nephritis. Curr Opin Rheumatol 14:498–503
86. Ferri C, La Civita L, Longombardo G, Zignego AL, Pasero G (1998) Mixed cryoglobulinaemia: a cross-road between autoimmune and lymphoproliferative disorders. Lupus 7:275–279
87. Cacoub P, Costedoat-Chalumeau N, Lidove O, Alric L (2002) Cryoglobulinemia vasculitis. Curr Opin Rheumatol 14:29–35
88. Nanki T, Nagasaka K, Hayashida K, Saita Y, Miyasaka N (2001) Chemokines regulate IL-6 and IL-8 production by fibroblast-like synoviocytes from patients with rheumatoid arthritis. J Immunol 167:5381–5385
89. Buckley CD (2003) Why does chronic inflammatory joint disease persist? Clin Med 3:361–366
90. Muehlinghaus G, Cigliano L, Huehn S, Peddinghaus A, Leyendeckers H, Hauser AE, Hiepe F, Radbruch A, Arce S, Manz RA (2005) Regulation of CXCR3 and CXCR4 expression during terminal differentiation of memory B cells into plasma cells. Blood 105:3965–3971

91. Langenkamp A, Casorati G, Garavaglia C, Dellabona P, Lanzavecchia A, Sallusto F (2002) T cell priming by dendritic cells: thresholds for proliferation, differentiation and death and intraclonal functional diversification. Eur J Immunol 32:2046–2054
92. Baggiolini M (1998) Chemokines and leukocyte traffic. Nature 392:565–568
93. Cooper PG, Caton JG, Polson AM (1983) Cell populations associated with gingival bleeding. J Periodontol 54:497–502
94. Luzina IG, Atamas SP, Storrer CE, daSilva LC, Kelsoe G, Papadimitriou JC, Handwerger BS (2001) Spontaneous formation of germinal centers in autoimmune mice. J Leukoc Biol 70:578–584
95. Souto-Carneiro MM, Burkhardt H, Muller EC, Hermann R, Otto A, Kraetsch HG, Sack U, Konig A, Heinegard D, Muller-Hermelink HK, Krenn V (2001) Human monoclonal rheumatoid synovial B lymphocyte hybridoma with a new disease-related specificity for cartilage oligomeric matrix protein. J Immunol 166:4202–4208
96. De Boer BA, Voigt I, Kim HJ, Camacho SA, Lipp M, Forster R, Berek C (2000) Affinity maturation in ectopic germinal centers. Curr Top Microbiol Immunol 251:191–195
97. Magalhaes R, Stiehl P, Morawietz L, Berek C, Krenn V (2002) Morphological and molecular pathology of the B cell response in synovitis of rheumatoid arthritis. Virchows Arch 441:415–427

Genetics of Autoimmune Diseases: A Multistep Process

M. Johannesson · M. Hultqvist · R. Holmdahl (✉)

Medical Inflammation Research, Lund University, BMC I11, Sölvegatan 19,
22184 Lund, Sweden
rikard.holmdahl@med.lu.se

1	Introduction	260
2	Definition of Autoimmune Disease: Physiology Versus Pathology	260
3	From Genes to Disease: The Basic Science Approach	262
4	From Disease to Genes: The Monogenic Success and the Polygenic Failure	262
5	The Use of Animal Models in a Disease-to-Gene Approach	264
6	Positional Cloning of *Ncf1*, a Genetic Polymorphism Explaining a Major Quantitative Trait Locus Controlling Chronic Inflammation	265
7	The Ncf1 Protein and the NADPH Complex	267
8	Pathway Analysis	268
9	Therapeutic Possibilities Can Be Immediately Explored	270
10	Analyses of a QTL Containing Interacting Genes	270
11	Conclusions	273
	References	273

Abstract It has so far been difficult to identify genes behind polygenic autoimmune diseases such as rheumatoid arthritis (RA), multiple sclerosis (MS), and type I diabetes (T1D). With proper animal models, some of the complexity behind these diseases can be reduced. The use of linkage analysis and positional cloning of genes in animal models for RA resulted in the identification of one of the genes regulating severity of arthritis in rats and mice, the *Ncf1* gene. The *Ncf1* gene encodes for the Ncf1 protein that is involved in production of free oxygen radicals through the NADPH oxidase complex, which opens up a new pathway for therapeutic treatment of inflammatory diseases. In most cases, however, a quantitative trait locus (QTL) is the sum effect of several genes within and outside the QTL, which make positional cloning difficult. Here we will discuss the possibilities and difficulties of gene identification in animal models of autoimmune disorders.

1
Introduction

The major autoimmune diseases such as rheumatoid arthritis (RA), multiple sclerosis, (MS) and type I diabetes (T1D) as well as related inflammatory disorders such as asthma, psoriasis, and atherosclerosis are complex, and it has been difficult to understand their fundamental genetic and environmental causes. With proper animal models genetic and environmental factors can be better controlled and also manipulated. This enables genetic approaches that lead to an insight not possible to achieve with direct human studies only. The possibility of combining the genetic knowledge with direct animal studies will enhance the understanding of these diseases and shorten the time needed to develop new therapies with higher efficiency and limited side-effects. We will discuss these possibilities, mainly using examples from recent studies of models for RA.

2
Definition of Autoimmune Disease: Physiology Versus Pathology

Identification of genes controlling autoimmune diseases requires that we have a clear definition of what an autoimmune disease is. Over the years, this definition has been shifting and also varies depending on whether it is seen from a clinical point of view or from a basic science point of view.

From a clinical point of view, these diseases are inflammatory diseases of unknown origin, which cannot be explained by any obvious cause such as infection or allergen exposure. To strengthen the classification they should be chronic, i.e. they should last for a period that exceeds a normal acute inflammatory phase of usually 3–4 weeks. The occurrence of autoantibodies targeting some relevant tissue antigen is often, but not always, included as an additional criteria . However, the pathogenic relevance of such antibodies is not always clear. These definitions have led us to classify a number of commonly occurring chronic diseases as classical autoimmune, for example MS, RA, T1D, and systemic lupus erythematosus (SLE). A borderline group is made up of inflammatory diseases with a possible but not proven infectious cause such as spondyloarthropathies and inflammatory bowel diseases. Another borderline group comprises diseases in which an inflammatory component has emerged as one of the major driving factors, for example, psoriasis and atherosclerosis. It is obvious that from this perspective autoimmune diseases compose a highly heterogeneous group, even within each disease classification, as there are not yet means to link diagnosis with disease mechanisms. Rather we are bound to description of the more obvious pathologic end-result, such as the lack of insulin in T1D or the neurological deficit in MS.

From the basic science standpoint, autoimmune recognition is often the phenomenon of interest for definition of autoimmune diseases. It stems from a tradition of viewing autoimmunity as forbidden self or "horror autotoxicus," as Burnett described it. The view has been broadened over the years with inclusion of innate immune recognition, more colorfully expressed as "danger," as a factor not only in combat of infections but also in playing a role in the development of autoimmunity. The immune recognition is seen as the essential key for understanding both regulatory/suppressor and helper/effector mechanisms. Autoimmunity is defined through autoimmune recognition by lymphocytes, an event that is physiologic but results in an autoimmune disease when such lymphocytes are pathogenic. Proof for autoimmunity can be tested in animal models but not in humans, which has led to the development of animal models for autoimmune diseases. The models are mainly of two types: one that is induced and one where the disease develops spontaneously. Of the induced models, many are induced through immunization with an autoantigen, and the pathogenicity of autoreactive lymphocytes can be clearly shown. In general, only the acute phase of the first inflammatory response is studied. Examples of induced models are collagen-induced arthritis (CIA) as a model for RA [1, 2] and experimental autoimmune encephalomyelitis (EAE) as a model for MS [3]. Other models develop "spontaneously" due to genetic aberrations. In the spontaneous models, as in humans, the pathogenicity of specific autoimmune recognition is often difficult to document and the disease course is often chronic. But in contrast to human disease, these models are often monogenic, highly penetrant and less influenced by environmental factors. Examples of spontaneous models are the transgenic models for arthritis (TNFα [4], IL1Rα deficiency [5], anti-glucose-6-phosphoisomeras T cell receptor [6]), various spontaneous lupus models (NZB xNZW, MRL/lpr, BXSB) [7] and diabetes in the NOD mouse [8].

Clearly, discrepancies between results from studies of autoimmune diseases between human and mouse are not only influenced by the species differences but are in most cases due to different disease definitions and methods. A better definition of the human diseases and also more appropriate, well-characterized animal models are therefore needed.

3
From Genes to Disease: The Basic Science Approach

The weakness of the basic science approach is the difficulties to clearly define the pathology of the phenomenon. In search of the pathologic effect of the mechanisms, numerous experiments has been carried out in animal models for human diseases where basically any disturbance of the physiology after knocking out a hypothesized gene is described as pathological. Clearly, in a complex system such as the immune system, the result will be pathologic in most cases, but the question remains, what is relevant for a naturally selected disease as occurring in humans? And how do we know that the postulated genes, proteins, mechanisms, or pathways are indeed relevant and essential for an autoimmune disease in humans? One way to find out is to first identify the genes involved in the disease development. Then, when we have defined the most critical genes and thereby the most critical pathways, the basic approaches to studying the molecular interacting pathways will be crucial for understanding the disease.

4
From Disease to Genes: The Monogenic Success and the Polygenic Failure

The cause of autoimmune diseases seems to be easily delivered by genetics. Why not just define the genes carried by diseased individuals and then determine their functional genetics? Is this not just a question of adding resources into the human genetic project and its prolongations in the form of various strategic research platforms? The human genome project has indeed been fruitful and we have had enormous success with hundreds of monogenic diseases. One example in the autoimmune field is the identification of the *AIRE* (autoimmune regulator) gene causing the APECED syndrome [9, 10]. The APECED syndrome is a familiar disease characterized by a combination of fungal infections and autoimmune inflammation of various endocrine organs. It is a monogenic disease with high penetrance and caused by mutations in the *AIRE* gene. This discovery did not only identify the gene behind APECED but also led to a renewed understanding of autoimmunity as the *AIRE* gene plays an important role in the induction of central tolerance through its expression in the thymic epithelial cells [11]. However, polymorphism in AIRE could not explain the major autoimmune diseases that are more complex and polygenic in nature. Genetic linkage analysis of large familiar cohorts has been relatively unsuccessful. A few, relatively highly penetrant genes, such as *NOD2* [12] and *PTPN22* [13], have been replicated in several association studies, but these are likely to represent only the tip of the iceberg. What we need is a more complete picture of the genetic architecture, with all the genes involved, high- as well as low-penetrant, and to know how they interact with each other and with the environment. However, even when the association with a gene or haplotype is known, it can still be difficult to find the actual function. One example of the difficulties is the MHC complex. Most autoimmune diseases have been known for decades to be associated with various strongly conserved MHC haplotypes. However, it has not been possible in any disease to clearly identify the gene(s) within the haplotypes, although there is circumstantial evidence for the importance of certain class II genes (DR4/DR1 with the shared epitope) in RA [14] and class I genes (B27) in spondyloarthropathies [15].

It is likely that more of the genetic secrets in humans will be revealed by adding resources, as done through the HapMap project and other efforts. However, the approach requires substantial resources and the question is whether we can make shortcuts and what complementary approaches we can use. The use of improved animal models for human diseases would be a major advantage in several aspects. The environmental factors could be controlled and we have inbred strains simplifying the genetics and the linkage analysis, strains that can be genetically manipulated and thereby allow us to test our hypotheses (Fig. 1).

The advantages of using animal models are mainly;

- The animals can be genetically controlled. Laboratory mouse and rat strains are inbred which dramatically facilitate genetic studies.

- The environment can be better controlled for animals than for humans. The influence of environment on disease phenotype can be studied i.e. immunization, infection or stress.

- Manipulative experiments can be made. The genome of inbred strains can be changed by mutations, insertions and deletions.

- It is more ethical to use animals instead of humans for experimental research purpose.

Fig. 1 The advantages of using animal models for genetic studies

5
The Use of Animal Models in a Disease-to-Gene Approach

Experience from studies on animal models of autoimmune diseases show that they are much more efficient and appropriate for linkage analysis than human cohorts. The process of positional cloning involves five generic steps that intend to lead from phenotype to gene discovery (described in Fig. 2). In general, an F2 intercross of 100–400 animals will reveal loci explaining 10%–50% of a given disease trait and also allows for studying some of the genetic interactions involved. Thus, the power is much higher compared to human

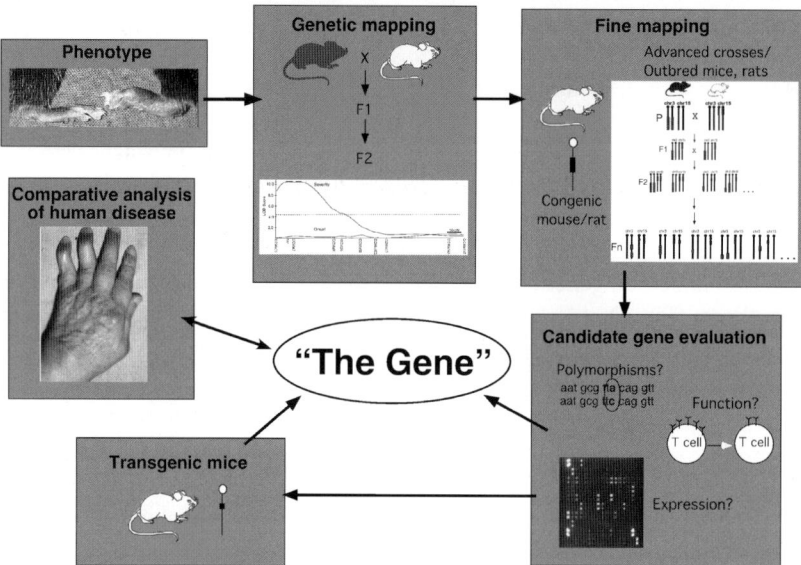

Fig. 2 The five generic steps in positional cloning of quantitative trait genes. The first step is to map QTLs to chromosomal segments, usually in an F2 intercross or N2 backcross. This also involves the selection of inbred strains different for the phenotype studied. The number of F2 or N2 progeny genotyped and phenotyped determines the size of the linked regions and also sets the detection limits for how weak QTLs that can be found. The second step is to genetically isolate single QTLs and to measure the phenotypic effect of each. This is usually done in a congenic strain. If the effect is reproduced in the congenic strain, then the third step is to reduce the size of the critical region as much as possible. Before molecular studies can be undertaken for gene identification, the linked region must be reduced to a few Mb, preferably less. The fourth step is then to identify and evaluate candidate genes with different methods, all dependent on the identity of the genes. The fifth and final step is to establish proof of identity of the candidate genes with, for example, gene targeting, transgenic mice, or other functional tests

studies. What we have learned from animal models for autoimmune diseases so far is that there are a multitude of genes of variable penetrance controlling a disease, and in addition, there are complex genetic interactions and also interactions with the environment. It is important to remember that, depending on the phenotype, the number of loci, their relative effects, and how they interact with each other and the environment varies considerably. Most likely, the complexity revealed in the genetic studies of animal models will also apply for humans. Therefore, the definition of both genetic and environmental interactions are critical for finding the underlying genes causing and controlling autoimmune diseases, a task that is also difficult in animal models, here illustrated by two examples: the positional cloning of the *Pia4* gene *Ncf1* and the complex structure and interactions of the *Eae3* and *Eae2* loci.

6
Positional Cloning of *Ncf1*, a Genetic Polymorphism Explaining a Major Quantitative Trait Locus Controlling Chronic Inflammation

Pristane-induced arthritis (PIA) in rats is a model mimicking RA. Arthritis is induced by a subcutaneous injection of the adjuvant oil pristane at the base of the tail and signs of arthritis appear after about 14 days. The subsequent development of arthritis is chronic and relapsing in the susceptible DA strain, with an erosive and symmetric destruction of peripheral joints and the disease fulfils the classical RA criteria [16, 17]. PIA is T cell-dependent and there is no evidence for an influence of B cells or arthritogenic antibodies in contrast to CIA, the primarily used arthritis model in mice, in which arthritogenic antibodies to CII play a significant role [18].

To identify the genes contributing to the disease, the arthritis-susceptible DA strain was crossed with the arthritis-resistant E3 strain [19, 20]. In a number of both intercrosses and backcrosses involving more than 1,000 rats, the major quantitative trait loci (QTLs) could be identified (Fig. 3). These loci could clearly be separated to control specific phases of the disease course, i.e. onset, severity, and chronicity (Fig. 4). One of the QTLs, *Pia4* located on chromosome 12, was found to be associated with severity of PIA. By insertion of the genetic fragment of interest from the resistant strain (in this case E3) into the genome of the susceptible DA strain through conventional backcross breeding (more than ten generations), we created a congenic strain. At this stage, the congenic fragment was 20 cM and we found that the congenic rat developed a milder arthritis than the parental DA strain. In fact, the difference was significant using fewer than ten rats in each group, which is a criterion for going further to clone the underlying gene/s. In other words, the prerequisite

Identified quantitative trait loci for PIA in rats

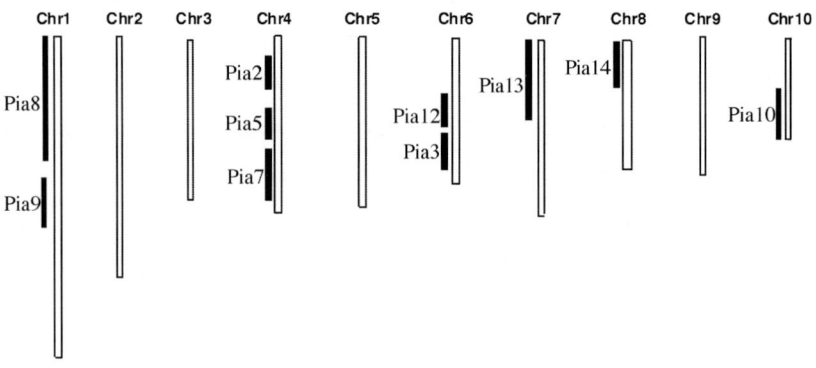

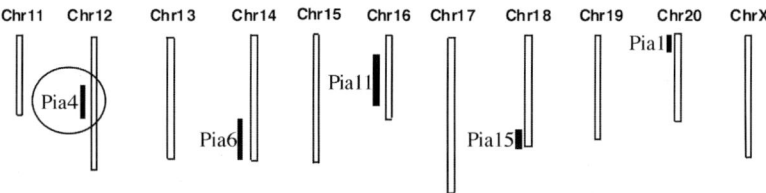

Fig. 3 Known regions in the rat genome linked to PIA

was that we had transformed the trait to be more Mendelian. On this basis, we started a process of collecting and testing small cohorts of animals having recombinations within this fragment in order to establish subcongenic strains [21]. Each new subcongenic strain was screened for the presence of the disease-associated genes by testing them for PIA susceptibility. With this method, the fragment could be reduced to contain only two genes, *Ncf1* and *Gtf2i*. No differential expression of either Ncf1 or Gtf2i could be detected and only *Ncf1* (alias *p47phox*) had polymorphism alterations in the coding sequence leading to changes in amino acid sequence in the translated protein, suggesting that Ncf1 was essential for arthritis susceptibility. One of the alterations was at position 106 ATG/GTG and resulted in a Met/Val alteration, the other one was at position 153 ATG/ACG and resulted in a Met/Thr alteration. Brown Norway (BN) rats, which are resistant to arthritis, share all genotypes but one with DA, the alteration in position 153, suggesting that this alteration is important for the Ncf1 function. Consequently, this approach allowed us to

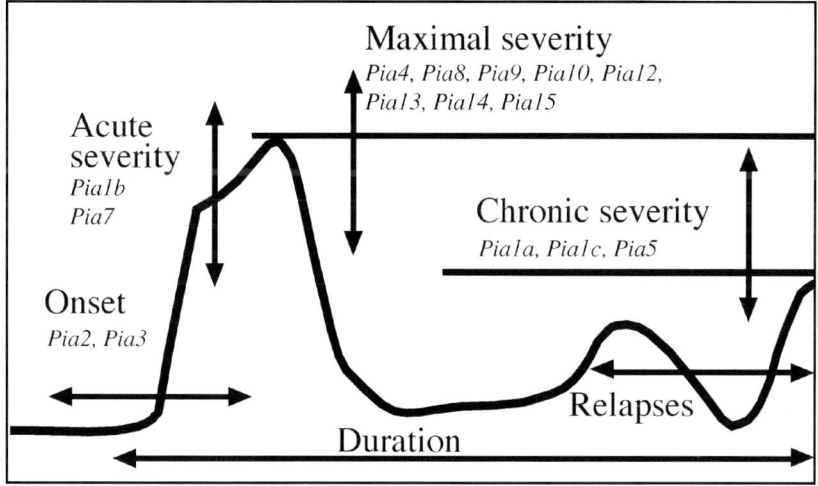

Fig. 4 Different loci control separate phases of PIA

identify a causative gene, which could now be subjected for further functional analysis and studies of this new pathogenic pathway associated with arthritis severity.

7
The Ncf1 Protein and the NADPH Complex

How could the *Ncf1* gene be involved in the development of arthritis? To our advantage, a huge effort in investigation and characterization had already been made regarding the *Ncf1* gene and the encoded Ncf1 protein. The fact that a lot of information was already available simplified the process of finding phenotypes associated with the genotype. The Ncf1 protein is part of the NADPH oxidase complex expressed in phagocytic cells. The complex is composed of five subunits, of which two, Cyba (gp91phox) and Cybb (p22 phox), resides in the membrane where they form a heterodimeric flavohemoprotein—cytochrome b_{558}. The other three subunits—Ncf1, Ncf2 (p67phox) and Ncf4 (p40phox)—are in the resting state forming a complex in the cytosol, but when activated by any of a wide variety of stimuli, the Ncf1 protein gets heavily phosphorylated and the complex migrates to the membrane to form the activated complex [22]. The Ncf1 protein is the subunit responsible for transporting the cytosolic complex to the endosomal membrane or the cell membrane during activation [23]. The NADPH oxidase complex functions as an electron donor in the oxidative burst process activated in response to pathogenic invaders, ultimately generating reactive oxygen species (ROS) [24]. To investigate the functional consequences of the identified *Ncf1* polymorphism, we tested the ability of rat peritoneal cells to produce ROS. The surprising results showed that the arthritis-susceptible DA rat had a *lower* burst than the resistant DA. $Ncf1^{E3}$ congenic rat [21]. One allele containing the functional *Ncf1* was enough to correct for the deficiency in oxidative burst and protect from disease since the congenic heterozygous for the $Ncf1^{E3}$ allele had a milder disease than the homozygous DA rat. These results contradict the general belief that oxidative burst promotes inflammation and suggest that the oxidative burst is involved in a previously unknown pathway controlling inflammation. In fact, transfer of spleen-derived T cells from the congenic DA. $Ncf1^{E3}$ rat to the parental DA and vice versa showed that the *Ncf1* polymorphism operated before activation of the T cells, indicating that it plays a role in the control of autoimmune activation.

8
Pathway Analysis

Natural selection does not operate on single genes but rather on molecular pathways. Thus, the discovery of a genetic polymorphism, like in *Ncf1*, regulating a disease trait, opens up the possibility for the identification of a new pathway leading to arthritis. The pathways are likely to be shared between different species; however, the exact nucleotide variant in the rat *Ncf1* gene is probably specific. Thus, for further studies it can be assumed that the pathway will operate similarly in rats, mice, and humans.

To investigate this possibility we looked to the mouse. In the mouse there is an arthritis QTL identified that contains the *Ncf1* gene. However, we found that *Ncf1* was not polymorphic and we did not find an effect on the oxidative burst using a congenic strain with a fragment derived from C3H on a B10.Q background (P. Olofsson et al., unpublished data). Another mouse that was made deficient for *Ncf1* was not possible to use for our purpose, as the mutation results in a complete destruction of the gene. Moreover, the *Ncf1*-targeted mutation also contains a genetically linked 129-derived fragment [25], known to contain other polymorphic genes of importance for arthritis [26]. However, a worldwide search through available mouse strains identified a variant of a C57B1/6 strain with mutations in both the leptin receptor and the *Ncf1* gene [27]. The point mutation in the *Ncf1* gene is located at position −2 in exon 8 and results in an aberrant splicing of the *Ncf1* mRNA transcripts. One of the transcripts resulting from this mutation gives rise to low levels of a protein that is truncated, lacking eight amino acids in the second SH3 domain that are important for interaction with the Ncf2 protein, thus resulting in absence of detectable NADPH oxidase activity. Consequently, we now had another mutation that presumably should affect the same pathway as was discovered in the rat. The C57Bl/6 mouse with the mutation in the *Ncf1* gene was therefore backcrossed to the arthritis-susceptible B10.Q strain. The mice were tested for susceptibility to CIA, where arthritis is induced by an intradermal injection of rat collagen type II (CII) emulsified in complete Freund's adjuvant. The B10.Q mice homozygous for the mutation in *Ncf1* developed severe arthritis with chronic development, i.e., similar to the low oxidative burst responder DA rat strain [28]. Mice heterozygous for the mutation were found to develop a less severe arthritis than *Ncf1*-mutated mice resembling the situation in rats where one functional *Ncf1* allele is enough to correct both oxidative burst and disease severity. Interestingly, both the delayed type hypersensitivity and antibody response to CII were higher in the *Ncf1* mutated mice, indicating an increased activity of CII reactive T cells. We also found that some female *Ncf1* mutated mice in the breeding colony spontaneously developed arthritis. In an experiment, 3 out of 12 female mice developed severe arthritis a few days after partus, confirming earlier findings that there is a high risk for arthritis susceptibility during the postpartum period [29]. The arthritis was severe and chronic, as in CIA, and the mice with spontaneous arthritis also had a higher level of antibodies against CII with the same fine-specificity as in CIA [28].

The overall data clearly suggest another role of NADPH oxidase-derived ROS than just elimination of pathogens, adding a complexity to the redox status of the cell. ROS response has been reported not only in phagocytes but also in antigen-presenting cells (APCs), such as dendritic cells (DCs) [30]. Also, T cells have been reported to express Ncf1 during antigen presentation and activation [31], adding further complexity to the process of finding the mechanisms behind the phenotype.

The immune regulatory effect of ROS could be involved in one or more of the different stages of the interactions of the immune system. There are a number of pathways that are proposed to be affected by free radicals and state of oxidation. On the antigen-presenting level, it has been shown that by inhibiting ROS production, the proliferation of T cells in response to antigen presentation of DCs is prevented [30], suggesting that the burst response in an APC could modulate the antigen presentation capacity of that cell. The level of radicals could also directly act on T cells. ROS could possibly be transferred over the synapse from APC to T cell and thereby alter the oxidation state of the recipient cell. It has been suggested that the level of oxidation on membranes of cells, influenced by interacting cells, are important for function [32]. Extracellular ROS has also been shown to act as an immune regulator through its interaction with the T cell proliferation regulator NO [33]. The oxidation could also possibly act by affecting other important structures on the cell surface and thereby alter their status. It has been shown that oxidation on T cell receptor signaling pathways, such as the linker for activation of T cells (LAT) molecule, modulates the function of T cells [34]. It is also possible that ROS by itself acts as a modulator of the system. It is known that ROS in low concentrations serves as a second messenger in the initiation and amplification of signaling at the antigen receptor in lymphocyte activation (reviewed in [32]). Another possibility is that ROS is involved in feedback mechanisms. Direct cell–cell contact between an activated T cell and human PMN has been shown to induce intracellular ROS production in the PMN, which then could act as an intracellular messenger [35]. Further studies are needed in order to clarify which effect is of importance for the development of arthritis.

9
Therapeutic Possibilities Can Be Immediately Explored

Taken together these data show that it is possible to identify the underlying genes of a QTL. It also shows that the importance of this finding is the identification of new pathogenic pathways and that these pathways are conserved between species. The NADPH oxidase complex proved to be an important regulator of the immune system and the pathway appears to involve autoreactive T cells, but it is not yet fully understood. This new pathway for modulating inflammatory diseases is, however, expected to open up new possibilities for generating drugs to target chronic inflammatory autoimmune diseases such as arthritis. Most importantly, using the animal model platform including the congenic strains, methods are then already prepared for testing proof of concepts of the different therapeutic possibilities. This will contribute to shorten the time from the target identification to validation.

10
Analyses of a QTL Containing Interacting Genes

Several factors affected the successes of the positional cloning of *Ncf1*. First of all, it is a gene with a large effect size, accounting for about 20% of the total phenotypic variation [19]. Moreover, the mutation has a dominant effect on a well-characterized phenotype and also, the rest of the genome in the DA background allows the functional expression of the allele. However, in many cases a QTL effect is the sum effect of several positionally linked genes and their interactions with other genes both within and outside the QTL. This certainly makes positional cloning more difficult.

One such example is two of the first QTLs reported to control an animal model of an autoimmune disease: the *Eae2* and *Eae3* loci associated with experimental autoimmune encephalomyelitis [36]. *Eae2* and *Eae3* are located on chromosomes 3 and 15, respectively, and these loci have an interacting effect on the disease [36]. We made congenic strains with these fragments from the resistant RIIIS/J strain on the susceptible B10.RIII background. The effect on disease in these mice was mild, far from being Mendelian and therefore not suitable for positional cloning of the underlying genes. Clearly both the environmental and genetic conditions needed to be better defined in order to increase the effect of the RIIIS/J alleles [37, 38]. Firstly we found that both loci also controlled CIA. Moreover, studying environmental factors affecting the arthritis phenotype we found that inducing the disease without tubercle antigens in the adjuvant increased the penetrance of the congenic effect in both chromosome 15 and chromosome 3 congenics. We also utilized the observation that these loci interacted and developed a strategy to define the genetic interactions. The congenics were intercrossed for more than eight generations, resulting in a partial advanced intercross cohort of roughly 1,000 mice. This accumulated both the recombination density and statistical power to dissect the loci into several subloci and to identify the interactions between them. Within the previous QTL on chromosome 3 (*Eae3*), we were able to identify three separate loci (*Cia5*, *Cia21*, and *Cia22*) and within the previous QTL on chromosome 15 (*Eae2*) we found four loci (*Cia26*, *Cia30*, *Cia31*, and *Cia32*). Most of these loci interacted with each other (Fig. 5) and RIIIS/J alleles at the different loci could be either disease-promoting or disease-decreasing. For example; *Cia5* affected the onset and early severity of arthritis in additive interaction with *Cia30* on chromosome 15, whereas the *Cia21* and *Cia22* affected severity during the chronic phase of the disease in epistatic interaction with *Cia31* on chromosome 15. The definition of the environmental conditions and the genetic interactions was a prerequisite to dissect the *Eae2* and *Eae3* QTLs. Human studies will have the same problem, but they are more readily seen and analyzed in animal model studies. In the case of the *Eae2/Eae3* project, the interactions between the QTLs could be detected in the F2 intercross with no more than approximately 100 animals. However, the breakdown of the two QTLs into seven and detecting the specific interactions among them was only possible by collecting a larger number of recombinations in approximately 1,000 mice. What we learned was that by analyzing the genetic interactions in the F2 intercross we could get information

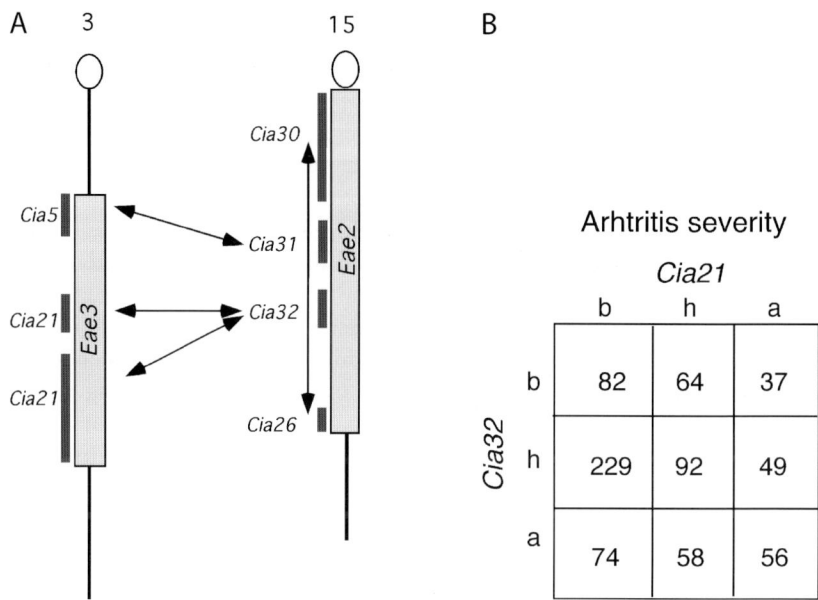

Fig. 5A,B **A** A schematic view of the genetic interactions between the *Eae2* and *Eae3* loci affecting arthritis. **B** The sum of arthritis score in female mice depending on their genotypes at *Cia21* and *Cia32*

on how to design congenic strains with the optimal effect on the phenotype. The knowledge of the genetic interactions is then not only useful in the positional cloning process but also once the gene is identified and studied in humans.

The interactions within a QTL are another situation and they pose both new problems and possibilities. The problems are the difficulties in splitting up a tightly linked haplotype. This is an apparent problem in human studies, for example in addressing conserved haplotypes within the MHC region. In animal models, haplotypes can be intentionally broken up through the search of recombinations. Such recombinations will often lead to new and changed effects on the phenotype, possibly caused by a balancing interaction between closely positioned genes. It will be a challenging task to investigate in detail such clusters but it is also important to remember that the minimal congenic fragment, containing such conserved haplotypes, are likely to have been selected for a balanced control of a specific pathway. Such congenic strains will therefore be of value for studies of pathophysiologic pathways and thereby for understanding the fundamental laws determining the possibility of developing drugs with efficiency and with limited side-effects.

The possibility of genetically modifying mouse strains through transgene and embryonic stem cell-based technologies is a major advantage in the further dissection of the critical genes and haplotypes. Studies on the role of MHC genes are an excellent example of this. The establishment of H-2 (i.e., mouse MHC) congenic strains was the basis for the identification of the MHC regions and such strains are still useful for studies of the role of MHC. It has, however, been difficult to split this region in order to isolate each gene and thereby understand its function. Instead, transgenic experiments have been conducted with which it has been possible to insert both specific murine class II genes [39, 40] and their human counterparts [41–44], and thereby prove the role of these genes for the development of autoimmune disease such as RA and MS. These studies also show the risk in transgenic technology as overexpression of class II genes may also lead to an artifactual toxicity in B cells [45, 46], which is the most likely explanation for a suppressive effect by transgenic class II genes, as has been reported in diabetes in the NOD mouse.

11
Conclusions

It is essential to backtrack the work of nature, and disease-causing factors need to be searched for in the balance between a naturally but historically selected genome and newly introduced environmental factors. Due to the complexity of the major diseases, it has been difficult to follow an approach to make a direct search for the genetic and environmental factors causing autoimmune diseases. We have been arguing for the usefulness of proper animal models, with which it is possible to make a shortcut for the identifications of the major genetically selected pathways leading to autoimmune disease. Once identified the strength of the well-developed tools for experimental studies can be used. In combination this will shorten the time and efforts to develop new types of treatment addressing the disease-causing mechanisms.

Acknowledgements Grant supporters were the Craaford foundation, the Lundberg foundation, the Kock and Österlund foundations, the Swedish Association Against Rheumatism, the Swedish Medical Research Council, the Swedish Foundation for Strategic Research, Arexis AB, and the European Union Grant EUROME QLG1-CT2001–01407.

References

1. Trentham DE, Townes AS, Kang AH (1977) Autoimmunity to type II collagen an experimental model of arthritis. JExp Med 146:857

2. Courtenay JS, Dallman MJ, Dayan AD, Martin A, Mosedale B (1980) Immunisation against heterologous type II collagen induces arthritis in mice. Nature 283:666
3. Holmdahl R (1999) Genetic control of experimental models of multiple sclerosis. In: H Links (ed) Advances in multiple sclerosis. Clinical research and therapy. Martin Dunitz, London, p 15
4. Keffer J, Probert L, Cazlaris H, Georgopoulos S, Kaslaris E, Kioussis D, Kollias G (1991) Transgenic mice expressing human tumour necrosis factor: a predictive genetic model of arthritis. EMBO J 10:4025
5. Horai R, Saijo S, Tanioka D, Nakae S, Sudo K, Okahara A, Ikuse T, Asano M, Iwakura Y (2000) Development of chronic inflammatory arthropathy resembling rheumatoid arthritis in interleukin 1 receptor antagonist-deficient mice. J Exp Med 191:313
6. Kouskoff V, Korganow AS, Duchatelle V, Degott C, Benoist C, Mathis D (1996) Organ-specific disease provoked by systemic autoimmunity. Cell 87:811
7. Theofilopoulos AN, Dixon FJ (1985) Murine models of systemic lupus erythematosus. Adv Immunol 37:269
8. Delovitch TL, Singh B (1997) The nonobese diabetic mouse as a model of autoimmune diabetes: immune dysregulation gets the NOD. Immunity 7:727
9. Nagamine K, Peterson P, Scott HS, Kudoh J, Minoshima S, Heino M, Krohn KJ, Lalioti MD, Mullis PE, Antonarakis SE, Kawasaki K, Asakawa S, Ito F, Shimizu N (1997) Positional cloning of the APECED gene. Nat Genet 17:393
10. Aaltonen J, Björses P, Perheentupa J, Horelli-Kuitunen N, Palotie A, Peltonen L, Lee YS, Francis F, Hennig S, Thiel C, Lehrach H, Yapso M-L (1997) An autoimmune disease APECED, caused by mutations in a novel gene featuring two PHD-type zinc-finger domains. Nat Genet 17:399
11. Liston A, Lesage S, Wilson J, Peltonen L, Goodnow CC (2003) Aire regulates negative selection of organ-specific T cells. Nat Immunol 4:350
12. Hugot JP, Chamaillard M, Zouali H, Lesage S, Cezard JP, Belaiche J, Almer S, Tysk C, O'Morain CA, Gassull M, Binder V, Finkel Y, Cortot A, Modigliani R, Laurent-Puig P, Gower-Rousseau C, Macry J, Colombel M Sahbatou JF, Thomas G (2001) Association of NOD2 leucine-rich repeat variants with susceptibility to Crohn's disease. Nature 411:599
13. Begovich AB, Carlton VE, Honigberg LA, Schrodi SJ, Chokkalingam AP, Alexander HC, Ardlie Q Huang KG, Smith AM, Spoerke JM, Conn MT, Chang M, Chang SY, Saiki RK, Catanese JJ, Leong DU, Garcia VE, McAllister LB, Jeffery DA, Lee AT, Batliwalla F, Remmers E, Criswell LA, Seldin MF, Kastner DL, Amos CI, Sninsky JJ, Gregersen PK (2004) A missense single-nucleotide polymorphism in a gene encoding a protein tyrosine phosphatase (PTPN22) is associated with rheumatoid arthritis. Am J Hum Genet 75:330
14. Gregersen PK, Silver J, Winchester RJ (1987) The shared epitope hypothesis. An approach to understanding the molecular genetics of susceptibility to rheumatoid arthritis. Arthritis Rheum 30:1205
15. Benjamin R, Parham P (1990) Guilt by association: HLA-B27 and ankylosing spondylitis. Immunol Today 11:137

16. Vingsbo C, Sahlstrand P, Brun JG, Jonsson R, Saxne T, Holmdahl R (1996) Pristane-induced arthritis in rats: a new model for rheumatoid arthritis with a chronic disease course influenced by both major histocompatibility complex and non-major histocompatibility complex genes. Am J Pathol 149:1675
17. Arnett FC, Edworthy SM, Bloch DA et al (1988) The American Rheumatism Association 1987 revised criteria for the classification of rheumatoid arthritis. Arthritis Rheum 31:315
18. Holmdahl R, Rubin K, Klareskog L, Larsson E, Wigzell H (1986) Characterization of the antibody response in mice with type II collagen-induced arthritis, using monoclonal anti-type II collagen antibodies. Arthritis Rheum 29:400
19. Vingsbo-Lundberg C, Nordquist N, Olofsson P, Sundvall M, Saxne T, Pettersson U, Holmdahl R (1998) Genetic control of arthritis onset, severity and chronicity in a model for rheumatoid arthritis in rats. Nat Genet 20:401
20. Olofsson P, Holmberg J, Pettersson U, Holmdahl R (2003) Identification and isolation of dominant susceptibility loci for pristane-induced arthritis. J Immunol 171:407
21. Olofsson P, Holmberg J, Tordsson J, Lu S, Akerstrom B, Holmdahl R (2003) Positional identification of Ncf1 as a gene that regulates arthritis severity in rats. Nat Genet 33:25
22. Groemping Y, Lapouge K, Smerdon SJ, Rittinger K (2003) Molecular basis of phosphorylation-induced activation of the NADPH oxidase. Cell 113:343
23. Heyworth PG, Curnutte JT, Nauseef WM, Volpp BD, Pearson DW, Rosen H, Clark RA (1991) Neutrophil nicotinamide adenine dinucleotide phosphate oxidase assembly. Translocation of p47-phox and p67-phox requires interaction between p47-phox and cytochrome b558. J Clin Invest 87:352
24. Babior BM (2000) Phagocytes and oxidative stress. Am J Med 109:33
25. Jackson SH, Gallin JI, Holland SM (1995) The p47phox mouse knock-out model of chronic granulomatous disease. J Exp Med 182:751
26. Blom T, Franzen A, Heinegard D, Holmdahl R (2003) Comment on "The influence of the proinflammatory cytokine, osteopontin, on autoimmune demyelinating disease". Science 299:1845; author reply 1845
27. Huang CK, Zhan L, Hannigan MO, Ai Y, Leto TL (2000) P47(phox)-deficient NADPH oxidase defect in neutrophils of diabetic mouse strains C57BL/6J-m db/db and db/+. J Leukoc Biol 67:210
28. Hultqvist M, Olofsson P, Holmberg J, Backstrom BT, Tordsson J, Holmdahl R (2004) Enhanced autoimmunity, arthritis, and encephalomyelitis in mice with a reduced oxidative burst due to a mutation in the Ncf1 gene. Proc Natl Acad Sci U S A 101:12646
29. Mattsson R, Mattsson A, Holmdahl R, Whyte A, Rook GA (1991) Maintained pregnancy levels of oestrogen afford complete protection from post-partum exacerbation of collagen-induced arthritis. Clin Exp Immunol 85:41
30. Matsue H, Edelbaum D, Shalhevet D, Mizumoto N, Yang C, Mummert ME, Oeda J, Masayasu H, Takashima A (2003) Generation and function of reactive oxygen species in dendritic cells during antigen presentation. J Immunol 171:3010
31. Jackson SH, Devadas S, Kwon J, Pinto LA, Williams MS (2004) T cells express a phagocyte-type NADPH oxidase that is activated after T cell receptor stimulation. Nat Immunol 5:818

32. Reth M (2002) Hydrogen peroxide as second messenger in lymphocyte activation. Nat Immunol 3:1129
33. Van der Veen RC, Dietlin TA, Karapetian A, Holland SM, Hofman FM (2004) Extracellular superoxide promotes T cell expansion through inactivation of nitric oxide. J Neuroimmunol 153:183
34. Gringhuis SI, Breedveld FC, Verweij CL (2002) Linker for activation of T cells: sensing redox imbalance. Methods Enzymol 352:248
35. Cettour-Rose P, Nguyen TX, Serrander L, Kaufmann MT, Dayer JM, Burger D, Roux-Lombard P (2005) T cell contact-mediated activation of respiratory burst in human polymorphonuclear leukocytes is inhibited by high-density lipoproteins and involves CD18. J Leukoc Biol 77:52
36. Sundvall M, Jirholt J, Yang HT, Jansson L, Engstrom A, Pettersson U, Holmdahl R (1995) Identification of murine loci associated with susceptibility to chronic experimental autoimmune encephalomyelitis. Nat Genet 10:313
37. Karlsson J, Johannesson M, Lindvall T, Wernhoff P, Holmdahl R, Andersson A (2005) Genetic interactions in Eae2 control collagen-induced arthritis and the CD4+/CD8+ T cell ratio. J Immunol 174:533
38. Johannesson M, Karlsson J, Wernhoff P, Nandakumar KS, Lindqvist AK, Olsson L, Cook AD, Andersson A, Holmdahl R (2005) Identification of epistasis through a partial advanced intercross reveals three arthritis loci within the Cia5 QTL in mice. Genes Immun 6:175
39. Brunsberg U, Gustafsson K, Jansson L, Michaelsson E, Ahrlund-Richter L, Pettersson RMattsson S, Holmdahl R (1994) Expression of a transgenic class IIAb gene confers susceptibility to collagen-induced arthritis. Eur J Immunol 24:1698
40. Kjellen P, Jansson L, Vestberg M, Andersson A, Mattsson R, Holmdahl R (2001) The H2-Ab gene influences the severity of experimental allergic encephalomyelitis induced by proteolipoprotein peptide 103–116. J Neuroimmunol 120:25
41. Rosloniec EF, Brand DD, Myers LK, Whittington KB, Gumanovskaya M, Zaller DM, WoodsA, Altmann DM, Stuart JM, Kang AH (1997) An HLA-DR1 transgene confers susceptibility to collagen-induced arthritis elicited with human type II collagen. J Exp Med 185:1113
42. Rosloniec EF, Brand DD, Myers LK, Esaki Y, Whittington KB, Zaller DM, Woods A, Stuart JM, Kang AH (1998) Induction of autoimmune arthritis in HLA-DR4 (DRB1*0401) transgenic mice by immunization with human and bovine type II collagen. J Immunol 160:2573
43. Andersson EC, Svendsen P, Svejgaard A, Holmdahl R, Fugger L (2000) A molecule basis for the HLA association in rheumatoid arthritis. Rev Immunogenet 2:81
44. Madsen LS, Andersson EC, Jansson L, Krogsgaard M, Andersen CB, Engberg J, Strominger, Svejgaard A, Hjorth JP, Holmdahl R, Wucherpfennig KW, Fugger L (1999) A humanized model for multiple sclerosis using HLA-DR2 and a human T-cell receptor. Nat Genet 23:343
45. Singer SM, Umetsu DT, McDevitt HO (1996) High copy number I-Ab transgenes induce production of IgE through an interleukin 4-dependent mechanism. Proc Natl Acad Sci U S A 93:2947
46. Labrecque N, Madsen L, Fugger L, Benoist C, Mathis D (1999) Toxic MHC class II beta chains. Immunity 11:515

Subject Index

absence of persistent microbial 112
adrenalitis 54
affinity maturation 169
Aire 28, 29
allelic exclusion 36
allergy 56
altered peptide ligand 33
annexin-V 166
antibiotics 114
antigen presentation 33, 34, 36
antigen-presenting cells 41
APC 26, 30, 33, 34, 36, 37, 40, 41
APL 33
apoptosis 41, 162
– DNA fragmentation 162
arenas 117
astrocytes 27, 28, 35, 40, 43
autoantibody 31, 33, 43, 44
autoantibody-dependent 44
autoantigen 26–32, 36, 37, 39, 40, 44, 169
autoantigen presentation 37
autoantigenic 27, 33
autoimmune 106
autoimmune diseases 52
autoimmune gastritis 54
autoimmune myocarditis 61
autoimmune neuritis 61
autoimmunity 162
autoinflammatory 148
autoinflammatory disease 128

B cell 26, 30, 31, 34, 36, 38, 44
B cell receptor 30, 31
B cell receptor editing 30
back-up mechanism 165

BBB 26, 40
biologicals 205
biomarkers 171
Blau syndrome (BS)/early-onset sarcoidosis (EOS) 128, 140, 141, 148
– NOD2/CARD15 139–141
blood–brain barrier 26, 44
bone marrow 26, 30–32, 41

C-reactive protein 164
CD25 53
CD34 170
CD4 37–39
CD4 mature 30
CD40 57
$CD4^+$ 35
$CD4^+CD25^+$ 38
CD8 39
central nervous system 26
chromatin 163
CIDP (chronic inflammatory demyelinating polyneuropathy) 61
class II 33, 34, 40, 41
clearance 162
– heterogeneous 170
– intrinsic defect 170
CNS 26–28, 30, 32, 33, 35–41
complement 164
– C1q 165
– C3 165
– C4 165
CR2/CD21 170
Crohn's disease 107

cryopyrinpathies   132, 135, 138,
    139, 141, 148
- anakinra treatment   139
- caterpiller 1.1   135
- chronic infantile neurological,
    cutaneous, and articular
    syndrome (CINCA)   136,
    137, 139
- cryopyrin   135
- familial cold autoinflammatory
    syndrome (FCAS)   135, 136, 139,
    141, 142
- Muckle-Wells syndrome (MWS)
    136, 138, 139, 141, 142
- NALP3   135, 138
- neonatal onset multisystem
    inflammatory disease (NOMID)
    136, 137, 139
- PYPAF1   135
CTLA-4   55
cyclosporin A (CsA)   59

DC   26, 28, 30, 41
defective neutrophil   109
dendritic cell   26, 41, 116
determinant spreading   41
diabetes/insulitis   54
disease may have instigated
    autoimmunity   107
DNase I   165
downregulatory mechanisms   115

EAE   27, 31, 33–41, 43, 44
elevation in IgD common   148
etiopathogenesis   171
experimental autoimmune
    encephalomyelitis   27

familial mediterranean fever (FMF)
    130, 131, 133, 136, 142, 145, 148
- amyloidosis   130
- colchicine   130
- colchicine prophylaxis   130
- cryopyrin   137
- IL-1β   131, 132, 134, 137–139
- marenostrin   130
- MEFV mediterranean fever   130

- NF-κB   133, 137, 139
- NF-κB activation   133
- pyrin   130–135, 137
- systemic amyloidosis   130
follicular dendritic cells   169
Foxp3   55
Freund's adjuvant   32, 37, 38

germinal centers   168
GFP   40
giant cell myocarditis   61
GITR   57
glycoprotein   166
granulocytes   170

HLA-DR4   199
hyperimmunoglobulinemia D with
    periodic fever syndrome (HIDS)
    142, 145, 147, 148
- mevalonate   147
- mevalonate kinase (MK)   145
- MK   147
- MVK   145
- serum IgD   145

IL-2 receptor   55
IL-2Rα (CD25)   56
IL-2Rβ (CD122)   56
immune privilege   26
immunoglobulin   30, 31, 44
immunopathology   106
impedes   118
infections unlikely   108
inflammation   162
inflammatory bowel disease
    (IBD)   54
innate   34
innate immune   37
innate immune response   37
IPEX (immune dysregulation,
    polyendocrinopathy, enteropathy,
    X-linked syndrome)   55

lectins   167
- frucose   167
- mannose   167
- N-actelyglucosamine   167

Subject Index

Lewis rat   43, 44
lymph node   168
lysophosphatidylcholine   164

MAb   31, 32, 37, 44
macrophage   40, 41, 43, 44, 170
MBP   27, 28, 33, 35, 37–39, 43, 44
medulla   28–30
medullary   28
MFG-E8
– "eat me" signal   163
MHC   26, 27, 29, 30, 33, 34, 37, 39–41, 60
microenvironment   32, 36, 37
microglia   40, 41
MOG   28, 30, 31
molecular mimicry   32
MS   27, 35, 40
multiple sclerosis   27, 45
myelin basic protein   27

necrosis   162
– ATP   163
– chromatin   165
– nuclei   164
neonatal thymectomy   53
neurotrophin   45

oligodendrocytes   28, 40, 44
oophoritis   54
opsonin   164
orchitis   54

pentraxin PTX3   167
phagocytes   163, 165
phagocytosis   164
phosphatidylserine   163
– "eat me" signal   163
– lateral mobility   166
polyendocrinopathy   56
pyogenic arthritis, pyoderma gangrenosum and acne (PAPA)   128, 134, 148
– CD2-PSTPIP1   135
– CD2BP1   133
– PSTPIP1   133, 135

receptor editing   30, 31
regulatory mechanisms   115
regulatory T cell   29, 38, 39, 52
rheumatic inflammation   202
– pregnancy   202
– T cell clone   203
– Th1 cell   203, 204
rheumatoid   52
rubella   59

secondary necrotic cells   162
self-tolerance   29, 31, 52
shared epitope   199
sialadenitis   54
somatic mutation   170
spondyloarthritides   112
stem cells   170
superantigen   32, 34, 35
superantigenic   35
suppressor   32, 38
survival signal   170
systemic lupus erythematosus   163

T cell   27–30, 32–34
– $\alpha\beta$ T cell   196, 198
– CD4 T cell   196
    effector function   200
    rheumatic inflammation   199
    Th1 cell   200
    Th2 cell   201
– CD8 T cell   196, 197
    rheumatic inflammation   197
    tissue damage   197
– cytotoxic T cell   196
– differentiation   198, 201
– effector cell   198
– $\gamma\delta$ T cell   197
    rheumatic inflammation   197
– helper T cell   196
– memory T cell   198
– naïve T cell   198
– T cell-directed therapy   200, 204
– Th1 cell
    autoimmune disease   202
    rheumatic inflammation   202
    rheumatoid arthritis   202

T cell-directed therapy 200, 204
- biologicals 205
- CTLA-4-IgG1 206
- DMARDs 205
- LFA-3-IgG1 206
- mAbs to CD4 206
- mAbs to ICAM-1 206
- mAbs to LFA-1 206
- Th1/Th2 shift 205
TCR 34–37
TCR$^{+/+}$ 38
therapeutic targets 171
thymus 26–28, 36
thyroiditis 54
tingible body macrophages 168
tolerance 170
Tregs 38, 52

triggering infection 113
tumor necrosis factor receptor-associated periodic syndrome (TRAPS) 141–145, 148
- CD120a 142
- etanercept 145
- p55 142, 144
- TNF receptor p55 protein 142
- TNFRI 142
- TNFRSF1 142
- TNFRSF1A 142, 144
type 1 diabetes 52

vaccine development 118

X irradiation 59

Current Topics in Microbiology and Immunology

Volumes published since 1989 (and still available)

Vol. 261: **Trono, Didier (Ed.):** Lentiviral Vectors. 2002. 32 figs. X, 258 pp. ISBN 3-540-42190-4

Vol. 262: **Oldstone, Michael B.A. (Ed.):** Arenaviruses I. 2002. 30 figs. XVIII, 197 pp. ISBN 3-540-42244-7

Vol. 263: **Oldstone, Michael B. A. (Ed.):** Arenaviruses II. 2002. 49 figs. XVIII, 268 pp. ISBN 3-540-42705-8

Vol. 264/I: **Hacker, Jörg; Kaper, James B. (Eds.):** Pathogenicity Islands and the Evolution of Microbes. 2002. 34 figs. XVIII, 232 pp. ISBN 3-540-42681-7

Vol. 264/II: **Hacker, Jörg; Kaper, James B. (Eds.):** Pathogenicity Islands and the Evolution of Microbes. 2002. 24 figs. XVIII, 228 pp. ISBN 3-540-42682-5

Vol. 265: **Dietzschold, Bernhard; Richt, Jürgen A. (Eds.):** Protective and Pathological Immune Responses in the CNS. 2002. 21 figs. X, 278 pp. ISBN 3-540-42668X

Vol. 266: **Cooper, Koproski (Eds.):** The Interface Between Innate and Acquired Immunity, 2002. 15 figs. XIV, 116 pp. ISBN 3-540-42894-X

Vol. 267: **Mackenzie, John S.; Barrett, Alan D. T.; Deubel, Vincent (Eds.):** Japanese Encephalitis and West Nile Viruses. 2002. 66 figs. X, 418 pp. ISBN 3-540-42783X

Vol. 268: **Zwickl, Peter; Baumeister, Wolfgang (Eds.):** The Proteasome-Ubiquitin Protein Degradation Pathway. 2002. 17 figs. X, 213 pp. ISBN 3-540-43096-2

Vol. 269: **Koszinowski, Ulrich H.; Hengel, Hartmut (Eds.):** Viral Proteins Counteracting Host Defenses. 2002. 47 figs. XII, 325 pp. ISBN 3-540-43261-2

Vol. 270: **Beutler, Bruce; Wagner, Hermann (Eds.):** Toll-Like Receptor Family Members and Their Ligands. 2002. 31 figs. X, 192 pp. ISBN 3-540-43560-3

Vol. 271: **Koehler, Theresa M. (Ed.):** Anthrax. 2002. 14 figs. X, 169 pp. ISBN 3-540-43497-6

Vol. 272: **Doerfler, Walter; Böhm, Petra (Eds.):** Adenoviruses: Model and Vectors in Virus-Host Interactions. Virion and Structure, Viral Replication, Host Cell Interactions. 2003. 63 figs., approx. 280 pp. ISBN 3-540-00154-9

Vol. 273: **Doerfler, Walter; Böhm, Petra (Eds.):** Adenoviruses: Model and Vectors in VirusHost Interactions. Immune System, Oncogenesis, Gene Therapy. 2004. 35 figs., approx. 280 pp. ISBN 3-540-06851-1

Vol. 274: **Workman, Jerry L. (Ed.):** Protein Complexes that Modify Chromatin. 2003. 38 figs. XII, 296 pp. ISBN 3-540-44208-1

Vol. 275: **Fan, Hung (Ed.):** Jaagsiekte Sheep Retrovirus and Lung Cancer. 2003. 63 figs., XII, 252 pp. ISBN 3-540-44096-3

Vol. 276: **Steinkasserer, Alexander (Ed.):** Dendritic Cells and Virus Infection. 2003. 24 figs., X, 296 pp. ISBN 3-540-44290-1

Vol. 277: **Rethwilm, Axel (Ed.):** Foamy Viruses. 2003. 40 figs. X, 214 pp. ISBN 3-540-44388-6

Vol. 278: **Salomon, Daniel R.; Wilson, Carolyn (Eds.):** Xenotransplantation. 2003. 22 figs., IX, 254 pp. ISBN 3-540-00210-3

Vol. 279: **Thomas, George; Sabatini, David; Hall, Michael N. (Eds.):** TOR. 2004. 49 figs., X, 364 pp. ISBN 3-540-00534X

Vol. 280: **Heber-Katz, Ellen (Ed.):** Regeneration: Stem Cells and Beyond. 2004. 42 figs., XII, 194 pp. ISBN 3-540-02238-4

Vol. 281: **Young, John A. T. (Ed.):** Cellular Factors Involved in Early Steps of Retroviral Replication. 2003. 21 figs., IX, 240 pp. ISBN 3-540-00844-6

Vol. 282: **Stenmark, Harald (Ed.):** Phosphoinositides in Subcellular Targeting and Enzyme Activation. 2003. 20 figs., X, 210 pp. ISBN 3-540-00950-7

Vol. 283: **Kawaoka, Yoshihiro (Ed.):** Biology of Negative Strand RNA Viruses: The Power of Reverse Genetics. 2004. 24 figs., IX, 350 pp. ISBN 3-540-40661-1

Vol. 284: **Harris, David (Ed.):** Mad Cow Disease and Related Spongiform Encephalopathies. 2004. 34 figs., IX, 219 pp. ISBN 3-540-20107-6

Vol. 285: **Marsh, Mark (Ed.):** Membrane Trafficking in Viral Replication. 2004. 19 figs., IX, 259 pp. ISBN 3-540-21430-5

Vol. 286: **Madshus, Inger H. (Ed.):** Signalling from Internalized Growth Factor Receptors. 2004. 19 figs., IX, 187 pp. ISBN 3-540-21038-5

Vol. 287: **Enjuanes, Luis (Ed.):** Coronavirus Replication and Reverse Genetics. 2005. 49 figs., XI, 257 pp. ISBN 3-540-21494-1

Vol. 288: **Mahy, Brain W. J. (Ed.):** Foot-and-Mouth-Disease Virus. 2005. 16 figs., IX, 178 pp. ISBN 3-540-22419X

Vol. 289: **Griffin, Diane E. (Ed.):** Role of Apoptosis in Infection. 2005. 40 figs., IX, 294 pp. ISBN 3-540-23006-8

Vol. 290: **Singh, Harinder; Grosschedl, Rudolf (Eds.):** Molecular Analysis of B Lymphocyte Development and Activation. 2005. 28 figs., XI, 255 pp. ISBN 3-540-23090-4

Vol. 291: **Boquet, Patrice; Lemichez Emmanuel (Eds.)** Bacterial Virulence Factors and Rho GTPases. 2005. 28 figs., IX, 196 pp. ISBN 3-540-23865-4

Vol. 292: **Fu, Zhen F (Ed.):** The World of Rhabdoviruses. 2005. 27 figs., X, 210 pp. ISBN 3-540-24011-X

Vol. 293: **Kyewski, Bruno; Suri-Payer, Elisabeth (Eds.):** CD4+CD25+ Regulatory T Cells: Origin, Function and Therapeutic Potential. 2005. 22 figs., XII, 332 pp. ISBN 3-540-24444-1

Vol. 294: **Caligaris-Cappio, Federico, Dalla Favera, Ricardo (Eds.):** Chronic Lymphocytic Leukemia. 2005. 25 figs., VIII, 187 pp. ISBN 3-540-25279-7

Vol. 295: **Sullivan, David J.; Krishna Sanjeew (Eds.):** Malaria: Drugs, Disease and Post-genomic Biology. 2005. 40 figs., XI, 446 pp. ISBN 3-540-25363-7

Vol. 296: **Oldstone, Michael B. A. (Ed.):** Molecular Mimicry: Infection Induced Autoimmune Disease. 2005. 28 figs., VIII, 167 pp. ISBN 3-540-25597-4

Vol. 297: **Langhorne, Jean (Ed.):** Immunology and Immunopathogenesis of Malaria. 2005. 8 figs., XII, 236 pp. ISBN 3-540-25718-7

Vol. 298: **Vivier, Eric; Colonna, Marco (Eds.):** Immunobiology of Natural Killer Cell Receptors. 2005. 27 figs., VIII, 286 pp. ISBN 3-540-26083-8

Vol. 299: **Domingo, Esteban (Ed.):** Quasispecies: Concept and Implications. 2006. 44 figs., XII, 401 pp. ISBN 3-540-26395-0

Vol. 300: **Wiertz, Emmanuel J.H.J.; Kikkert, Marjolein (Eds.):** Dislocation and Degradation of Proteins from the Endoplasmic Reticulum. 2006. 19 figs., VIII, 168 pp. ISBN 3-540-28006-5

Vol. 301: **Doerfler, Walter; Böhm, Petra (Eds.):** DNA Methylation: Basic Mechanisms. 2006. 24 figs., VIII, 324 pp. ISBN 3-540-29114-8

Vol. 302: **Robert N. Eisenman (Ed.):** The Myc/Max/Mad Transcription Factor Network. 2006. 28 figs. XII, 278 pp. ISBN 3-540-23968-5

Vol. 303: **Thomas E. Lane (Ed.):** Chemokines and Viral Infection. 2006. 14 figs. XII, 154 pp. ISBN 3-540-29207-1

Vol. 304: **S.A. Plotkin (Ed.):** Mass Vaccination: Global Aspects – Progress and Obstacles. 2006. 40 figs. X, 235 pp. ISBN 3-540-29382-5

Printing: Krips bv, Meppel
Binding: Stürtz, Würzburg